"十四五"国家重点出版物
The "14th Five-Year Plan" National Key Publications

腧穴层次解剖学图谱

（汉英对照）

Atlas of Layered Anatomy of Acupoints

(Chinese-English Edition)

主　编　邵水金　程明亮
Chief Editors　Shao Shuijin　Cheng Mingliang
主　译　单宝枝
Chief Translator　Shan Baozhi

全国百佳图书出版单位
中国中医药出版社
·北　京·
National Top 100 Book Publishing Units
China Press of Chinese Medicine
Beijing PRC

图书在版编目（CIP）数据

腧穴层次解剖学图谱：汉英对照 / 邵水金，程明亮主编；单宝枝主译．-- 北京：中国中医药出版社，2025. 6

ISBN 978-7-5132-9513-0

Ⅰ. R224.2-64

中国国家版本馆 CIP 数据核字第 2025CC2882 号

中国中医药出版社出版

北京经济技术开发区科创十三街 31 号院二区 8 号楼

邮政编码　100176

传真　010-64405721

东港股份有限公司印刷

各地新华书店经销

开本 787×1092　1/16　印张 16　字数 584 千字

2025 年 6 月第 1 版　2025 年 6 月第 1 次印刷

书号　ISBN 978 – 7 – 5132 – 9513 – 0

定价　129.00 元

网址　www.cptcm.com

服务热线　010-64405510

购书热线　010-89535836

维权打假　010-64405753

微信服务号　zgzyycbs

微商城网址　https://kdt.im/LIdUGr

官方微博　http://e.weibo.com/cptcm

天猫旗舰店网址　https://zgzyycbs.tmall.com

如有印装质量问题请与本社出版部联系（010-64405510）

《腧穴层次解剖学图谱（汉英对照）》
编委会

主　编　邵水金　程明亮

副主编　国海东　牟芳芳　郑　燕　董贤慧　刘起颖　张振华　包　莉　赵　顺
徐迎坤　马　冉

编　委　朱　晶　孟婉婷　郭春霞　黄振超　贺小平　赵建伟　李桂军　贠跃进
邢现锋　吉晓磊　侯海光　姚　方　刘宝年　王兴兴　赵恬田　王　昊
王　欢　黄武帮

主　译　单宝枝

Editorial Board of *Atlas of Layered Anatomy of Acupoints*
(Chinese-English Edition)

Chief Editors Shao Shuijin Cheng Mingliang

Deputy Chief Editors Guo Haidong Mou Fanfan Zheng Yan Dong Xianhui
Liu Qiying Zhang Zhenhua Bao Li Zhao Shun
Xu Yingkun Ma Ran

Editorial Board Zhu Jing Meng Wanting Guo Chunxia Huang Zhenchao
He Xiaoping Zhao Jianwei Li Guijun Yuan Yuejin Xing Xianfeng
Ji Xiaolei Hou Haiguang Yao Fang Liu Baonian Wang Xingxing
Zhao Tiantian Wang Hao Wang Huan Huang Wubang

Chief Translator Shan Baozhi

主编主译介绍

About the Chief Editors and Chief Translator

邵水金

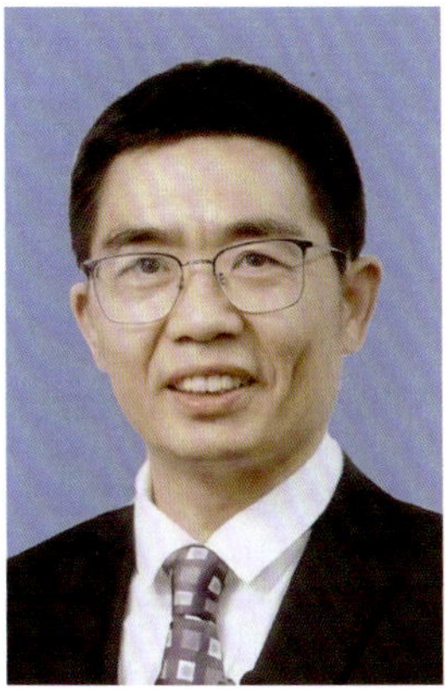

上海中医药大学博士、教授、博士研究生导师、博士后合作导师，人体解剖学教研室主任，经穴解剖实验室主任，“严振国名师工作室”传承人，上海市精品课程“腧穴解剖学”负责人。曾任上海中医药大学学术委员会委员。现任上海中医药大学教学督导组专家，中国解剖学会常务理事，中国解剖学会中医形态学分会主任委员，上海市解剖学会副理事长，中国中医药研究促进会中医微创专业委员会副主任委员。从事正常人体解剖学、腧穴解剖学、局部解剖学、正常人体学等课程教学近 30 年。出版专著、教材和图谱 130 余本，其中主编全国规划教材 18 本、“十一五”国家级规划教材 2 本。主要研究针灸治疗周围神经损伤的作用及其机制，主持国家自然科学基金、国家中医药管理局、上海市教委等课题 7 项。发表学术论文 140 余篇，其中 SCI 论文 20 余篇。授权专利 4 项。荣获全国宝钢优秀教师奖，上海中医药大学首届校园明星教师、我心目中的好老师、教学成果奖、优秀教学团队，上海市精品课程、上海市一流本科课程、上海市优秀教材奖、上海市精品教材、上海市教育科学研究优秀成果三等奖、上海市科学技术三等奖、上海市工人先锋号、上海市课程思政示范团队，以及教育部首批课程思政示范课程、教学团队和教学名师等 20 余项奖励和荣誉。

Shao Shuijin

Ph.D., professor, doctoral supervisor, postdoctoral collaborating supervisor of Shanghai University of Traditional Chinese Medicine, director of the Teaching and Research Office of Human Anatomy, director of the Acupoint Anatomy Laboratory, inheritor of “Yan Zhenguo Famous Teacher Studio”, and the person in charge of “Acupoint Anatomy” of the Shanghai excellent course. He was a member of the Academic Committee of Shanghai University of Traditional Chinese Medicine and is currently an expert in the Teaching Supervision Group of Shanghai University of Traditional Chinese Medicine, and executive director of the Chinese Society for Anatomical Sciences (CSAS), chairman of the Chinese Anatomy Society’s Traditional Chinese Medicine Morphology Branch, deputy chairman of the Shanghai Society for Anatomical Sciences, and deputy chairman of the Traditional Chinese Medicine Minimally Invasive Professional Committee of the China Association for the Promotion of Traditional Chinese Medicine Research.

He has been engaged in teaching courses such as normal human anatomy, acupoint anatomy, regional anatomy, etc. for nearly 30 years. He has published more than 130 monographs, textbooks and atlases, including 18 national-level planning textbooks and 2 national-level planning textbooks for the "11th Five-Year" Plan.

He mainly studies the role and mechanism of acupuncture in the treatment of peripheral nerve injury, and has presided over 7 projects of the National Natural Science Foundation of China, the State Administration of Traditional Chinese Medicine and Shanghai Municipal Education Commission, etc.

He has published over 140 academic papers, including over 20 SCI papers and has had 4 authorized patents. He has been conferred more than 20 awards and honorary titles such as the National Baogang Excellent Teacher Award, the First Campus Star Teacher of Shanghai University of Traditional Chinese Medicine, the My Ideal Teacher, the Teaching Achievement Award, the Excellent Teaching Team, Shanghai Excellent Curriculum, Shanghai First-Class Undergraduate Curriculum, Shanghai Excellent Textbook Award, the Third Prize of the Shanghai Excellent Achievements in Education and Scientific Research, the Third Prize of the Shanghai Science and Technology, Shanghai Workers' Pioneer, Shanghai Curriculum Ideological and Political Demonstration Team as well as the first batch of curriculum ideological and political demonstration courses, teaching teams, and teaching masters by the Ministry of Education of the PRC.

程明亮

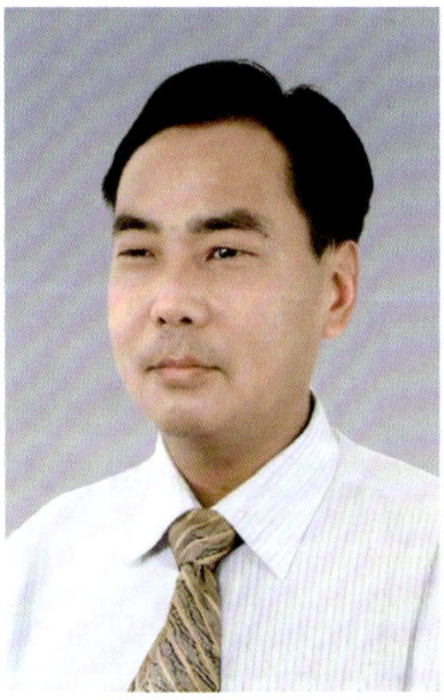

郑州卫生健康职业学院解剖学高级讲师，中国解剖学会职业教育解剖分会副主任委员，中国解剖学会科技开发和咨询工作委员会副主任委员。入选“河南省中原英才计划”，被河南省委组织部及省人社厅授予“2022 年度中原科技创业领军人才”，表彰在生物塑化标本研发、生命科学馆设计及建设、人体解剖虚拟仿真实验室开发等方面的突出成绩；主持研发的“断层包埋标本制备技术开发及应用”项目获 2023 年度“河南省技术发明三等奖”；主持制定的《人体生命科学馆建设规范》经专家组讨论认为可作为企业标准向全国推广；主编的《人体解剖学基础》（第 3 版）获“教育部‘十四五’职业教育国家规划教材”等。

Cheng Mingliang

Senior lecturer of Anatomy in Zhengzhou Health Vocational College, deputy chairman of the Vocational Education Anatomy Branch of the Chinese Society for Anatomical Sciences (CSAS), deputy chairman of the Science and Technology Development and Advisory Committee of CSAS.

He was selected as one of the talents of the “Henan Central Plains Talent Program”, and was awarded “2022 Leading Talent of the Central Plains Science and Technology Bussiness Startup” by the Organization Department of the Henan Provincial Committee of the Communist Party of China and the Department of Human Resources and Social Security of Henan Province for his outstanding achievements in bio-plasticized specimen development, life science museum design and construction, human anatomy virtual simulation laboratory development, etc. The project entitled *Development and Application of Sectional Embedded Specimen Preparation Technology* developed by him won the third prize of “Henan Provincial Technology Invention Award” in 2023 and the *Standards for the Construction of the Human Life Science Museum* presided over and formulated by him was discussed by the expert group who believed that it could be promoted to the whole country as an enterprise standard. The *Fundamentals of Human Anatomy* (the third edition) edited by him was selected as one of the “National Planning Textbook for Vocational Education of the 14th Five-Year Plan of the Ministry of Education” and so on.

单宝枝

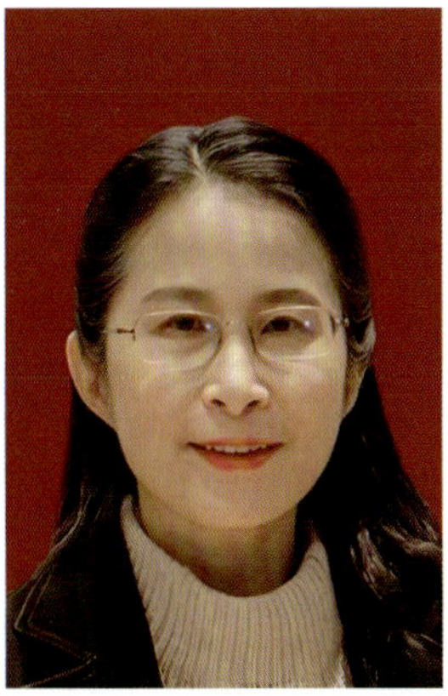

医学博士，中国中医药出版社编辑部主任、编审，江西中医药大学特聘教授、硕士研究生导师和江西中医药大学中医药文化国际传播研究中心主任，天津中医药大学客座教授，广东药科大学客座教授，欧洲针灸学院中方校长、特聘教授，（英国兰卡斯特大学）中医药人文与健康教育和传播中心主任和创始人，曾兼南京中医药大学非医专业中医典籍翻译联合博导和客座教授。世界中医药学会联合会（WFCMS）主席团执委、翻译专业委员会会长、中医人类学专业委员会副会长、教育指导委员会副会长兼副秘书长、代谢病专业委员会副会长，中国翻译协会医学翻译委员会副主任委员，中国针灸学会针灸文献专业委员会常务理事，《中医基础理论术语》国家标准修订项目英文专家组组长；*Chinese Medicine and Natural Products* 副主编、*Acupuncture and Herbal Medicine* 常务编委、*Evidence-Based Complementary and Alternative Medicine* 和 *Social Sciences & Humanities Open* 审稿人。主持国家出版基金、国家科技出版基金和国家中医药管理局中医药国际合作专项基金 6 项（计 220 万元）。“岐黄天下杯”世界中医翻译大赛策划 / 组织者和评审专家，人民日报社人民康养智库高级顾问专家，北京大学图书馆期刊评审专家库成员。曾执教江西中医药大学 5 年，从事临床 7 年，国际中医药教学 5 年。已编辑出版近 90 部中医英语和英文 / 汉英中医图书，为该类图书出版领军人才。发表学术论文 29 篇，参加科研课题 6 项，主编 / 副主编 / 参编 / 主译 / 主审图书 20 余部。第七届中医药国际贡献奖和第五届中国出版政府奖图书奖得主。研究方向：中医药传播和翻译、养生、针灸文献研究。

Shan Baozhi, Ph.D., Doctor of Medicine

- Professor of the editorship and director of the editorial department of the China Press of Chinese Medicine.
- Distinguished professor and master's supervisor of Jiangxi University of Chinese Medicine, director of the International Communication Research Centre of Traditional Chinese Medicine Culture of Jiangxi University of Chinese Medicine, visiting professor of Tianjin University of Traditional Chinese Medicine, visiting professor of Guangdong Pharmaceutical University, Chinese principal and distinguished professor of the European Institute of Acupuncture (EIA), director and founder of the Network for Traditional Chinese Medicine Humanities and Health Education & Dissemination (University of Lancaster, UK), and former doctoral co-supervisor and visiting professor of Nanjing University of Chinese Medicine.
- Team leader of the English expert group for the revision project of the National Standard for Terms in Basic Theories of Traditional Chinese Medicine, planner/organizer and review expert of the "Qihuang Tianxia Cup" World Traditional Chinese Medicine Translation Competition, senior consultant expert of the People's Health & Wellness-Keeping Think-Tank of the People's Daily, member of the Journal Review Expert Pool of the Peking University Library.
- Executive member of the presidential council of the World Federation of Chinese Medicine Societies (WFCMS); president of the Specialty Committee of Translation, WFCMS; deputy president of the Committee of Chinese Medicine Anthropology, WFCMS; deputy secretary-general and vice-president of the Educational Instruction Committee (EIC), WFCMS; deputy president of the Specialty Committee of Metabolic Diseases, WFCMS; deputy president of the Committee of Medical Translation of the Translators Association of China; executive director of the Professional Committee of Acupuncture Literature of the China Association of Acupuncture-Moxibustion; associate editor-in-chief of the Journal of *Chinese Medicine and Natural Products*; standing editor of the Journal of *Acupuncture and Herbal Medicine*; and reviewer of such journals as *Evidence-Based Complementary and Alternative Medicine*, and *Social Sciences & Humanities Open*.
- She taught at Jiangxi University of Chinese Medicine for 5 years, engaged in clinical practice for 7 years, and international teaching of traditional Chinese medicine for 5 years. She has edited and published nearly 90 books on English for Traditional Chinese Medicine (TCM) as well as English Version/Chinese-English TCM books, and is a leading figure in publishing such books.
- She has presided over six projects funded by the National Publishing Fund, the National

Science and Technology Publishing Fund, and the Special Fund for International Cooperation of Traditional Chinese Medicine of the National Administration of Traditional Chinese Medicine, with a total funding of 2.2 million yuan. She has published 29 academic papers, participated in 6 scientific research projects, and served as chief editor, associate chief editor, co-author, chief translator, or chief reviewer for more than 20 books.

- She is the winner of the 7th International Contribution Award for Traditional Chinese Medicine and the Book Award of the 5th China Publishing Government Award.
- Her research areas include the dissemination and translation of traditional Chinese medicine, health preservation, and research on the literature of acumoxology.

编写说明

《腧穴层次解剖学图谱（汉英对照）》是解剖学与腧穴学相结合的跨学科专著，以适应中西医结合、基础与临床相融合的发展需要。书中腧穴插图全部是实体标本照片，而且全部是由浅入深的层次图片，完全从另一个角度反映穴位的解剖结构，将填补腧穴层次解剖类图书的空白，能更好地指导针灸临床应用，是国内外从事针灸学习和研究的教师、学生、医生必读之作，可供中医院校师生、针灸医生、针灸爱好者、国外针灸医生、出国人员、留学生使用。

本书的特色主要有：①全书 219 幅插图为实物标本照片，插图中腧穴采用黑色字体显示，解剖结构则以蓝色字体显示，这样容易区分和查阅。因精装全彩印刷，图谱将更加精美和实用。②应用层次解剖的手段，对 152 个常用腧穴的层次结构进行了研究，内容主要包括定位、操作、主治、进针层次、针刺意外与预防，简明扼要，重点突出，便于学习和掌握。③本书在编排上一改按经络循行次序的传统方法，按人体各部位编排腧穴，这样有利于发现邻近腧穴之间的结构差别与联系，做到真正掌握腧穴的位置和解剖结构，为提高临床针灸疗效和避免针刺意外事故发生提供保障。④全书汉英对照，英文译文专业、流畅，便于中医更好地走向世界。

本书在编写过程中，得到了中国中医药出版社和河南中博科技有限公司的大力支持。由于我们的水平有限，书中若有不足之处，希望在使用过程中能得到读者的批评指正，以便再版时修订和完善。

编委会

2025 年 1 月 18 日

Instructions for Compilation

The *Atlas of Layered Anatomy of Acupoints* (*Chinese-English Edition*) is an interdisciplinary monograph that combines anatomy and acupoint science to meet the development needs of the integration of traditional Chinese and Western medicine, as well as the integration of basic and clinical medicine. The illustrations of acupoints in this book are all photos of physical specimens, and all of them are hierarchical pictures from the simple to the profound. They completely reflect the anatomical structure of acupoints from another perspective, and will fill the gap in the hierarchical anatomy books of acupoints, which can better guide the clinical application of acupuncture and moxibustion. It is a must-read work for teachers, students and doctors engaged in acupuncture learning and research at home and abroad. It can be used by teachers and students of traditional Chinese medicine colleges and universities, acupuncturists, acupuncture enthusiasts, foreign acupuncturists, professionals going abroad and international students.

The main features of this book are: ①219 illustrations in the book are physical specimen photos. In the illustrations, the acupoints are displayed in black font, and the anatomical structure is displayed in blue font, which is easy to distinguish and search. Due to hardcover full-color printing, the atlas will be more exquisite and practical. ②Using the means of hierarchical anatomy, the hierarchical structure of 152 commonly used acupoints has been studied. The contents mainly include location, operation, indications, needle-inserting layers or stratified anatomy, acupuncture accidents and prevention or cautions. It is concise, focused, and easy to learn and master. ③This book changes the traditional method of order of meridians and collaterals, and arranges acupoints according to all parts of the human body, which is conducive to discovering the structural differences and connections between adjacent acupoints, so as to truly grasp the position and anatomical structure of acupoints, and provide a guarantee for improving the efficacy of clinical acupuncture and avoiding accidents. ④This atlas is a Chinese-English version, with a professional and fluent English translation, which facilitates the better integration of traditional Chinese medicine into the world.

During the writing process, this atlas received strong support from China Press of Traditional Chinese Medicine and Henan Zhongbo Technology Co., Ltd. Due to our limited level, if there are any shortcomings in this atlas, we hope to receive criticism and recommendation from readers during the process of use, so that it can be revised and improved when reprinting.

Editorial board

January 18, 2025

目　录

CONTENTS

第一章　头部腧穴层次解剖

Chapter 1　Layered Anatomy of Acupoints on the Head

第一节　头前面腧穴

Section 1　Acupoints on the anterior aspect of the head

一、印堂

【定位】两眉毛内侧端中间的凹陷中。

【操作】向下斜刺或平刺 0.5 ～ 1 寸，或点刺出血。

【主治】头痛，眩晕，失眠，小儿急、慢惊风，鼻渊，目痛。

【进针层次】①皮肤；②皮下组织（内有滑车上神经的分支、滑车上动脉的分支和滑车上静脉的属支）；③降眉间肌（图 1-1 ～图 1-3）。

1. Yintang (GV 29)

【Location】In the depression of the midpoint of the inner end of the eyebrows.

【Method】Puncture obliquely downward or subcutaneously 0.5-1 cun, or prick to cause bleeding.

【Indications】Headache, dizziness, insomnia, acute and chronic infantile convulsions, sinusitis, and eye pain.

【Stratified anatomy】①Skin; ②Subcutaneous tissue (There are branches of the supratrochlear n., branches or tributaries of the supratrochlear a. & v..); ③Procerus (Fig.1-1 ~ Fig.1-3).

二、素髎

【定位】鼻尖的正中央。

【操作】向上斜刺 0.3 ～ 0.5 寸，或点刺出血。

【主治】鼻塞，鼻渊，酒渣鼻，齿痛，昏迷，晕厥。

【进针层次】①皮肤；②皮下组织（内有筛前神经的鼻外支、面动脉的鼻背支和面静脉的鼻背支）；③鼻中隔软骨和鼻外侧软骨（图 1-1 ～图 1-3）。

2. Suliao (GV 25)

【Location】In the centre of the tip of the nose.

【Method】Puncture obliquely upward 0.3-0.5 cun, or prick to cause bleeding.

【Indications】Stuffy nose, sinusitis, rosacea, toothache, coma, and faint.

【Stratified anatomy】①Skin; ②Subcutaneous tissue (There are external nasal branch of the anterior ethmoidal n., dorsal nasal branch of the facial a. & v..); ③Laminae septi and lateral nasal cartilage (Fig.1-1 ~ Fig.1-3).

三、水沟

【定位】人中沟的上 1/3 与下 2/3 交点处。

【操作】向上斜刺 0.3 ～ 0.5 寸，或用指甲按掐。

【主治】昏迷，晕厥，中风，牙关紧闭，癫痫，抽搐，齿痛，闪挫腰痛。

【进针层次】①皮肤；②皮下组织（内有眶下神经的分支、上唇动脉和上唇静脉）；③口轮匝肌（图 1–1 ～图 1–3）。

3. Shuigou (GV 26)

【Location】At the junction of the upper 1/3 and lower 2/3 of the philtrum.

【Method】Puncture obliquely upward 0.3-0.5 cun, or pinch with fingernail.

【Indications】Coma, loss of consciousness, stroke, closed teeth, epilepsy, convulsions, toothache, and sprain lumbago.

【Stratified anatomy】①Skin; ②Subcutaneous tissue (There are branches of the infraorbital n., superior labial a. & v..); ③Orbicularis oris (Fig.1-1 ~ Fig.1-3).

四、承浆

【定位】颏唇沟的正中凹陷处。

【操作】斜刺 0.3 ～ 0.5 寸。

【主治】口喎，唇紧，齿痛，齿衄，流涎，口舌生疮，暴喑，面肿。

【进针层次】①皮肤；②皮下组织（内有颏神经、颏动脉和颏静脉）；③口轮匝肌；④降下唇肌；⑤颏肌（图 1–1 ～图 1–3）。

4. Chengjiang (CV 24)

【Location】In the depression of the centre of the mentolabial sulcus.

【Method】Puncture obliquely 0.3-0.5 cun.

【Indications】Deviated mouth, lockjaw, toothache, gingival bleeding, salivation, sore of tongue and mouth, sudden loss of voice, and face edema.

【Stratified anatomy】①Skin; ②Subcutaneous tissue (There are mental n., a. & v..); ③Orbicularis oris; ④Depressor labii inferioris m.; ⑤Mentalis m. (Fig.1-1 ~ Fig.1-3).

五、攒竹

【定位】眉头凹陷中，额切迹处。

【操作】向下斜刺 0.3 ～ 0.5 寸，可平刺或透刺鱼腰穴 1 ～ 1.5 寸。

【主治】目赤肿痛，目视不明，迎风流泪，眼睑瞤动，眼睑下垂，头痛，眉棱骨痛，面痛，口眼喎斜，呃逆，急性腰痛。

【进针层次】①皮肤；②皮下组织（内有滑车上神经的分支、滑车上动脉的分支和滑车上静脉的属支）；③眼轮匝肌；④皱眉肌（图 1–1 ～图 1–3）。

【针刺意外与预防】①若向下斜刺，有可能刺中滑车上动、静脉，可引起局部血肿。②若向外侧透刺鱼腰穴，有可能刺中眶上动、静脉等，可引起局部血肿。

5. Cuanzhu (BL 2)

【Location】In the depression of the medial extremity of the eyebrow, and at the frontal notch.

【Method】Puncture obliquely downward 0.3-0.5 cun, or puncture subcutaneously or through Yuyao (EX-HN 4) 1-1.5cun.

【Indications】Pain and swelling in the eyes, dim vision, tearing against wind, twitching of eyelids, ptosis of the eyelids, headache, pain in the supraorbital bone, facial pain, deviated mouth and eyes, hiccup, and acute lumbago.

【Stratified anatomy】①Skin; ②Subcutaneous tissue (There are branches of the supratrochlear n., branches or tributaries of supratrochlear a. & v..); ③Orbicularis oculi m.; ④Corrugator supercilii (Fig.1-1 ~ Fig.1-3).

【Cautions】①It is possible to stab the supratrochlear a. & v. resulting in local hematoma if puncturing obliquely downward is used; ②It is possible to stab the supraorbital a. & v. resulting in local hematoma if piercing through Yuyao (EX-HN 4) acupoint outward is applied.

六、睛明

【定位】目内眦内上方，眶内侧壁凹陷中。

【操作】嘱患者闭目，医者押手拇指将眼球轻推向外侧固定，刺手持针沿眼眶边缘缓缓刺入 0.3 ～ 0.5 寸，不提插，少捻转。

【主治】目赤肿痛，目视不明，迎风流泪，内眦痒痛，近视，夜盲。

【进针层次】①皮肤；②皮下组织（内有滑车上神经的分支、内眦动脉的分支和内眦静脉的属支）；③眼轮匝肌；④眶脂体；⑤内直肌与筛骨眶板之间（图 1–1 ～图 1–3）。

【针刺意外与预防】①若针刺超过 0.8 寸，且贴近眶内侧壁处，则易刺伤筛前、后动脉，可造成上、下眼睑的皮下淤血。②若进针时未按压眼球或过于贴近眼球，则有可能刺中眼球；特别是眼球“赤道”处最薄，仅为 0.4 ～ 0.5mm，若刺中此处，则有可能刺入眼球。③若针刺超过 1.8 寸时，在进针的直后方则易刺中总腱环和视神经；刺中总腱环，则针感黏滞；刺中视神经，患者主诉眼冒金星（视神经受刺激）、头痛头昏（硬脑膜受刺激），严重者可有恶心、呕吐等重症出现。④若朝后外方向刺入 2 寸以上，则针尖可直达眶上裂，不仅可能刺中通过眶上裂的神经和血管，进而可透过眶上裂而伤及颅中窝的海绵窦，甚至刺中大脑颞叶前端，造成颅内出血，引起剧烈头昏、头痛、恶心、呕吐，甚至休克、死亡。

6. Jingming (BL 1)

【Location】In the depression of the medial wall of the orbit above the inner canthus of the eye.

【Method】Ask the patient to close his eyes. The acupuncturist gently pushes the eyeball to the outside to fix it with his thumb, and slowly needles 0.3-0.5 cun along the edge of the orbit with his needling hand, with no lifting and thrusting and less twirling manipulation.

【Indications】Pain and swelling in the eyes, dim vision, tearing against wind, itching and pain in the inner canthus, myopia, and night blindness.

【Stratified anatomy】①Skin; ②Subcutaneous tissue (There are branches of the supratrochlear n., branches or tributaries of the angular a. & v..); ③Orbicularis oculi m.; ④Adipose body of orbit; ⑤Between the rectus medialis and the orbital plate of ethmoid bone (Fig.1-1 ~ Fig.1-3).

【Cautions】①If the depth of insertion exceeds 0.8 cun and is close to the inner wall of the orbit, it is easy to puncture the anterior and posterior ethmoidal a., causing subcutaneous congestion of the upper and lower eyelids. ②If the needle is inserted without pressing the eyeball or too close to the eyeball, it may pierce the eyeball, especially at the "equator"of the eyeball Where it is the thinnest part, only 0.4-0.5mm in thickness. If piercing here, it is possible to pierce the eyeball. ③If the depth of insertion exceeds 1.8 cun, it is easy to puncture the common tendon ring or optic n. which locates directly behind the needle. Piercing the common tendon ring will cause a sticky sensation. When the optic nerve is stabbed, the patient complains of flaming eyes (the optic nerve is stimulated), headache and dizziness (dura mater is stimulated). In severe cases, nausea, vomiting and other severe diseases may occur. ④If the depth of insertion exceeds 2 cun in a backward and outward direction, the tip of the needle can go directly to the superior orbital fissure, which may not only pierce the nerves and blood vessels through the superior orbital fissure, but also hurt the cavernous sinus of the midcranial fossa through the superior orbital fissure, and even pierce the front of the temporal lobe of the brain, causing intracranial hemorrhage, severe dizziness, headache, nausea, vomiting, and even shock and death.

七、迎香

【定位】鼻翼外缘中点旁，鼻唇沟中。

【操作】向内上斜刺或平刺 0.3 ～ 0.5 寸。

【主治】鼻塞，鼻衄，鼻渊，鼻息肉，口㖞，面痒。

【进针层次】①皮肤；②皮下组织（内有眶下神经的分支、面动脉的分支和面静脉的属支）；③提上唇肌（图 1-1 ～图 1-3）。

7. Yingxiang (LI 20)

【Location】Next to the midpoint of the outer edge of the nosewing, and in the nasolabial groove.

【Method】Puncture obliquely inward and upward or subcutaneously 0.3-0.5 cun.

【Indications】Stuffy nose, epistaxis, sinusitis, nasal polyp, deviated mouth, and itching on the face.

【Stratified anatomy】①Skin; ②Subcutaneous tissue (There are branches of infraorbital n., branches or tributaries of facial a. & v..); ③Levator labii superioris (Fig.1-1 ~ Fig.1-3).

八、阳白

【定位】瞳孔直上，眉上 1 寸。

【操作】平刺 0.5 ～ 0.8 寸。

【主治】头痛，眩晕，目痛，视物模糊，眼睑瞤动，口眼㖞斜。

【进针层次】①皮肤；②皮下组织（内有眶上神经的外侧支、眶上动脉的分支和眶上静脉的属支）；③枕额肌额腹（图 1–1，图 1–2）。

8. Yangbai (GB 14)

【Location】Directly above the pupil, and 1 cun above the midpoint of the eyebrow.

【Method】Puncture subcutaneously 0.5-0.8 cun.

【Indications】Headache, dizziness, eye pain, blurred vision, twitching of eyelids, and deviated mouth and eye.

【Stratified anatomy】①Skin; ②Subcutaneous tissue (There are lateral branch of the supraorbital n., branches or tributaries of the supraorbital a. & v..); ③Frontal belly of occipitofrontalis (Fig.1-1, Fig.1-2).

九、承泣

【定位】瞳孔直下，眼球与眶下缘之间。

【操作】嘱患者闭目，医者押手拇指向上轻推眼球固定，刺手持针紧靠眶下缘缓慢直刺 0.5 ～ 0.7 寸，不提插，少捻转。

【主治】目赤肿痛，流泪，眼睑瞤动，夜盲，近视，口眼㖞斜。

【进针层次】①皮肤；②皮下组织（内有眶下神经的分支、面神经的颧支、眶下动脉的分支和眶下静脉的属支）；③眼轮匝肌；④眶脂体；⑤下斜肌（图 1–1 ～图 1–3）。

【针刺意外与预防】①若进针过于紧贴眶下壁且深度超过 0.4 寸时，有可能刺中眶下沟中的眶下动、静脉，可造成下眼睑的皮下淤血。②若进针过于贴紧眼球，有可能经下直肌刺中眼球壁，严重时可刺入眼球内部。③若针刺深度超过 1.9 寸，可能刺中总腱环、视神经、眶上裂及其深部结构，症状详见睛明穴。

9. Chengqi (ST 1)

【Location】Directly below the pupil, and between the eyeball and the infraorbital ridge.

【Method】Ask the patient to close his eyes. The acupuncturist gently pushes the eyeball up to fix it with the thumb of his pressing hand. He slowly needles perpendicularly 0.5-0.7 cun along the lower edge of the orbit with his needling hand with no lifting and thrusting and less twirling manipulation.

【Indications】Pain and swelling in the eyes, lacrimation, twitching of eyelids, night blindness, myopia, and deviated mouth and eye.

【Stratified anatomy】①Skin; ②Subcutaneous tissue (There are branches of the infraorbital n., zygomatic branches of facial n., branches or tributaries of the infraorbital a. & v..); ③Orbicularis oculi m.; ④Adipose body of orbit; ⑤Inferior oblique m. (Fig.1-1 ~ Fig.1-3).

【Cautions】①If the insertion is too close to the suborbital wall and the depth exceeds 0.4 cun, it may stab the suborbital arteries and veins in the suborbital groove, which can cause subcutaneous congestion in the lower eyelid. ②If the insertion is too close to the eyeball, it may pierce the eyeball wall through the infrarectus, and if it is serious, it can pierce the inside of the eyeball. ③If the depth of insertion exceeds 1.9 cun, the common tendinous ring, optic n., superior orbital fissure and its deep structure can be injured and for details of the symptoms, please refer to the Jingming (BL 1) acupoint.

十、四白

【定位】瞳孔直下，眶下孔凹陷处。

【操作】直刺 0.3 ～ 0.5 寸，或向下斜刺 1 寸。

【主治】目赤肿痛，眼睑瞤动，流泪，近视，口眼㖞斜，面痛，头痛，眩晕。

【进针层次】①皮肤；②皮下组织（内有眶下神经的分支、面神经颧支、面动脉的分支、面静脉的属支、眶下动脉的分支和眶下静脉的属支）；③眼轮匝肌和提上唇肌；④眶下孔或上颌骨（图 1–1 ～图 1–3）。

【针刺意外与预防】若直刺过深，则经眶下孔进入眶下管，极易刺中眶下管内的眶下动、静脉，可造成眼睑下方的皮下淤血。

10. Sibai (ST 2)

【Location】Directly below the pupil, and in the depression of the infraorbital foramen.

【Method】Puncture perpendicularly 0.3-0.5 cun, or puncture obliquely downward 1 cun.

【Indications】Pain and swelling in the eyes, twitching of eyelids, lacrimation, myopia, deviated mouth and eye, facial pain, headache, and vertigo.

【Stratified anatomy】①Skin; ②Subcutaneous tissue (There are branches of the infraorbital n., zygomatic branches of facial n., branches or tributaries of the facial and infraorbital a. & v..); ③Orbicularis oculi m. and levator labii superioris; ④Infraorbital foramen or maxilla (Fig.1-1 ~ Fig.1-3).

【Cautions】If the perpendicular needling is too deep, the tip of the needle will enter the suborbital canal through the suborbital foramina, which is very easy to pierce the infraorbital a. & v. in the suborbital canal, which can cause subcutaneous congestion below the eyelids.

十一、颧髎

【定位】颧骨下缘，目外眦直下的凹陷中。

【操作】直刺 0.3 ～ 0.5 寸，或斜刺 0.5 ～ 1 寸。

【主治】口㖞，眼睑瞤动，齿痛，面痛，颊肿。

【进针层次】①皮肤；②皮下组织（内有眶下神经的分支、面横动脉和面横静脉）；③颧肌；④咬肌；⑤颞肌（图 1–1，图 1–2）。

11. Quanliao (SI 18)

【Location】Directly below the outer canthus, and in the depression of the lower border of the zygoma.

【Method】Puncture perpendicularly 0.3-0.5 cun, or puncture obliquely 0.5-1 cun.

【Indications】Deviated mouth, twitching of eyelids, toothache, facial pain, and swelling in the cheek.

【Stratified anatomy】①Skin; ②Subcutaneous tissue (There are branches of the infraorbital n., transverse facial a. & v..); ③Zygomaticus major and zygomaticus minor; ④Masseter; ⑤Temporalis (Fig.1-1, Fig.1-2).

十二、地仓

【定位】口角外开 0.4 寸。

【操作】斜刺或平刺 0.5 ～ 0.8 寸，或向迎香、颊车方向透刺 1 ～ 2 寸。

【主治】口㖞，流涎，眼睑瞤动，唇缓不收，齿痛，颊肿。

【进针层次】①皮肤；②皮下组织（内有眶下神经的分支、颊神经的分支、面动脉的分支和面静脉的属支）；③口轮匝肌；④降口角肌或颊肌（图 1–1 ～图 1–3）。

12. Dicang (ST 4)

【Location】0.4 cun lateral to the corner of the mouth.

【Method】Puncture obliquely or subcutaneously 0.5-0.8 cun, or puncture subcutaneously 1-2 cun toward Yingxiang (LI 20) or Jiache (ST 6).

【Indications】Deviated mouth, salivation, twitching of eyelids, flabby lips, toothache, and swelling in the cheek.

【Stratified anatomy】①Skin; ②Subcutaneous tissue (There are branches of the infraorbital and buccal n., branches or tributaries of the facial a. & v..); ③Orbicularis oris; ④Depressor anguli oris or buccinator m. (Fig.1-1 ~ Fig.1-3).

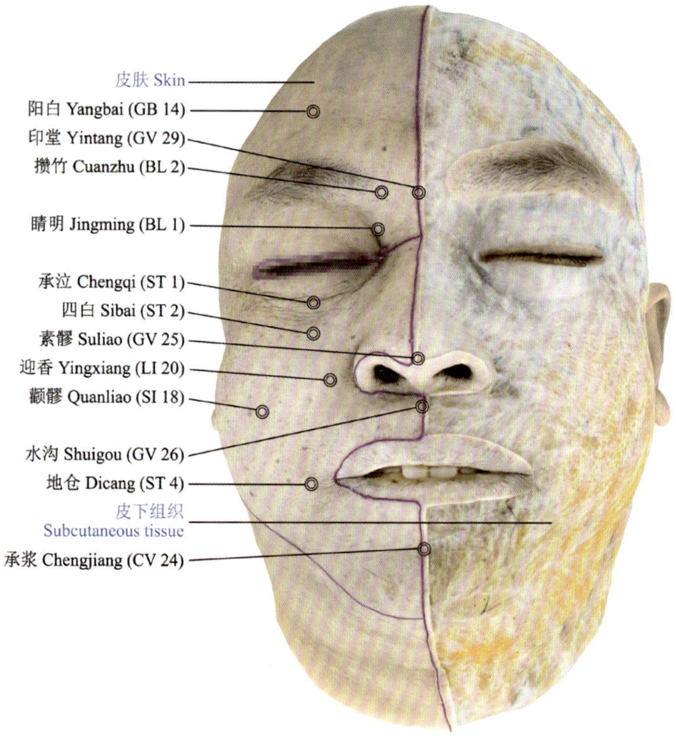
皮肤 Skin
阳白 Yangbai (GB 14)
印堂 Yintang (GV 29)
攒竹 Cuanzhu (BL 2)
睛明 Jingming (BL 1)
承泣 Chengqi (ST 1)
四白 Sibai (ST 2)
素髎 Suliao (GV 25)
迎香 Yingxiang (LI 20)
颧髎 Quanliao (SI 18)
水沟 Shuigou (GV 26)
地仓 Dicang (ST 4)
皮下组织
Subcutaneous tissue
承浆 Chengjiang (CV 24)

图 1–1　头前面腧穴层次解剖（1）

Fig.1-1 Layered anatomy of acupoints on the anterior aspect of the head (1)

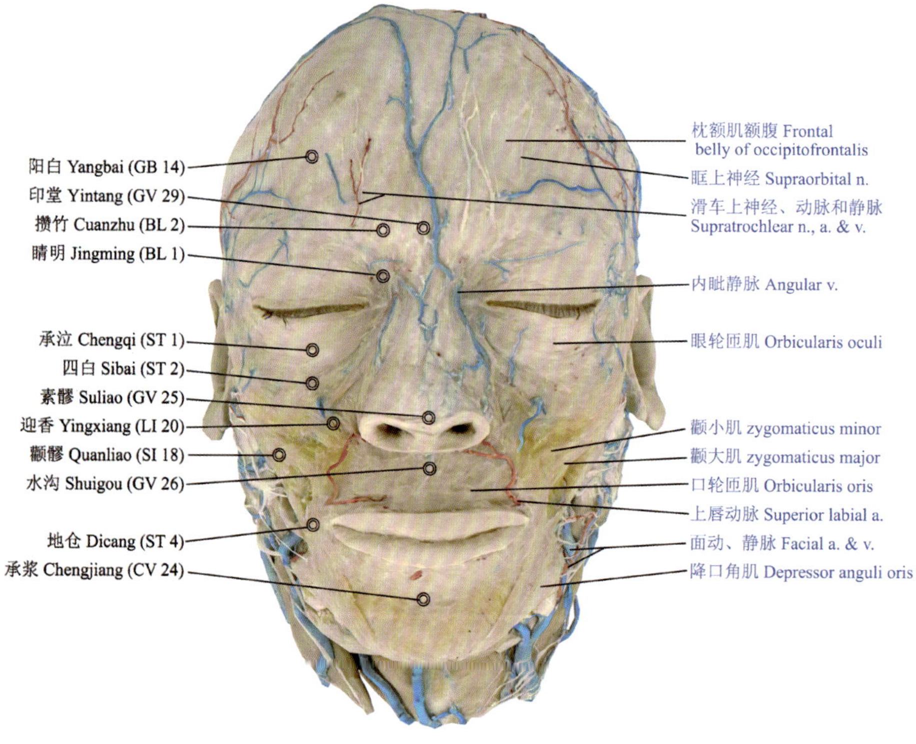
阳白 Yangbai (GB 14)
印堂 Yintang (GV 29)
攒竹 Cuanzhu (BL 2)
睛明 Jingming (BL 1)
承泣 Chengqi (ST 1)
四白 Sibai (ST 2)
素髎 Suliao (GV 25)
迎香 Yingxiang (LI 20)
颧髎 Quanliao (SI 18)
水沟 Shuigou (GV 26)
地仓 Dicang (ST 4)
承浆 Chengjiang (CV 24)
枕额肌额腹 Frontal belly of occipitofrontalis
眶上神经 Supraorbital n.
滑车上神经、动脉和静脉 Supratrochlear n., a. & v.
内眦静脉 Angular v.
眼轮匝肌 Orbicularis oculi
颧小肌 zygomaticus minor
颧大肌 zygomaticus major
口轮匝肌 Orbicularis oris
上唇动脉 Superior labial a.
面动、静脉 Facial a. & v.
降口角肌 Depressor anguli oris

图 1–2　头前面腧穴层次解剖（2）

Fig.1-2 Layered anatomy of acupoints on the anterior aspect of the head (2)

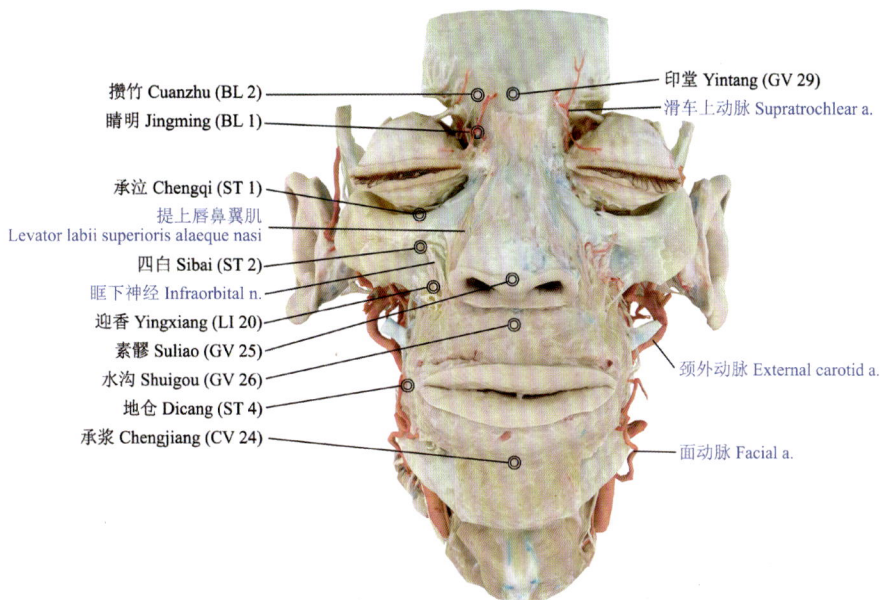

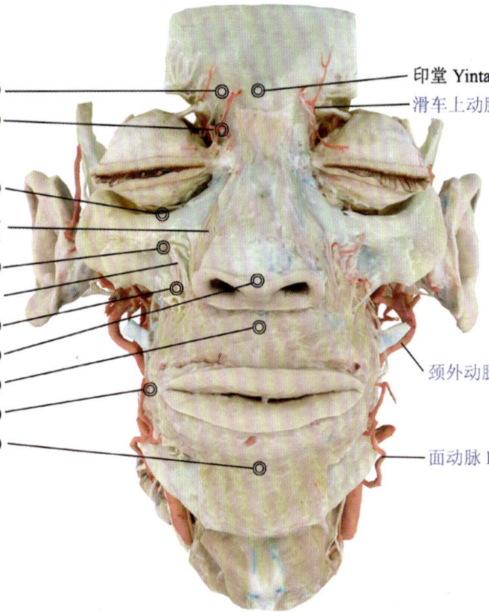

图 1–3　头前面腧穴层次解剖（3）

Fig.1-3 Layered anatomy of acupoints on the anterior aspect of the head (3)

第二节　头侧面腧穴

Section 2　Acupoints on the lateral aspect of the head

一、角孙

【定位】耳尖正对发际处。

【操作】平刺 0.3 ～ 0.5 寸。

【主治】耳部肿痛，目赤肿痛，齿痛，偏头痛，项强。

【进针层次】①皮肤；②皮下组织（内有耳颞神经的分支、颞浅动脉的分支和颞浅静脉的属支）；③耳上肌；④颞筋膜；⑤颞肌（图 1–4 ～图 1–10）。

1. Jiaosun (TE 20)

【Location】Directly above the ear apex within the hairline.

【Method】Puncture subcutaneously 0.3-0.5 cun.

【Indications】Swelling and pain in the ears, pain and swelling in the eyes, toothache, migraine, and stiffness in the nape.

【Stratified anatomy】①Skin; ②Subcutaneous tissue (There are branches of the auriculotemporal n., branches or tributaries of the superficial temporal a. & v..); ③Superior auricular m.; ④Temporal fascia; ⑤Temporalis (Fig.1-4 ~ Fig.1-10).

二、率谷

【定位】耳尖直上入发际 1.5 寸。

【操作】平刺 0.5 ～ 0.8 寸。

【主治】头痛，眩晕，耳鸣，耳聋，小儿急、慢惊风。

【进针层次】①皮肤；②皮下组织（内有耳颞神经的分支、颞浅动脉的分支和颞浅静脉的属支）；③耳上肌；④颞筋膜；⑤颞肌（图 1–4 ～图 1–11）。

2. Shuaigu (GB 8)

【Location】Above the ear apex within the hairline, and 1.5 cun above the hairline.

【Method】Puncture subcutaneously 0.5-0.8 cun.

【Indications】Headache, vertigo, tinnitus, deafness, and acute and chronic infantile convulsions.

【Stratified anatomy】①Skin; ②Subcutaneous tissue (There are branches of the auriculotemporal n., branches or tributaries of the superficial temporal a. & v..); ③Superior auricular m.; ④Temporal fascia; ⑤Temporalis (Fig.1-4 ~ Fig.1-11).

三、丝竹空

【定位】眉梢凹陷中。

【操作】平刺或斜刺 0.5 ～ 1 寸。

【主治】目眩，目赤肿痛，眼睑瞤动，头痛，癫狂痫。

【进针层次】①皮肤；②皮下组织（内有眶上神经的分支、颧神经的分支、颞浅动脉的分支和颞浅静脉的属支）；③眼轮匝肌（图 1–4 ～图 1–10）。

3. Sizhukong (TE 23)

【Location】In the depression at the lateral end of the eyebrow.

【Method】Puncture subcutaneously or obliquely 0.5-1 cun.

【Indications】Dizziness, pain and swelling in the eyes, twitching of eyelids, headache, insanity mania, and epilepsy.

【Stratified anatomy】①Skin; ②Subcutaneous tissue (There are branches of the supraorbital and zygomatic n., branches or tributaries of the superficial temporal a. & v..); ③Orbicularis oculi m. (Fig.1-4 ~ Fig.1-10).

四、瞳子髎

【定位】目外眦外侧 0.5 寸凹陷中。

【操作】平刺 0.3 ～ 0.5 寸，或点刺出血。

【主治】目赤肿痛，夜盲，口眼㖞斜，头痛。

【进针层次】①皮肤；②皮下组织（内有眶上神经的分支、颧神经的分支、颞浅动脉的分支和颞浅静脉的属支）；③眼轮匝肌；④颞筋膜；⑤颞肌（图 1–4 ～图 1–11）。

4. Tongziliao (GB 1)

【Location】0.5 cun lateral to outer canthus, and in the depression on the lateral aspect of the orbit.

【Method】Puncture subcutaneously 0.3-0.5 cun, or prick to cause bleeding.

【Indications】Pain and swelling in the eyes, night blindness, deviated mouth and eye, and headache.

【Stratified anatomy】①Skin; ②Subcutaneous tissue (There are branches of the supraorbital and zygomatic n., branches or tributaries of the superficial temporal a. & v..); ③Orbicularis oculi m.; ④Temporal fascia; ⑤Temporalis (Fig.1-4 ~ Fig.1-11).

五、太阳

【定位】眉梢与目外眦之间，向后约一横指的凹陷中。

【操作】直刺或斜刺 0.3 ～ 0.5 寸，或点刺出血。

【主治】头痛，目赤肿痛，目眩，口眼㖞斜，面痛。

【进针层次】①皮肤；②皮下组织（内有耳颞神经的分支、颞浅动脉的分支和颞浅静脉的属支）；③耳上肌；④颞筋膜；⑤颞肌（图 1–4 ～图 1–10）。

5. Taiyang (EX-HN 5)

【Location】Between the lateral end of the eyebrow and the outer canthus, and in the depression one finger-breadth posterior to them.

【Method】Puncture perpendicularly or obliquely 0.3-0.5 cun, or prick to cause bleeding.

【Indications】Headache, pain and swelling in the eyes, dizziness, deviated mouth and eye, and facial pain.

【Stratified anatomy】①Skin; ②Subcutaneous tissue (There are branches of the auriculotemporal n., branches or tributaries of the superficial temporal a. & v..); ③Orbicularis oculi m.; ④Temporal fascia; ⑤Temporalis (Fig.1-4 ~ Fig.1-10).

六、下关

【定位】颧弓下缘与下颌切迹之间凹陷中。

【操作】直刺或斜刺 0.5 ～ 1 寸。

【主治】耳鸣，耳聋，聤耳，齿痛，面痛，口㖞，牙关开合不利。

【进针层次】①皮肤；②皮下组织（内有耳颞神经的分支、面神经颧支、面横动脉的分支和面横静脉的属支）；③腮腺；④咬肌；⑤颞肌与下颌骨髁突之间；⑥上颌动、静脉；⑦翼外肌（图 1–4 ～图 1–11）。

【针刺意外与预防】若直刺过深，则可能刺中上颌动、静脉；若继续深刺，可刺中翼外肌的深面之下牙槽神经、舌神经和脑膜中动脉，若刺中脑膜中动脉，可引起严重出血。

6. Xiaguan (ST 7)

【Location】In the depression between the lower edge of the zygomatic arch and the mandibular notch.

【Method】Puncture perpendicularly or obliquely 0.5-1 cun.

【Indications】Tinnitus, deafness, otopyorrhea, toothache, facial pain, deviated mouth, and motor impairment of the jaw.

【Stratified anatomy】①Skin; ②Subcutaneous tissue (There are branches of the auriculotemporal n., zygomatic branches of the facial n., branches or tributaries of the transverse facial a. & v..); ③Parotid gland; ④Masseter; ⑤Between temporalis and condylar process of mandible; ⑥Maxillary a. & v.; ⑦Lateral pterygoid m. (Fig.1-4 ~ Fig.1-11).

【Cautions】If perpendicular insertion is too deep, the maxillary a. & v. may be injured. If stab deeper, it may prick the inferior alveolar n., lingual n. and middle meningeal a. under the deep surface of the lateral pterygoud m.. If the middle meningeal a is pricked, it can cause serious bleeding.

七、颊车

【定位】下颌角前上方一横指处。

【操作】直刺 0.3 ～ 0.5 寸，或向地仓方向透刺 1.5 ～ 2 寸。

【主治】口㖞，口噤，齿痛，颊肿。

【进针层次】①皮肤；②皮下组织（内有耳大神经的分支和面神经的下颌缘支）；③咬肌（图 1–4 ～图 1–11）。

7. Jiache (ST 6)

【Location】One finger-breadth anterosuperior to the angle of mandible.

【Method】Puncture perpendicularly 0.3-0.5 cun, or puncture subcutaneously 1.5-2 cun toward Dicang (ST 4).

【Indications】Deviated mouth, lockjaw, toothache, and swelling in the cheek.

【Stratified anatomy】①Skin; ②Subcutaneous tissue (There are branches of the great auricular n. and marginal mandibular branches of the facial n..); ③Masseter (Fig.1-4 ~ Fig.1-11).

八、大迎

【定位】下颌角前方，咬肌附着部的前缘凹陷中，面动脉搏动处。

【操作】避开面动脉直刺 0.3 ～ 0.5 寸，或向颊车方向斜刺 0.5 ～ 1 寸。

【主治】齿痛，颊肿，口噤，口㖞。

【进针层次】①皮肤；②皮下组织（内有耳大神经的分支、颊神经的分支、面神经的下颌缘支和颈阔肌）；③降口角肌；④面动、静脉（图 1–4 ～图 1–11）。

8. Daying (ST 5)

【Location】Anterior to the mandibular angle, and in the depression anterior to the attachment of the masseter, the pulsation site of facial a..

【Method】Avoid the facial a., puncture perpendicularly 0.3-0.5 cun, or puncture obliquely 0.5-1 cun toward Jiache (ST 6).

【Indications】Toothache, swelling in the cheek, lockjaw, and deviated mouth.

【Stratified anatomy】①Skin; ②Subcutaneous tissue (There are branches of the great auricular and buccal n., marginal mandibular branches of the facial n. and platysma.); ③Depressor anguli oris; ④Facial a. & v. (Fig.1-4 ~ Fig.1-11).

九、耳门

【定位】耳屏上切迹与下颌骨髁突之间的凹陷中。

【操作】微张口，直刺 0.5 ～ 1 寸。

【主治】耳聋，耳鸣，聤耳，齿痛。

【进针层次】①皮肤；②皮下组织（内有耳颞神经的分支、颞浅动脉的分支和颞浅静脉的属支）；③腮腺上缘（图 1–4 ～图 1–11）。

9. Ermen (TE 21)

【Location】In the depression between the upper notch of the tragus and condyloid process of the mandible.

【Method】Ask the patient to open mouth gently, puncture perpendicularly 0.5-1 cun.

【Indications】Deafness, tinnitus, otopyorrhea, and toothache.

【Stratified anatomy】①Skin; ②Subcutaneous tissue (There are branches of the auriculotemporal n., branches or tributaries of the superficial temporal a. & v..); ③Upper margin of the parotid gland (Fig.1-4 ~ Fig.1-11).

十、听宫

【定位】耳屏正中与下颌骨髁突之间的凹陷中。

【操作】微张口，直刺 0.5 ～ 1 寸。

【主治】耳鸣，耳聋，聤耳，齿痛，癫狂。

【进针层次】①皮肤；②皮下组织（内有耳颞神经的分支、颞浅动脉的分支和颞浅静脉的属支）；③外耳道软骨（图 1–4 ～图 1–11）。

10. Tinggong (SI 19)

【Location】In the depression between the centre of the tragus and the condyloid process of the mandible.

【Method】Ask the patient to open mouth gently, puncture perpendicularly 0.5-1 cun.

【Indications】Tinnitus, deafness, otopyorrhea, toothache, and insanity and mania.

【Stratified anatomy】①Skin; ②Subcutaneous tissue (There are branches of the auriculotemporal n., branches or tributaries of the superficial temporal a. & v..); ③External meatal cartilage (Fig.1-4 ~ Fig.1-11).

十一、听会

【定位】耳屏间切迹与下颌骨髁突之间的凹陷中。

【操作】微张口，直刺 0.5 ～ 0.8 寸。

【主治】耳鸣，耳聋，聤耳，齿痛，口㖞，面痛。

【进针层次】①皮肤；②皮下组织（内有耳颞神经的分支、颞浅动脉的分支和颞浅静脉的属支）；③腮腺（图 1–4 ～图 1–11）。

11. Tinghui (GB 2)

【Location】In the depression between the intertragic notch and the condyloid process of the mandible.

【Method】Ask the patient to open mouth gently, puncture perpendicularly 0.5-0.8 cun.

【Indications】Tinnitus, deafness, otopyorrhea, toothache, deviated mouth, and facial pain.

【Stratified anatomy】①Skin; ②Subcutaneous tissue (There are branches of the auriculotemporal n. and branches or tributaries of the superficial temporal a. & v..); ③Parotid gland (Fig.1-4 ~ Fig.1-11).

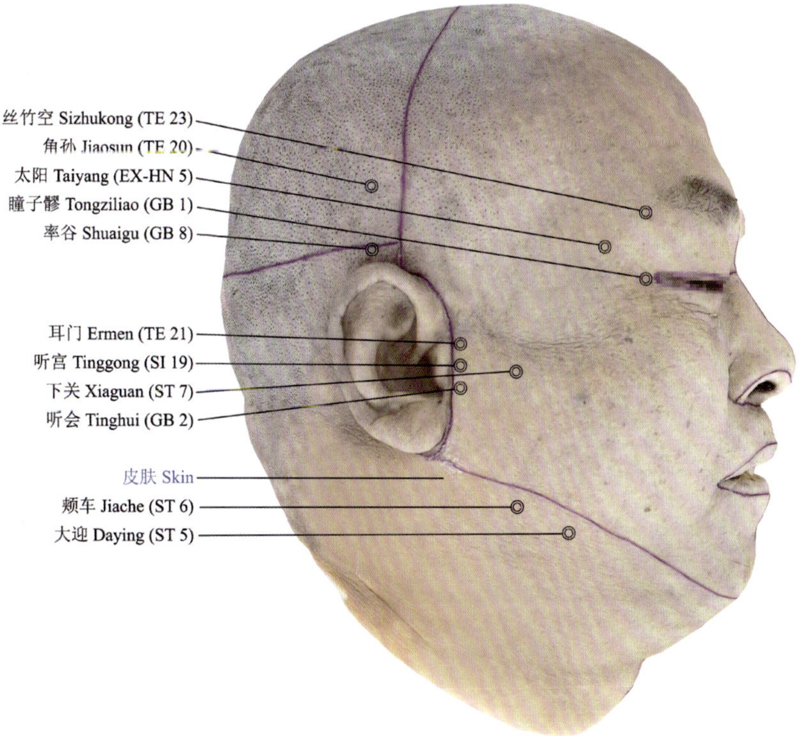
丝竹空 Sizhukong (TE 23)
角孙 Jiaosun (TE 20)
太阳 Taiyang (EX-HN 5)
瞳子髎 Tongziliao (GB 1)
率谷 Shuaigu (GB 8)
耳门 Ermen (TE 21)
听宫 Tinggong (SI 19)
下关 Xiaguan (ST 7)
听会 Tinghui (GB 2)
皮肤 Skin
颊车 Jiache (ST 6)
大迎 Daying (ST 5)

图 1-4 头侧面腧穴层次解剖（1）

Fig.1-4 Layered anatomy of acupoints on the lateral aspect of the head (1)

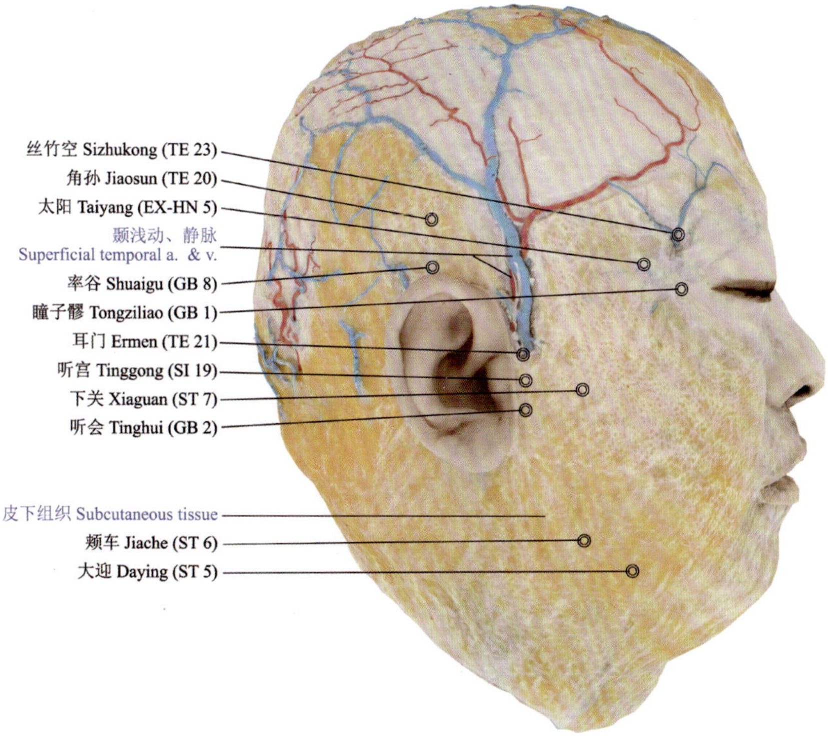
丝竹空 Sizhukong (TE 23)
角孙 Jiaosun (TE 20)
太阳 Taiyang (EX-HN 5)
颞浅动、静脉
Superficial temporal a. & v.
率谷 Shuaigu (GB 8)
瞳子髎 Tongziliao (GB 1)
耳门 Ermen (TE 21)
听宫 Tinggong (SI 19)
下关 Xiaguan (ST 7)
听会 Tinghui (GB 2)
皮下组织 Subcutaneous tissue
颊车 Jiache (ST 6)
大迎 Daying (ST 5)

图 1-5 头侧面腧穴层次解剖（2）

Fig.1-5 Layered anatomy of acupoints on the lateral aspect of the head (2)

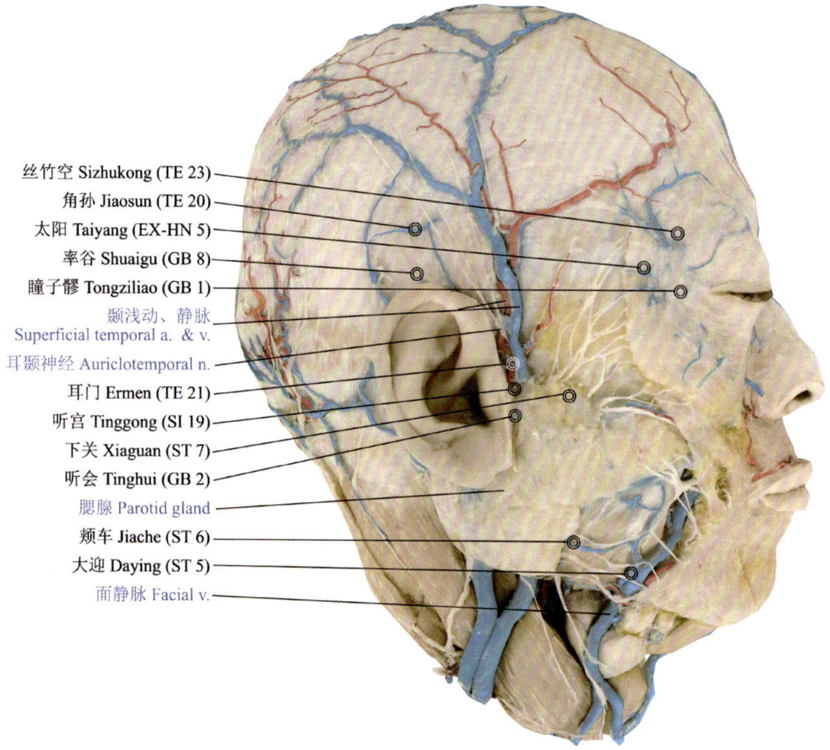

图 1–6　头侧面腧穴层次解剖（3）

Fig.1-6　Layered anatomy of acupoints on the lateral aspect of the head (3)

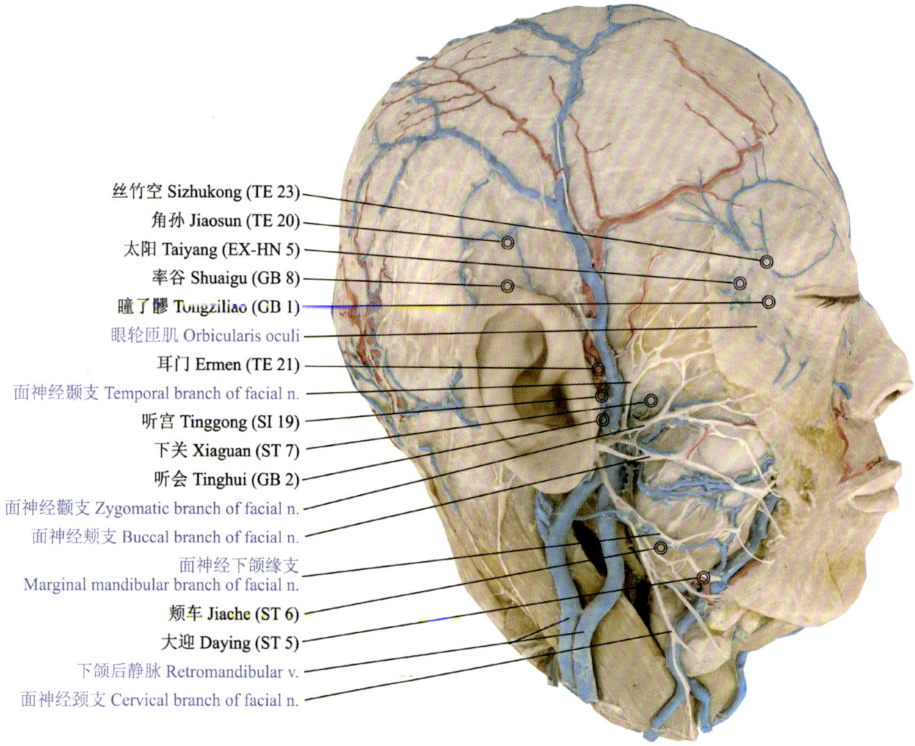

图 1–7　头侧面腧穴层次解剖（4）

Fig.1-7　Layered anatomy of acupoints on the lateral aspect of the head (4)

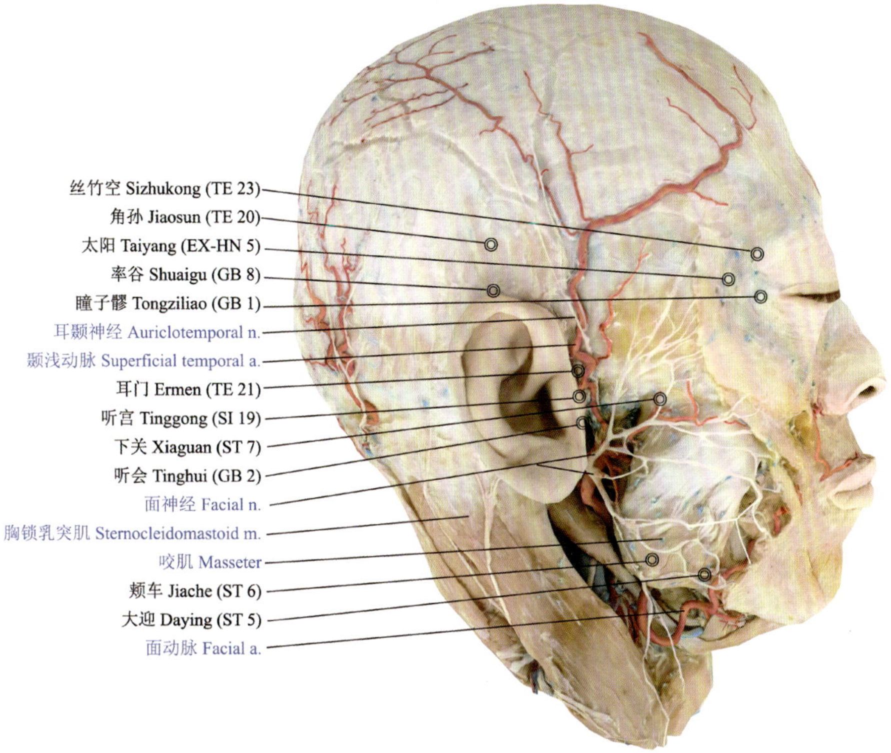
丝竹空 Sizhukong (TE 23)
角孙 Jiaosun (TE 20)
太阳 Taiyang (EX-HN 5)
率谷 Shuaigu (GB 8)
瞳子髎 Tongziliao (GB 1)
耳颞神经 Auriclotemporal n.
颞浅动脉 Superficial temporal a.
耳门 Ermen (TE 21)
听宫 Tinggong (SI 19)
下关 Xiaguan (ST 7)
听会 Tinghui (GB 2)
面神经 Facial n.
胸锁乳突肌 Sternocleidomastoid m.
咬肌 Masseter
颊车 Jiache (ST 6)
大迎 Daying (ST 5)
面动脉 Facial a.

图 1–8　头侧面腧穴层次解剖（5）

Fig.1-8　Layered anatomy of acupoints on the lateral aspect of the head (5)

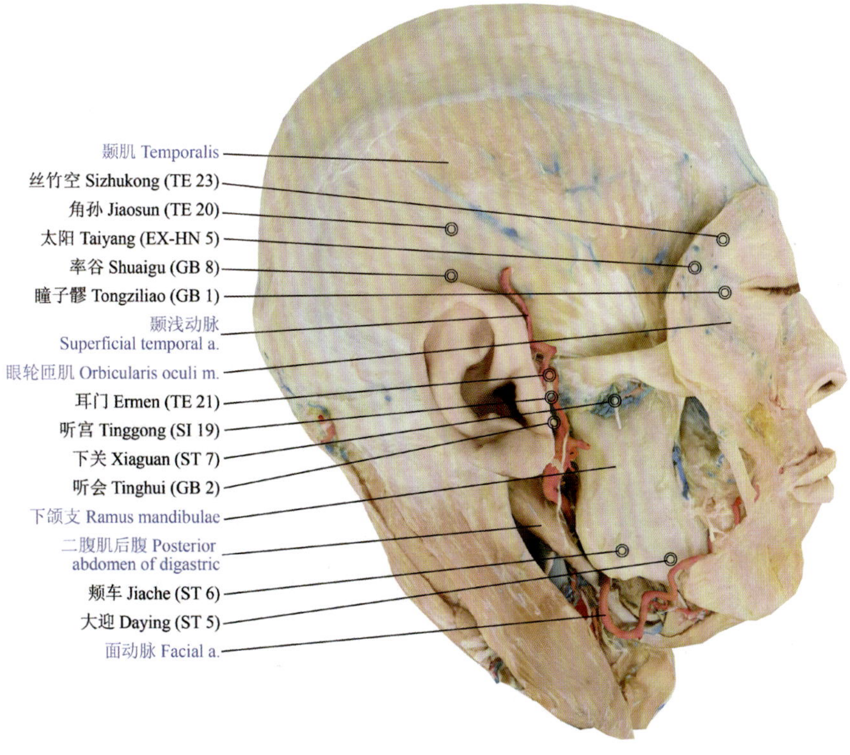
颞肌 Temporalis
丝竹空 Sizhukong (TE 23)
角孙 Jiaosun (TE 20)
太阳 Taiyang (EX-HN 5)
率谷 Shuaigu (GB 8)
瞳子髎 Tongziliao (GB 1)
颞浅动脉
Superficial temporal a.
眼轮匝肌 Orbicularis oculi m.
耳门 Ermen (TE 21)
听宫 Tinggong (SI 19)
下关 Xiaguan (ST 7)
听会 Tinghui (GB 2)
下颌支 Ramus mandibulae
二腹肌后腹 Posterior
abdomen of digastric
颊车 Jiache (ST 6)
大迎 Daying (ST 5)
面动脉 Facial a.

图 1–9　头侧面腧穴层次解剖（6）

Fig.1-9　Layered anatomy of acupoints on the lateral aspect of the head (6)

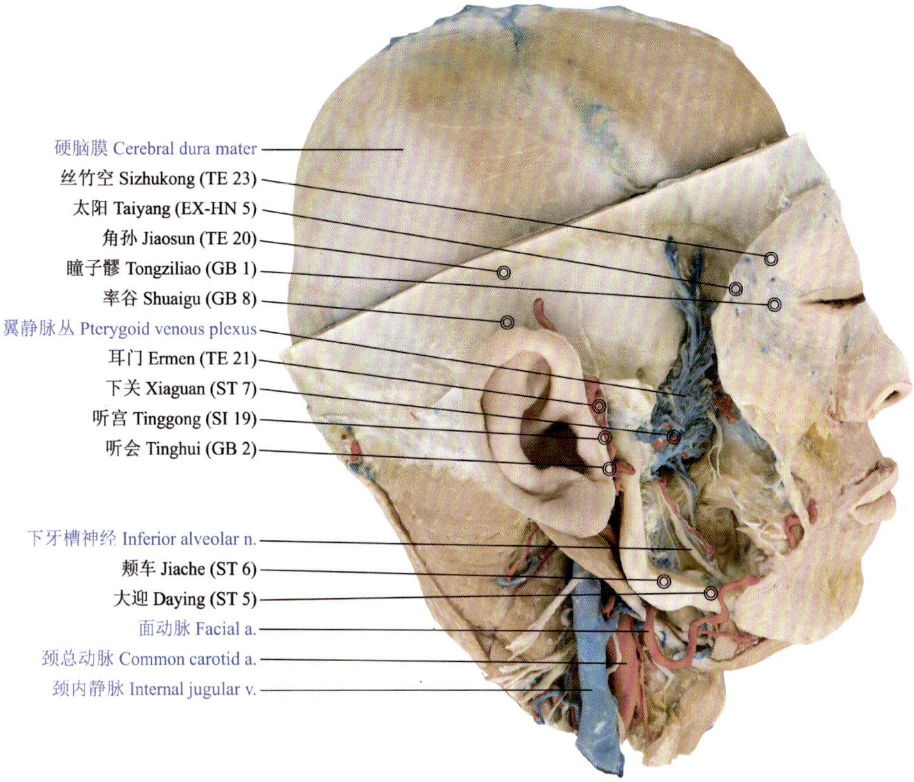
硬脑膜 Cerebral dura mater
丝竹空 Sizhukong (TE 23)
太阳 Taiyang (EX-HN 5)
角孙 Jiaosun (TE 20)
瞳子髎 Tongziliao (GB 1)
率谷 Shuaigu (GB 8)
翼静脉丛 Pterygoid venous plexus
耳门 Ermen (TE 21)
下关 Xiaguan (ST 7)
听宫 Tinggong (SI 19)
听会 Tinghui (GB 2)
下牙槽神经 Inferior alveolar n.
颊车 Jiache (ST 6)
大迎 Daying (ST 5)
面动脉 Facial a.
颈总动脉 Common carotid a.
颈内静脉 Internal jugular v.

图 1–10　头侧面腧穴层次解剖（7）

Fig.1-10　Layered anatomy of acupoints on the lateral aspect of the head (7)

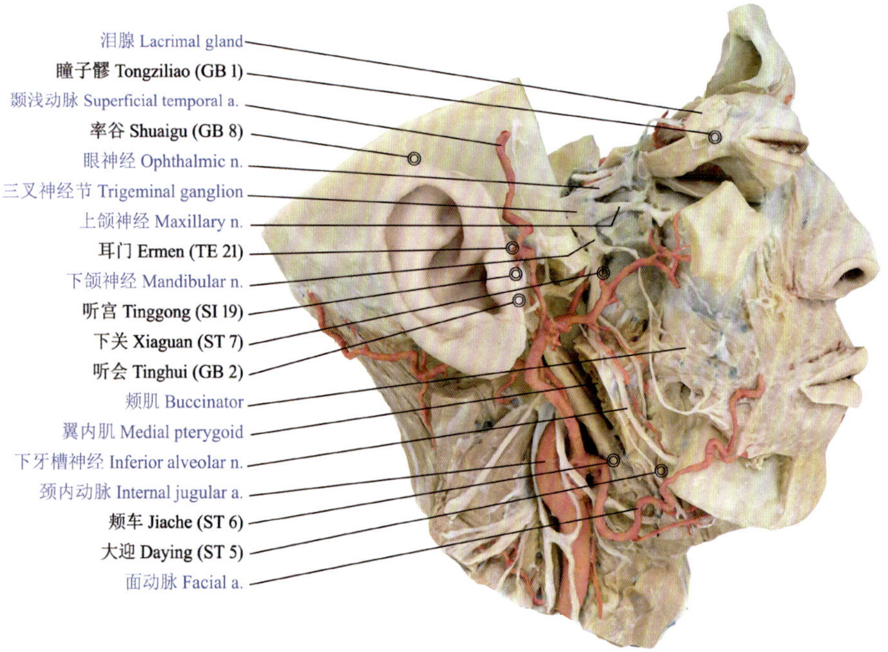
泪腺 Lacrimal gland
瞳子髎 Tongziliao (GB 1)
颞浅动脉 Superficial temporal a.
率谷 Shuaigu (GB 8)
眼神经 Ophthalmic n.
三叉神经节 Trigeminal ganglion
上颌神经 Maxillary n.
耳门 Ermen (TE 21)
下颌神经 Mandibular n.
听宫 Tinggong (SI 19)
下关 Xiaguan (ST 7)
听会 Tinghui (GB 2)
颊肌 Buccinator
翼内肌 Medial pterygoid
下牙槽神经 Inferior alveolar n.
颈内动脉 Internal jugular a.
颊车 Jiache (ST 6)
大迎 Daying (ST 5)
面动脉 Facial a.

图 1–11　头侧面腧穴层次解剖（8）

Fig.1-11　Layered anatomy of acupoints on the lateral aspect of the head (8)

第三节　头顶部腧穴

Section 3　Acupoints on the top of the head

一、百会

【定位】前发际正中直上 5 寸。

【操作】平刺 0.5 ～ 1 寸。

【主治】头痛，眩晕，昏厥，癫狂痫，中风失语，久泻，脱肛，阴挺，健忘，失眠。

【进针层次】①皮肤；②皮下组织（内有滑车上神经、枕大神经和耳颞神经，颞浅动脉和枕动脉的分支，颞浅静脉和枕静脉的属支）；③帽状腱膜；④腱膜下疏松结缔组织（图 1–12 ～图 1–16）。

【针刺意外与预防】针刺头顶部腧穴，如百会、神庭、上星、头临泣、头维等，通常将针平刺在腱膜下疏松结缔组织中，一般不提插，多采用持续捻转手法，亦可以电针代替手法捻转。若针刺入头皮（即皮肤、皮下组织和帽状腱膜三层），并继续刺入此层，针尖阻力加大，患者立感剧烈疼痛。由于皮下组织血管丰富，出针时，应缓慢退针，并用干棉球按压半分钟，以免出血。

1. Baihui (GV 20)

【Location】5 cun directly upward from the midpoint of the front hairline.

【Method】Puncture subcutaneously 0.5-1 cun.

【Indications】Headache, dizziness, coma, insanity, mania, epilepsy, aphasia due to apoplexy, prolonged diarrhea, prolapse of the rectum, prolapse of uterus, forgetfulness, and insomnia.

【Stratified anatomy】①Skin; ②Subcutaneous tissue (There are branches of the supratrochlear n., greater occipital n. and auriculotemporal n., branches or tributaries of the superficial temporal a. & v. and occiptal a. & v..); ③Epicranial aponeurosis; ④Subgaleal loose connective tissue (Fig.1-12 ~ Fig.1-16).

【Cautions】When puncture the acupoints on the top of the head, such as Baihui (GV 20), Shenting (GV 24), Shangxing (GV 23), Toulinqi (GB 15), and Touwei (ST 8), etc., the needle is usually inserted subcutaneously into the subgaleal loose connective tissue, with no lifting or thrusting, but continuous twisting is mostly used and it can be replaced by electroacupuncture. If the needle is stabbed into the scalp, the resistance of needle tip is increased, and the patient will feel terrible pain immediately. Due to the abundance of blood vessels in subcutaneous tissue, the needle should be slowly withdrawn and the pinhole should be pressed with a dry cotton ball for half a minute to avoid bleeding.

二、上星

【定位】前发际正中直上 1 寸。

【操作】平刺 0.5 ～ 0.8 寸。

【主治】头痛，眩晕，目赤肿痛，流泪，鼻渊，鼻衄。

【进针层次】①皮肤；②皮下组织（内有滑车上神经的分支、滑车上动脉的分支和滑车上静脉的属支）；③帽状腱膜；④腱膜下疏松结缔组织（图 1–12 ～图 1–16）。

2. Shangxing (GV 23)

【Location】1 cun directly upward from the midpoint of the front hairline.

【Method】Puncture subcutaneously 0.5-0.8 cun.

【Indications】Headache, vertigo, red, swollen and painful eyes, lacrimation, sinusitis, and epistaxis.

【Stratified anatomy】①Skin; ②Subcutaneous tissue (There are branches of the supratrochlear n., branches or tributaries of the supratrochlear a. & v..); ③Epicranial aponeurosis; ④Subgaleal loose connective tissue (Fig.1-12 ~ Fig.1-16).

三、神庭

【定位】前发际正中直上 0.5 寸。

【操作】平刺 0.3 ～ 0.5 寸。

【主治】头痛，眩晕，目赤肿痛，流泪，鼻渊，鼻衄，癫狂痫，失眠，健忘。

【进针层次】①皮肤；②皮下组织（内有滑车上神经的分支、滑车上动脉的分支和滑车上静脉的属支）；③左、右枕额肌额腹之间；④腱膜下疏松结缔组织（图 1–12 ～图 1–16）。

3. Shenting (GV 24)

【Location】0.5 cun directly upward from the midpoint of the front hairline.

【Method】Puncture subcutaneously 0.3-0.5 cun.

【Indications】Headache, vertigo, red, swollen and painful eyes, lacrimation, sinusitis, epistaxis, insanity, mania, epilepsy, insomnia, and forgetfulness.

【Stratified anatomy】①Skin; ②Subcutaneous tissue (There are branches of the supratrochlear n., branches or tributaries of the supratrochlear a. & v..); ③Between the left and right frontal belly of occipitofrontalis; ④Subgaleal loose connective tissue (Fig.1-12 ~ Fig.1-16).

四、头临泣

【定位】瞳孔直上，前发际上 0.5 寸。

【操作】平刺 0.5 ～ 0.8 寸。

【主治】头痛，目痛，目眩，鼻塞，鼻渊，小儿惊风。

【进针层次】①皮肤；②皮下组织（内有眶上神经的外侧支、眶上动脉的分支和眶上静脉的属支）；③帽状腱膜；④腱膜下疏松结缔组织（图 1–12 ～图 1–16）。

4. Toulinqi (GB 15)

【Location】0.5 cun upward from the front hairline straightly over the pupils.

【Method】Puncture subcutaneously 0.5-0.8 cun.

【Indications】Headache, eye pain, dizziness, nasal obstruction, sinusitis, and infantile convulsions.

【Stratified anatomy】①Skin; ②Subcutaneous tissue (There are lateral branch of the supraorbital n., branches or tributaries of the supraorbital a. & v..); ③Epicranial aponeurosis; ④Subgaleal loose connective tissue (Fig.1-12 ~ Fig.1-16).

五、头维

【定位】额角发际直上 0.5 寸，头正中线旁开 4.5 寸。

【操作】向后平刺 0.5 ～ 0.8 寸。

【主治】头痛，眩晕，目痛，流泪，眼睑瞤动。

【进针层次】①皮肤；②皮下组织（内有耳颞神经的分支、面神经的颞支、颞浅动脉的分支和颞浅静脉的属支）；③帽状腱膜；④腱膜下疏松结缔组织（图 1–12 ～图 1–16）。

5. Touwei (ST 8)

【Location】0.5 cun above the hairline of the frontal eminence, and 4.5 cun lateral to the midline of the head along the anteroposterior direction.

【Method】Puncture subcutaneously backwards 0.5-0.8 cun.

【Indications】Headache, vertigo, eye pain, lacrimation, and twitching of eyelids.

【Stratified anatomy】①Skin; ②Subcutaneous tissue (There are branches of the auriculotemporal n., temporal branches of facial n., branches or tributaries of the superficial temporal a. & v..); ③Epicranial aponeurosis; ④Subgaleal loose connective tissue (Fig.1-12 ~ Fig.1-16).

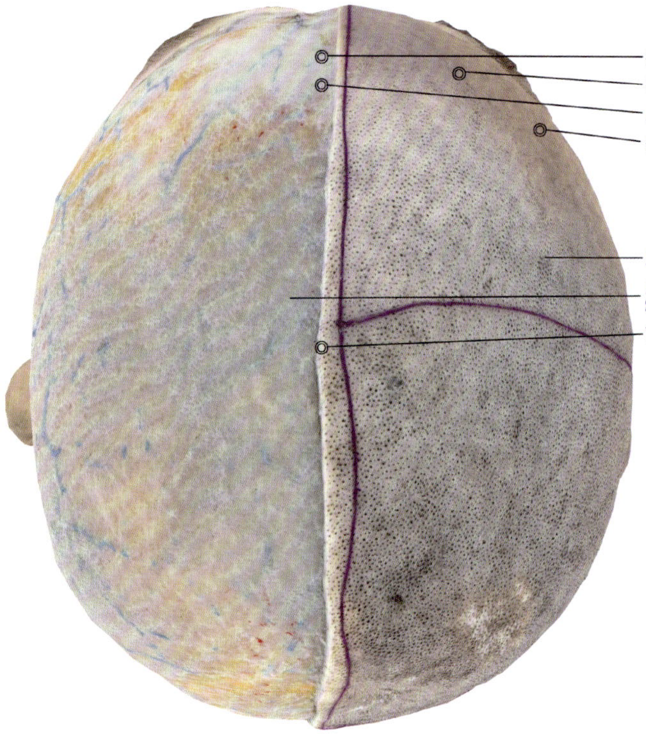
神庭 Shenting (GV 24)
头临泣 Toulinqi (GB 15)
上星 Shangxing (GV 23)
头维 Touwei (ST 8)
皮肤 Skin
皮下组织
Subcutaneous tissue
百会 Baihui (GV 20)

图 1–12　头顶部腧穴层次解剖（1）

Fig.1-12　Layered anatomy of acupoints on the top of the head (1)

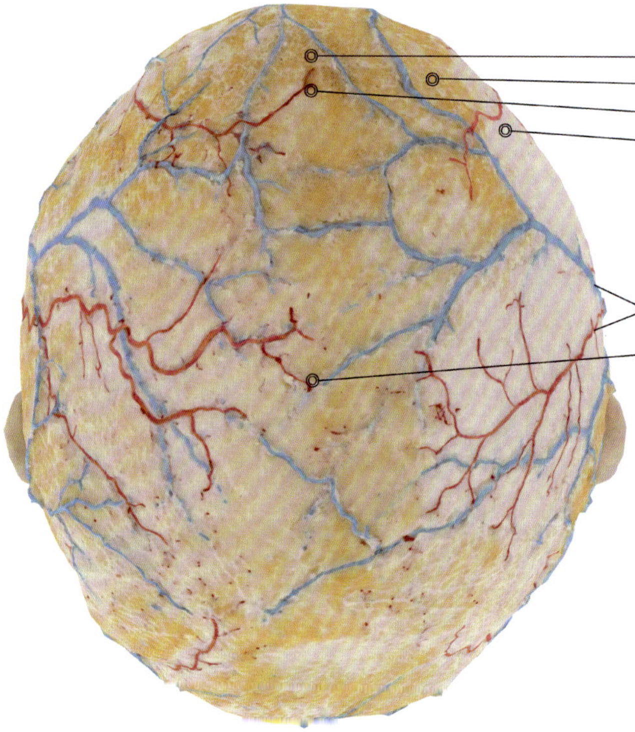
神庭 Shenting (GV 24)
头临泣 Toulinqi (GB 15)
上星 Shangxing (GV 23)
头维 Touwei (ST 8)
颞浅动、静脉
Superficial temporal a. & v.
百会 Baihui (GV 20)

图 1–13　头顶部腧穴层次解剖（2）

Fig.1-13　Layered anatomy of acupoints on the top of the head (2)

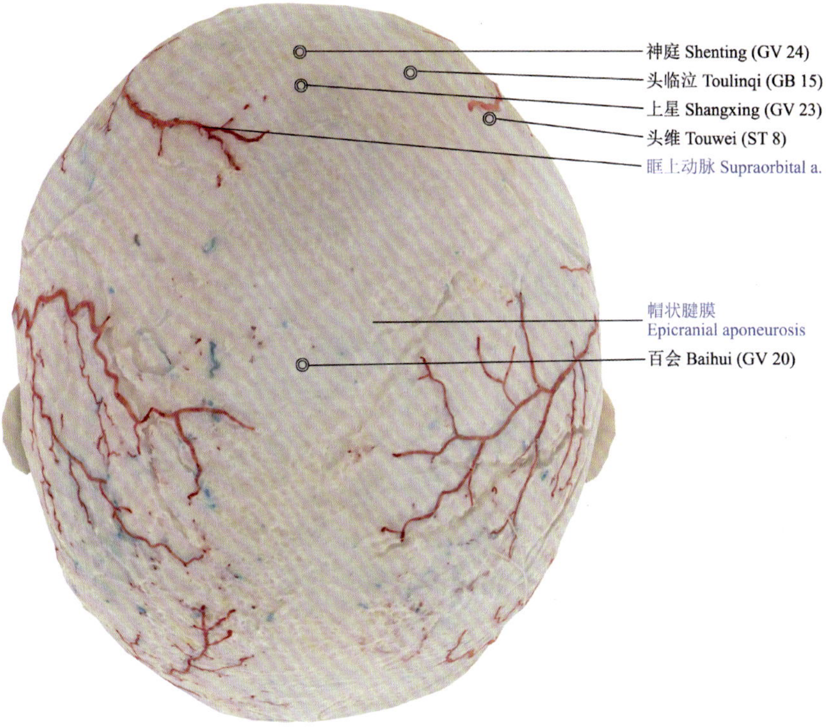
神庭 Shenting (GV 24)
头临泣 Toulinqi (GB 15)
上星 Shangxing (GV 23)
头维 Touwei (ST 8)
眶上动脉 Supraorbital a.
帽状腱膜
Epicranial aponeurosis
百会 Baihui (GV 20)

图 1–14　头顶部腧穴层次解剖（3）

Fig.1-14　Layered anatomy of acupoints on the top of the head (3)

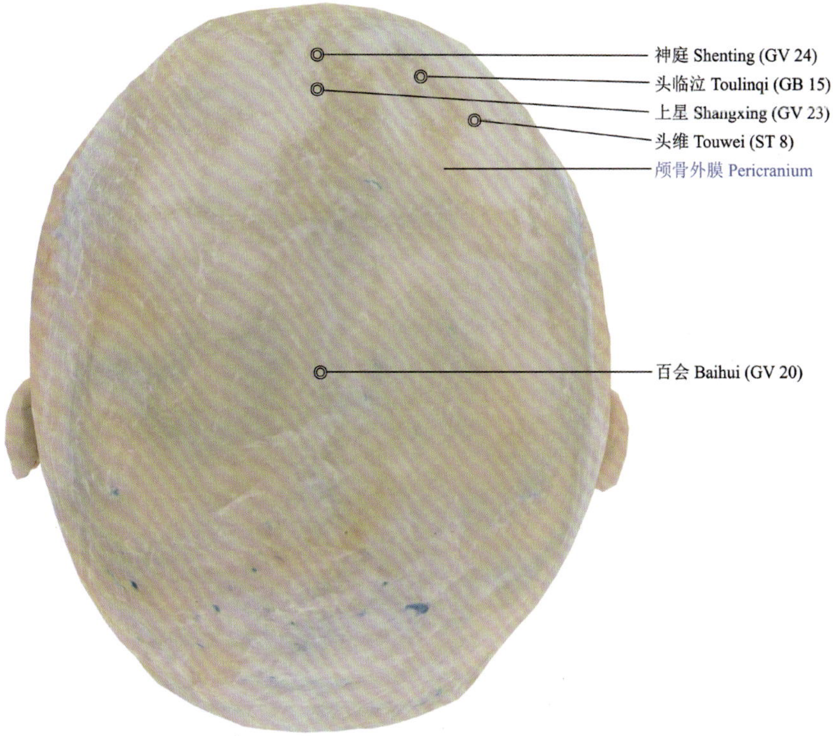
神庭 Shenting (GV 24)
头临泣 Toulinqi (GB 15)
上星 Shangxing (GV 23)
头维 Touwei (ST 8)
颅骨外膜 Pericranium
百会 Baihui (GV 20)

图 1–15　头顶部腧穴层次解剖（4）

Fig.1-15　Layered anatomy of acupoints on the top of the head (4)

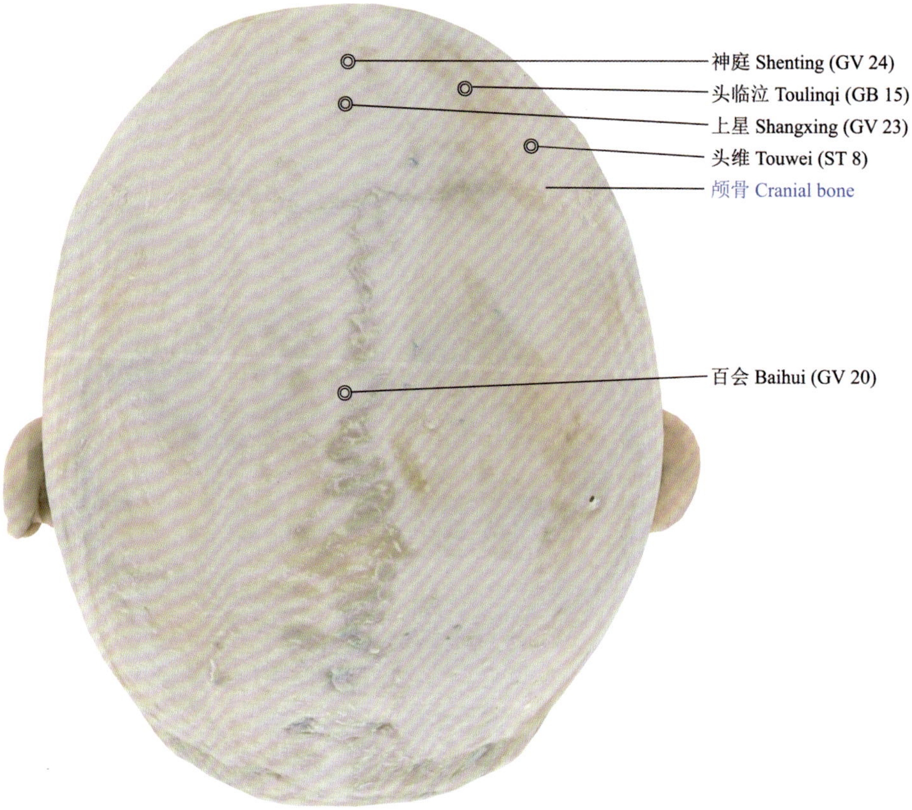
神庭 Shenting (GV 24)
头临泣 Toulinqi (GB 15)
上星 Shangxing (GV 23)
头维 Touwei (ST 8)
颅骨 Cranial bone
百会 Baihui (GV 20)

图 1-16　头顶部腧穴层次解剖（5）
Fig.1-16　Layered anatomy of acupoints on the top of the head (5)

第二章　颈项部腧穴层次解剖

Chapter 2　Layered Anatomy of Acupoints on the Neck

第一节　颈前面腧穴

Section 1　Acupoints on the anterior aspect of the neck

一、廉泉

【定位】喉结上方，舌骨上缘凹陷中，前正中线上。

【操作】向上斜刺 0.5 ～ 0.8 寸。

【主治】舌下肿痛，咽喉肿痛，舌缓流涎，舌干口燥，中风失语，暴喑，梅核气。

【进针层次】①皮肤；②皮下组织（内有颈横神经的分支、颈阔肌、颈前静脉和颏下淋巴结等）；③左、右二腹肌前腹之间；④下颌舌骨肌；⑤颏舌骨肌；⑥颏舌肌（图 2–1 ～图 2–9）。

1. Lianquan (CV 23)

【Location】On the anterior midline, superior to the laryngeal prominence, and in the depression of the upper edge of the hyoid bone.

【Method】Puncture obliquely upward 0.5-0.8 cun.

【Indications】Sublingual swelling and pain, sore throat, sluggish movement of the tongue, salivation, dry tongue and mouth, aphasia due to apoplexy, sudden loss of voice, and globus hystericus.

【Stratified anatomy】①Skin; ②Subcutaneous tissue (There are branches of the transverse cervical n., platysma, anterior jugular v. and submental lymph nodes, etc..); ③Between the left and right anterior belly of digastric m.; ④Mylohyoid m.; ⑤Geniohyoid m.; ⑥Genioglossus m. (Fig.2-1 ~ Fig.2-9).

二、天突

【定位】胸骨上窝中央，前正中线上。

【操作】先直刺 0.2 寸，然后沿胸骨柄后缘与气管前缘缓慢向下刺入 0.5 ～ 1 寸。

【主治】咳嗽，哮喘，咳唾脓血，暴喑，咽喉肿痛，噎膈，瘿气，梅核气。

【进针层次】①皮肤；②皮下组织（内有颈横神经的分支和颈静脉弓）；③左、右胸锁乳突肌；④颈静脉切迹上方；⑤左、右胸骨甲状肌之间；⑥气管前间隙（图 2–1 ～图 2–9）。

【针刺意外与预防】①若直刺超过 0.5 寸以上，则可刺中该穴深面的气管软骨环或相邻软骨环之间的韧带；若刺中气管软骨，针感坚韧不易刺穿，应略退针；刺入软骨环之间的韧带，若进入气管腔内，患者觉喉中作痒，引起剧烈的咳嗽，此时应立即退针。②若贴近气管深刺时，针尖偏后方易刺中主动脉弓，针尖偏向两侧易刺中左颈总动脉或头臂干；若针感搏动十分明显，应立即退针，以防损伤血管。③若针刺过深且达到胸骨角水平时，则易刺中胸膜前界和肺前缘，引起气胸。

2. Tiantu (CV 22)

【Location】On the anterior midline, and in the centre of the suprasternal fossa.

【Method】Puncture perpendicularly 0.2 cun and then insert the needle downward along the posteriror aspect of the sternum and the anterior aspect of the trachea slowly for 0.5-1 cun.

【Indications】Cough, asthma, spitting purulent bloody sputum, sudden loss of voice, sore throat, dysphagia, goiter, and globus hystericus.

【Stratified anatomy】①Skin; ②Subcutaneous tissue (There are branches of the transverse cervical n. and jugular venous arch.); ③Between left and right sternocleidomastoid m.; ④Above the jugular notch; ⑤Between the left and right sternothyroid m.; ⑥Pretracheal space (Fig.2-1 ~ Fig.2-9).

【Cautions】①If the depth of perpendicular insertion is more than 0.5 cun, the tracheal cartilage ring or the ligament between the adjacent tracheal cartilage rings in the deep site under the acupoint can be pricked. If the tracheal cartilage is pierced, the needle feels tough and not easy to pierce, and the needle should be slightly withdrawn. When the ligament between the tracheal cartilage rings is pierced, if the needle enters the tracheal cavity, the patient will feel itching in the throat resulting in severe cough, and the needle shall be removed immediately. ②If the needle is inserted deep close to the trachea, it is easy to pierce the aortic arch when the needle tip is tilted backward, and it is easy to pierce the left common carotid artery or brachiocephalic trunk when the needle tip is tilted to both sides. If the pulsation of the needle is very obvious, the needle should be immediately withdrawn for avoiding vascular injury. ③If the insertion is too deep and reaches the level of the sternum angle, it is easy to puncture the anterior boundary of the pleura and the anterior edge of the lungs, causing pneumothorax.

三、人迎

【定位】平喉结，胸锁乳突肌前缘，颈总动脉搏动处。

【操作】避开颈总动脉，直刺 0.3 ～ 0.8 寸。

【主治】咽喉肿痛，胸满喘息，瘰疬，瘿气，头痛，眩晕。

【进针层次】①皮肤；②皮下组织（内有颈横神经的分支和颈阔肌）；③颈筋膜浅层；④咽缩肌（图 2–1 ～图 2–9）。

【针刺意外与预防】①若针刺偏外侧，可能刺中颈总动脉，且有明显的搏动感，此时应立即退针。②若进针过于偏外侧，则可刺中颈内静脉，进而可刺中迷走神经；若提插捻转手法过重，或电针时通电流量过大、频率过快，均可引起患者心悸、胸闷、面色苍白等迷走神经反应症状，应立即退针，否则后果严重，甚至危及生命。

3. Renying (ST 9)

【Location】At the level of the Adam's apple, on the anterior border of the sternocleidomastoid m., and at the pulsation site of the common carotid a..

【Method】Avoid the common carotid a., and puncture perpendicularly 0.3-0.8 cun.

【Indications】Sore throat, fullness in the chest, panting, scrofula, goiter, headache, and vertigo.

【Stratified anatomy】①Skin; ②Subcutaneous tissue (There are branches of the transverse cervical n. and platysma.); ③Superficial layer of the cervical fascia; ④Pharyngeal constrictor m. (Fig.2-1 ~ Fig.2-9).

【Cautions】①If the insertion is lateralized, the common carotid a. may be punctured, and there is a clear sense of pulsation. At this time, the needle should be withdrawn immediately. ②If the needling direction is extremely lateral, the internal jugular v. and even the vagus n. can be pierced. If there are excessive manipulation of lifting, thrusting, twirling and rotating or with larger electrical current flow and faster frequency of electrical stimulation during eletroacupuncture treatment, the patient can have the vagus n. reactions such as palpitations, stuffy chest and pale complexion. The needle shall be removed immediately at this moment. Otherwise, there is a serious consequence even death.

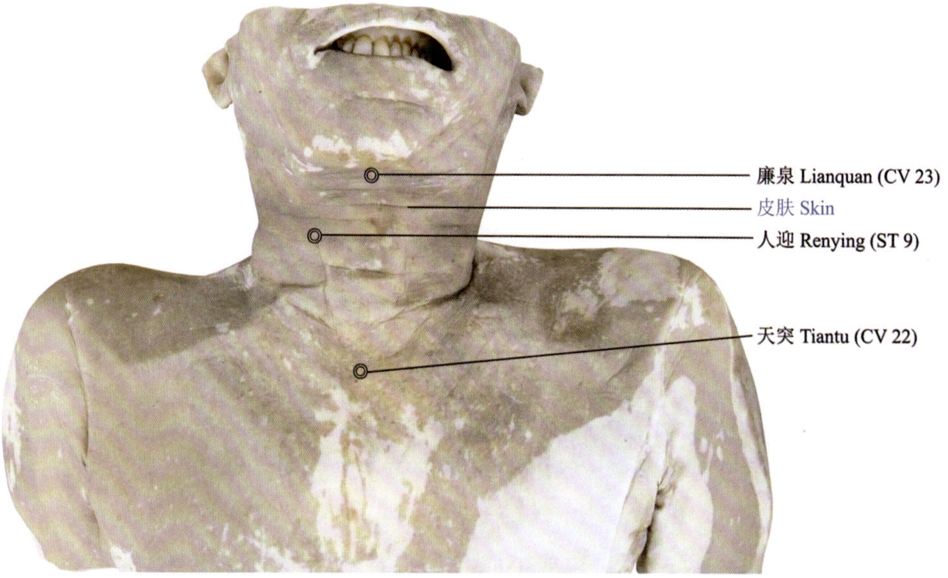

图 2–1　颈前面腧穴层次解剖（1）
Fig.2-1　Layered anatomy of acupoints on the anterior aspect of the neck (1)

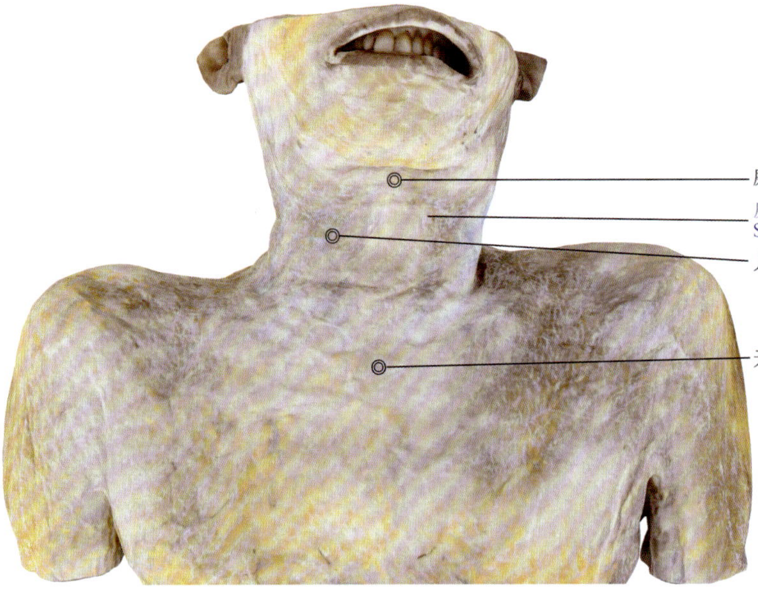

图 2-2　颈前面腧穴层次解剖（2）

Fig.2-2　Layered anatomy of acupoints on the anterior aspect of the neck (2)

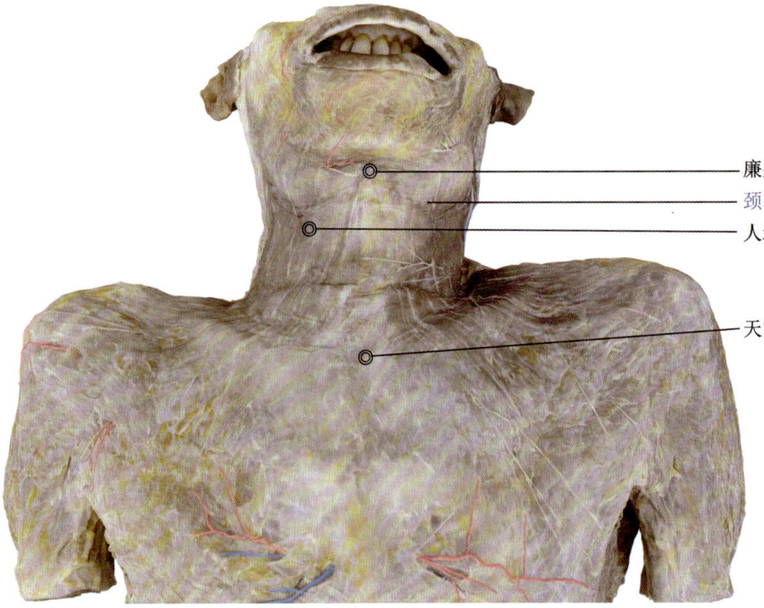

图 2-3　颈前面腧穴层次解剖（3）

Fig.2-3　Layered anatomy of acupoints on the anterior aspect of the neck (3)

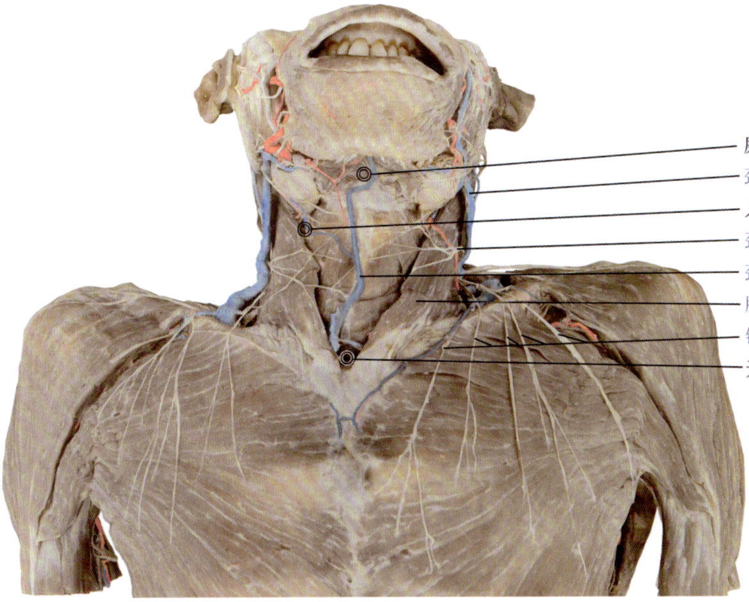
廉泉 Lianquan (CV 23)
颈外静脉 External jugular v.
人迎 Renying (ST 9)
颈横神经 Transverse cervical n.
颈前静脉 Anterior jugular v.
胸锁乳突肌 Sternocleidomastoid m.
锁骨上神经 Supraclavicular n.
天突 Tiantu (CV 22)

图 2–4　颈前面腧穴层次解剖（4）

Fig.2-4　Layered anatomy of acupoints on the anterior aspect of the neck (4)

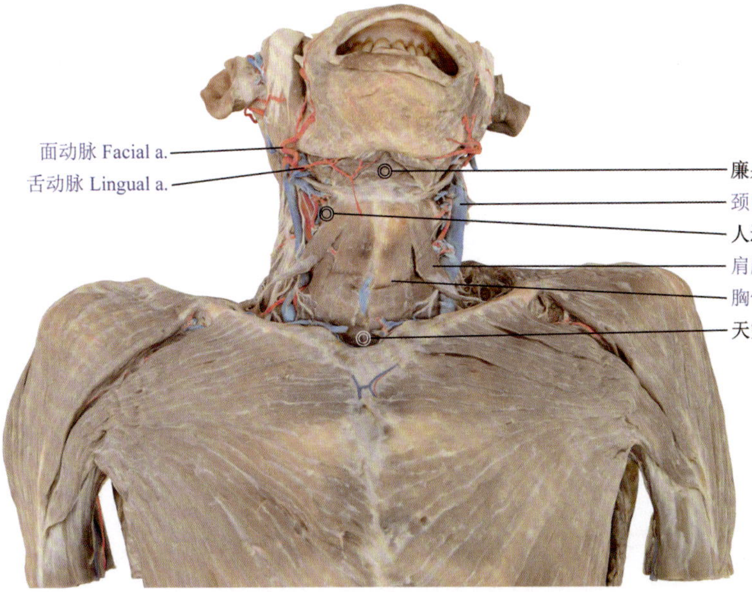
面动脉 Facial a.
舌动脉 Lingual a.
廉泉 Lianquan (CV 23)
颈内静脉 Internal jugular v.
人迎 Renying (ST 9)
肩胛舌骨肌 Omohyoid m.
胸骨舌骨肌 Sternohyoid m.
天突 Tiantu (CV 22)

图 2–5　颈前面腧穴层次解剖（5）

Fig.2-5　Layered anatomy of acupoints on the anterior aspect of the neck (5)

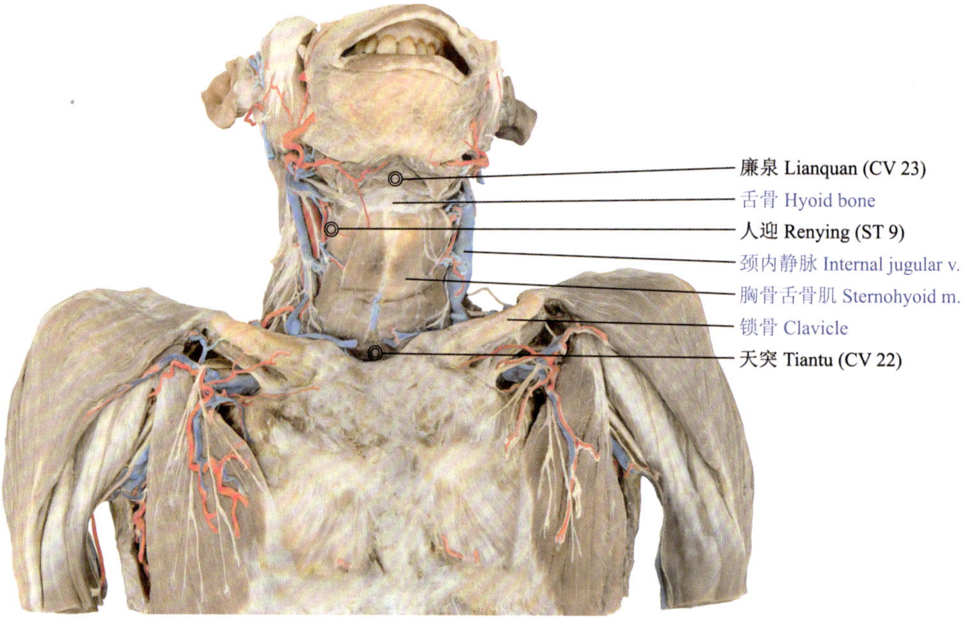
廉泉 Lianquan (CV 23)
舌骨 Hyoid bone
人迎 Renying (ST 9)
颈内静脉 Internal jugular v.
胸骨舌骨肌 Sternohyoid m.
锁骨 Clavicle
天突 Tiantu (CV 22)

图 2–6　颈前面腧穴层次解剖（6）

Fig.2-6　Layered anatomy of acupoints on the anterior aspect of the neck (6)

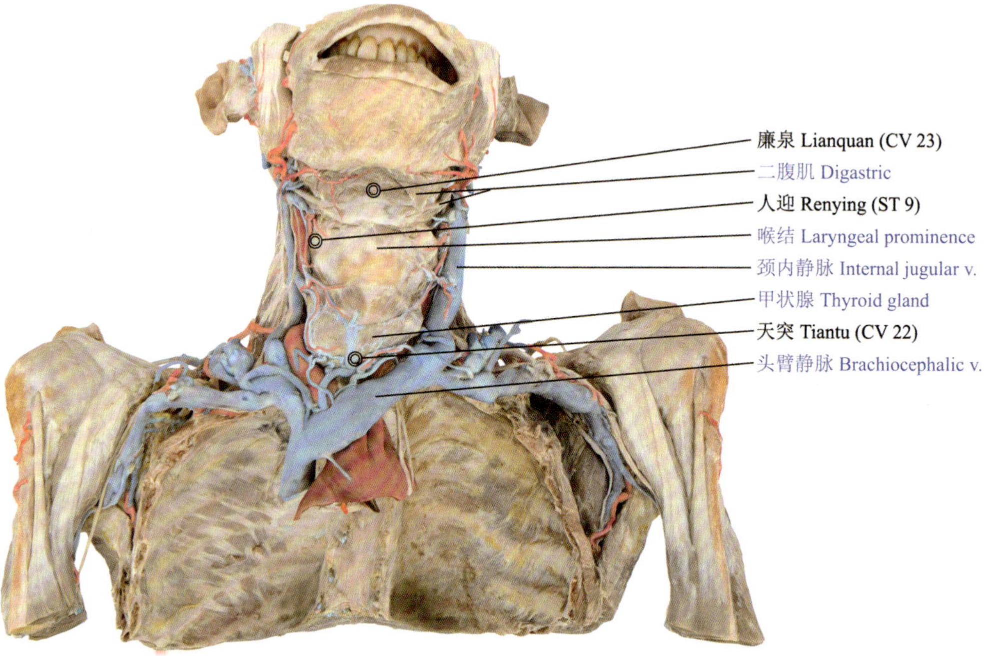
廉泉 Lianquan (CV 23)
二腹肌 Digastric
人迎 Renying (ST 9)
喉结 Laryngeal prominence
颈内静脉 Internal jugular v.
甲状腺 Thyroid gland
天突 Tiantu (CV 22)
头臂静脉 Brachiocephalic v.

图 2–7　颈前面腧穴层次解剖（7）

Fig.2-7　Layered anatomy of acupoints on the anterior aspect of the neck (7)

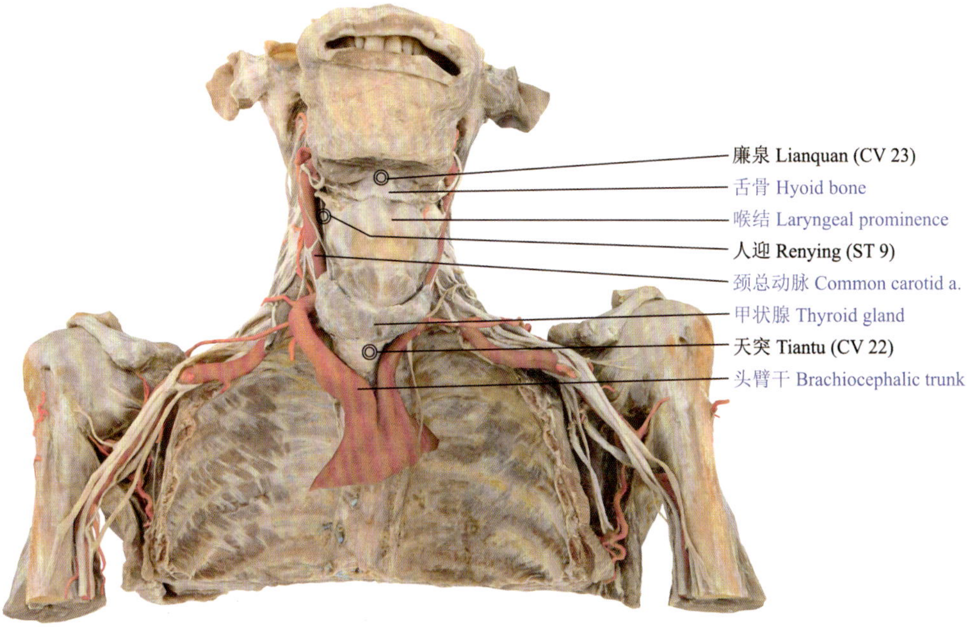
廉泉 Lianquan (CV 23)
舌骨 Hyoid bone
喉结 Laryngeal prominence
人迎 Renying (ST 9)
颈总动脉 Common carotid a.
甲状腺 Thyroid gland
天突 Tiantu (CV 22)
头臂干 Brachiocephalic trunk

图 2–8 颈前面腧穴层次解剖（8）

Fig.2-8 Layered anatomy of acupoints on the anterior aspect of the neck (8)

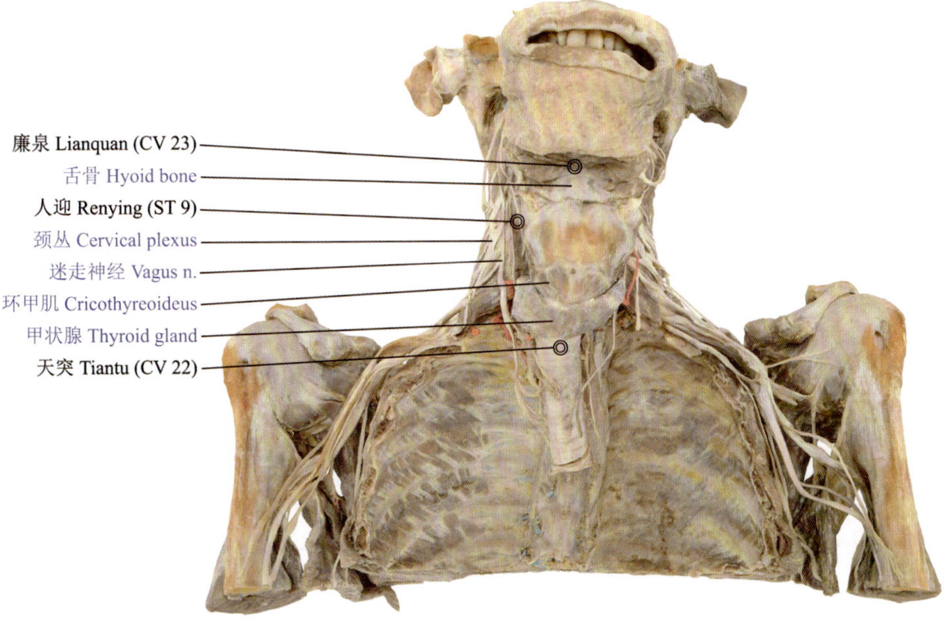
廉泉 Lianquan (CV 23)
舌骨 Hyoid bone
人迎 Renying (ST 9)
颈丛 Cervical plexus
迷走神经 Vagus n.
环甲肌 Cricothyreoideus
甲状腺 Thyroid gland
天突 Tiantu (CV 22)

图 2–9 颈前面腧穴层次解剖（9）

Fig.2-9 Layered anatomy of acupoints on the anterior aspect of the neck (9)

第二节　颈侧面腧穴

Section 2　Acupoints on the lateral aspect of the neck

一、翳风

【定位】耳垂后方，当乳突与下颌角之间的凹陷中。

【操作】直刺 0.8 ～ 1.2 寸。

【主治】耳鸣，耳聋，聤耳，口眼㖞斜，口噤，齿痛，颊肿，瘰疬。

【进针层次】①皮肤；②皮下组织（内有耳大神经的分支、耳后动脉的分支、耳后静脉的属支）；③腮腺；④面神经（图 2–10 ～图 2–15）。

【针刺意外与预防】①若针刺过深且偏向前方，有可能刺中颈内动脉、颈外动脉和颈内静脉。②若针刺过深且偏向后方，有可能刺中椎动脉。

1. Yifeng (TE 17)

【Location】Posterior to the ear lobe, and in the depression between the mastoid process and mandibular angle.

【Method】Puncture perpendicularly 0.8-1.2 cun.

【Indications】Tinnitus, deafness, otopyorrhea, deviated mouth and eye, lockjaw, toothache, swelling in the cheek, and scrofula.

【Stratified anatomy】①Skin; ②Subcutaneous tissue (There are branches of the great auricular n., branches or tributaries of the posterior auricular a. & v..); ③Parotid gland; ④Facial n. (Fig.2-10 ~ Fig.2-15).

【Cautions】①If the needle is inserted too deep and forward, it is possible to pierce the internal carotid a., external carotid a., and internal jugular v.. ②If the needle is inserted too deep and backward, it may pierce the vertebral artery.

二、扶突

【定位】平喉结，胸锁乳突肌前、后缘中间。

【操作】直刺 0.5 ～ 0.8 寸。

【主治】瘿气，暴喑，咽喉肿痛，咳嗽，气喘。

【进针层次】①皮肤；②皮下组织（内有颈横神经的分支、面神经的颈支和颈阔肌）；③胸锁乳突肌；④颈动脉鞘后缘（图 2–10 ～图 2–15）。

【针刺意外与预防】若向前内斜刺过深，易伤中颈内静脉、颈总动脉和迷走神经，迷走神经反应症状详见人迎穴。

2. Futu (LI 18)

【Location】At the level of the prominentia laryngea, and between the anterior and posterior borders of the sternocleidomastoid m..

【Method】Puncture perpendicularly 0.5-0.8 cun.

【Indications】Goiter, sudden loss of voice, sore throat, cough, and panting.

【Stratified anatomy】①Skin; ②Subcutaneous tissue (There are branches of the transverse cervical n., cervical branch of the facial n. and platysma.); ③Sternocleidomastoid m.; ④Posterior margin of carotid sheath (Fig.2-10 ~ Fig.2-15).

【Cautions】If the oblique insertion of the neede is too deep forward and inwards, it is easy to pierce the internal jugular v., common carotid a., and vagus n.. The symptoms of the vagus n. reaction are detailed in Renying (ST 9) acupoint.

三、缺盆

【定位】锁骨上大窝，锁骨上缘凹陷中，前正中线旁开 4 寸。

【操作】直刺或向后平刺 0.3 ～ 0.5 寸。

【主治】咳嗽，气喘，缺盆中痛，咽喉肿痛，瘰疬，颈肿。

【进针层次】①皮肤；②皮下组织（内有锁骨上神经的分支和颈阔肌）；③锁骨与肩胛舌骨肌下腹之间；④臂丛（图 2–10 ～图 2–15）。

【针刺意外与预防】若向下深刺，针尖可穿过前锯肌、第 1 肋间肌、壁胸膜进入胸膜腔，进而可刺中肺，引起气胸。

3. Quepen (ST 12)

【Location】At the centre of the supraclavicular fossa, in the depression at the upper edge of the clavicle and 4 cun lateral to the anterior midline.

【Method】Puncture perpendicularly or subcutaneously backwards 0.3-0.5 cun.

【Indications】Cough, panting, pain in the supraclavicular fossa, sore throat, scrofula, and neck swelling.

【Stratified anatomy】①Skin; ②Subcutaneous tissue (There are branches of the supraclavicular n. and platysma.); ③Between the clavicle and the inferior belly of omohyoid m.; ④Brachial plexus (Fig.2-10 ~ Fig.2-15).

【Cautions】If the needle is inserted too deep downward, the tip of the needle can pass through the serratus anterior m., the 1st intercostales m., the parital pleura, enter into the pleura cavity, and then pierce the lung and cause pneumothorax.

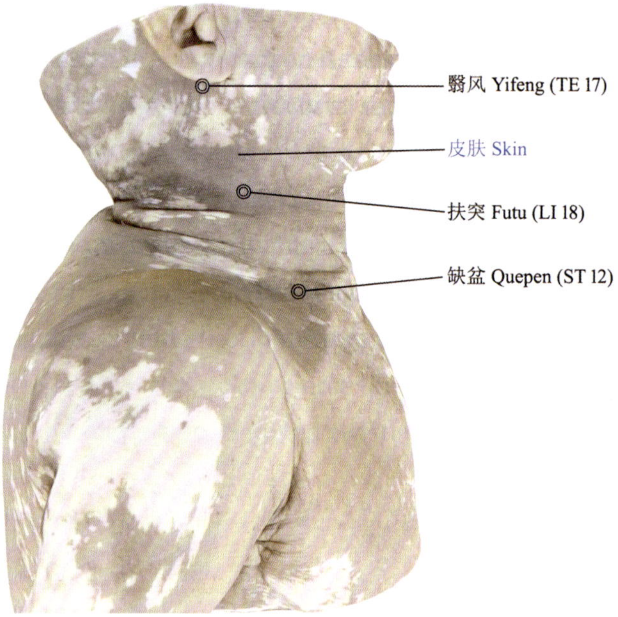

图 2–10　颈侧面腧穴层次解剖（1）

Fig.2-10　Layered anatomy of acupoints on the lateral aspect of the neck (1)

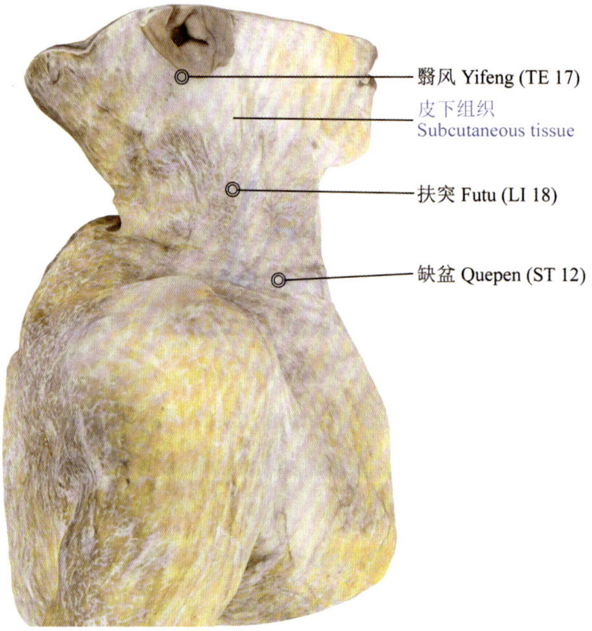

图 2–11　颈侧面腧穴层次解剖（2）

Fig.2-11　Layered anatomy of acupoints on the lateral aspect of the neck (2)

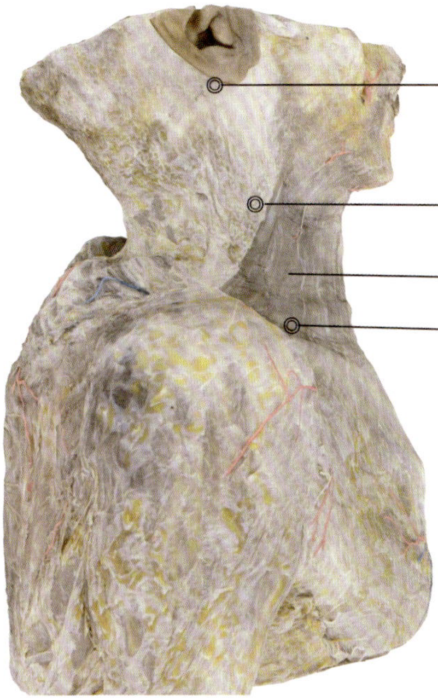
翳风 Yifeng (TE 17)
扶突 Futu (LI 18)
颈阔肌 Platysma
缺盆 Quepen (ST 12)

图 2–12 颈侧面腧穴层次解剖（3）
Fig.2-12 Layered anatomy of acupoints on the lateral aspect of the neck (3)

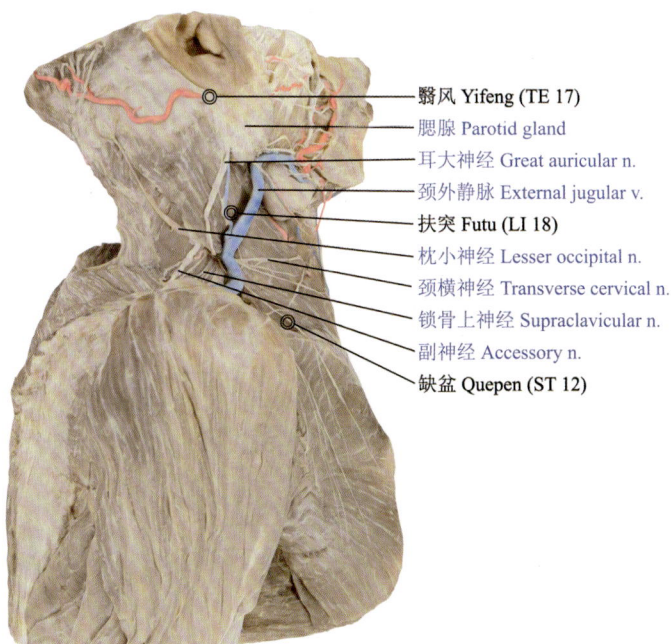

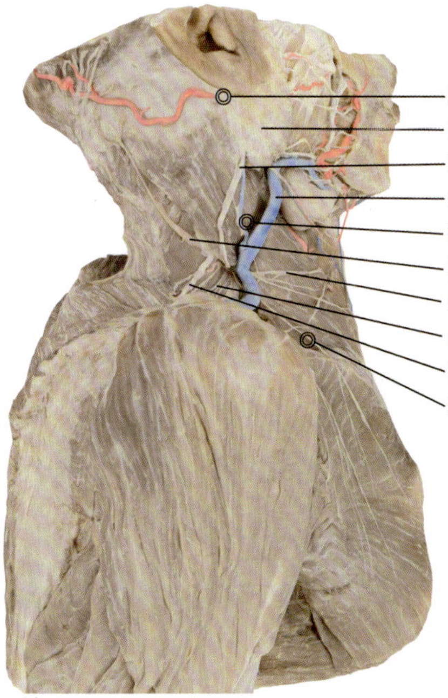
翳风 Yifeng (TE 17)
腮腺 Parotid gland
耳大神经 Great auricular n.
颈外静脉 External jugular v.
扶突 Futu (LI 18)
枕小神经 Lesser occipital n.
颈横神经 Transverse cervical n.
锁骨上神经 Supraclavicular n.
副神经 Accessory n.
缺盆 Quepen (ST 12)

图 2–13 颈侧面腧穴层次解剖（4）
Fig.2-13 Layered anatomy of acupoints on the lateral aspect of the neck (4)

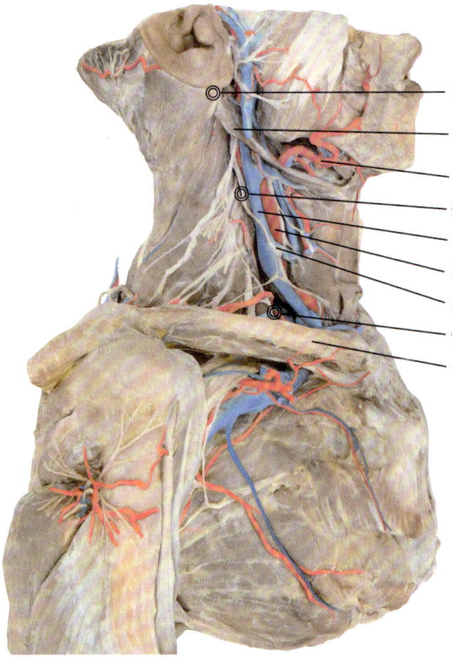
翳风 Yifeng (TE 17)
二腹肌后腹 Posterior abdomen of digastric
面动脉 Facial a.
扶突 Futu (LI 18)
颈内静脉 Internal jugular v.
颈总动脉 Common carotid a.
颈襻 Ansa cervicalis
缺盆 Quepen (ST 12)
锁骨 Clavicle

图 2–14　颈侧面腧穴层次解剖（5）

Fig.2-14　Layered anatomy of acupoints on the lateral aspect of the neck (5)

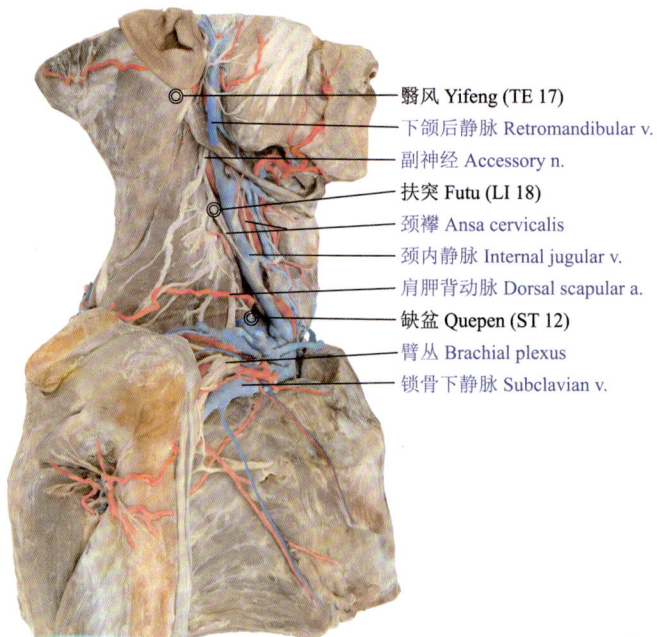

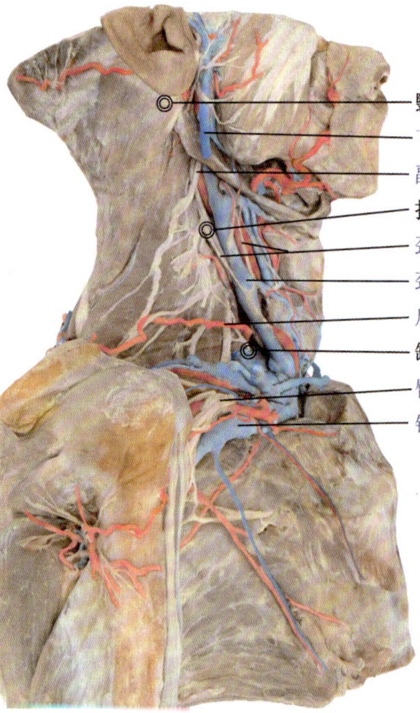
翳风 Yifeng (TE 17)
下颌后静脉 Retromandibular v.
副神经 Accessory n.
扶突 Futu (LI 18)
颈襻 Ansa cervicalis
颈内静脉 Internal jugular v.
肩胛背动脉 Dorsal scapular a.
缺盆 Quepen (ST 12)
臂丛 Brachial plexus
锁骨下静脉 Subclavian v.

图 2–15　颈侧面腧穴层次解剖（6）

Fig.2-15　Layered anatomy of acupoints on the lateral aspect of the neck (6)

第三节 项部腧穴

Section 3 Acupoints on the nape of the neck

一、风府

【定位】枕外隆凸直下，后发际正中直上 1 寸。

【操作】伏案正坐位，使头微前倾，朝下颌方向缓慢刺入 0.5 ～ 1 寸。

【主治】中风不语，半身不遂，癫狂痫，癔病，头痛，眩晕，项强，项背痛，目痛，鼻衄，咽喉肿痛。

【进针层次】①皮肤；②皮下组织（内有枕大神经和第 3 枕神经的分支，枕动脉的分支和枕静脉的属支）；③左、右斜方肌腱之间；④左、右头半棘肌之间；⑤项韧带；⑥左、右头后大直肌之间；⑦左、右头后小直肌之间（图 2–16 ～图 2–21）。

【针刺意外与预防】若针刺深度超过 1.5 寸以上，针尖可通过寰枕后膜、硬膜、蛛网膜而进入小脑延髓池，进而可刺中延髓。延髓损伤的患者，可有头痛、呼吸困难、语言不清、四肢瘫痪、神志模糊等症状，进而可出现深昏迷状态，应积极进行抢救；若大幅度提插捻转，延髓损伤更为严重，有可能在针刺过程中死亡。

1. Fengfu (GV 16)

【Location】Under the external occipital protuberance straightly, and 1 cun straightly above the posterior hairline.

【Method】Ask the patient to sit upright and bend over his desk with his head tilted forward slightly. Puncture slowly 0.5-1 cun in the direction of the mandible.

【Indications】Aphasia due to apoplexy, hemiplegia, insanity, mania, epilepsy, hysteria, headache, vertigo, stiffness in the neck, pain in the neck and back, eye pain, epistaxis, and sore throat.

【Stratified anatomy】①Skin; ②Subcutaneous tissue (There are branches of the greater occipital n. and the 3rd occipital n., branches or tributaries of the occipital a. & v..); ③Between the left and right trapezius tendon; ④Between the left and right semispinalis capitis; ⑤Ligamentum nuchae; ⑥Between the left and right rectus capitis posterior major; ⑦Between the left and right rectus capitis posterior minor (Fig.2-16 ~ Fig.2-21).

【Cautions】If the depth of insertion is more than 1.5 cun, the tip of the needle can enter the cerebellomedullary cistern through the posterior atlantooccipital membrane, dura mater and arachnoid mater, and then pierce the medulla oblongata. The patient with medulla oblongata injury may have headache, dyspnea, slurred speech, quadriplegia, blurred mind and other symptoms, and then may develop a deep coma, and should be actively rescued. If the insertion is significantly lifted and thrusted or twisted, the medulla oblongata damage will be more serious, and the patient may die during the acupuncture intervention.

二、风池

【定位】胸锁乳突肌与斜方肌上端之间的凹陷中，平风府。

【操作】伏案正坐位，使头微前倾，朝鼻尖方向缓慢刺入 0.8 ～ 1.2 寸。

【主治】头痛，眩晕，不寐，目赤肿痛，鼻渊，耳鸣，项强，中风，口眼㖞斜，感冒。

【进针层次】①皮肤；②皮下组织（内有枕小神经的分支，枕动脉的分支和枕静脉的属支）；③斜方肌与胸锁乳突肌之间；④头夹肌；⑤头半棘肌之间；⑥头后大直肌与头上斜肌之间（图 2–16 ～图 2–21）。

【针刺意外与预防】①若向内侧针刺 1.5 寸以上，针尖依次通过枕下三角、寰枕后膜、硬膜和蛛网膜进入小脑延髓池，进而刺中延髓；延髓损伤症状详见风府穴。②若向外侧针刺 1.5 寸以上，针尖可刺入枕下三角，有可能刺中椎动脉；若大幅度提插捻转，损伤将更为严重，甚至有生命危险。

2. Fengchi (GB 20)

【Location】At the level of Fengfu (GV 16), in the depression between the sternocleidomastoid m. and the upper area of the trapezius m..

【Method】Ask the patient to sit upright and bend over his desk with his head tilted forward slightly. Puncture slowly 0.8-1.2 cun in the direction of the nasal tip.

【Indications】Headache, vertigo, insomnia, pain and swelling in the eyes, sinusitis, tinnitus, stiffness in the neck, wind stroke, deviated mouth and eye, and common cold.

【Stratified anatomy】①Skin; ②Subcutaneous tissue (There are branches of the lesser occipital n., branches or tributaries of the occipital a. & v..); ③Between trapezius m. and sternocleidomastoid m.; ④Splenius capitis; ⑤Semispinalis capitis; ⑥Between the rectus capitis posterior major and the obliquus capitis superior (Fig.2-16 ~ Fig.2-21).

【Cautions】①If the depth of inward-insertion is more than 1.5 cun, the tip of the needle can enter the cerebellomedullary cistern through the suboccipital triangle, posterior atlantooccipital membrane, dura mater and arachnoid mater, and then pierce the medulla oblongata. The symptoms of medullary injury are detailed in Fengfu (GV 16) acupoint. ②If the depth of insertion is more than 1.5cun, the tip of the needle can enter the suboccipital triangle and may pierce vertebral a.. If the insertion is significantly lifted and thrusted or twisted, the damage will be more serious and even life-threatening.

三、哑门

【定位】第 2 颈椎棘突上际凹陷中，或后发际正中直上 0.5 寸。

【操作】伏案正坐位，使头微前倾，朝下颌方向缓慢刺入 0.5 ～ 1 寸。

【主治】舌强不语，暴喑，癫痫，头痛，项强，半身不遂。

【进针层次】①皮肤；②皮下组织（内有枕大神经和第 3 枕神经的分支，枕动脉的分支的枕静脉的属支）；③左、右斜方肌腱之间；④项韧带；⑤左、右头夹肌；⑥左、右头半棘肌之间（图 2–16 ～图 2–21）。

【针刺意外与预防】①若针刺深度超过 1.5 寸以上，针尖可通过寰枢后膜、硬膜外隙、硬脊膜、脊髓蛛网膜进入蛛网膜下隙，进而可刺中脊髓颈段。脊髓损伤轻者，可出现头痛、头晕等症状；损伤较重者，可有剧烈头痛、呕吐、昏迷、四肢瘫痪，应及时治疗。②若朝鼻背方向针刺过深，针尖可通过寰椎后结节上方的寰枕后膜等结构，进而刺中延髓；延髓损伤症状详见风府穴。

3. Yamen (GV 15)

【Location】In the depression of the superior spinous process of the 2nd cervical vertebra, or 0.5 cun directly above the posterior hairline.

【Method】Ask the patient to sit upright and bend over his desk with his head tilted forward slightly. Puncture slowly 0.5-1 cun in the direction of the mandible.

【Indications】Aphasia with stiff tongue, sudden loss of voice, epilepsy, headache, stiffness in the neck, and hemiplegia.

【Stratified anatomy】①Skin; ②Subcutaneous tissue (There are branches of the greater occipital n. and the 3rd occipital n., branches or tributaries of the occipital a. & v..); ③Between the left and right trapezius tendons; ④Ligamentum nuchae; ⑤Between the left and right splenius capitis; ⑥Between the left and right semispinalis capitis (Fig.2-16 ~ Fig.2-21).

【Cautions】①If the depth of insertion of the needle is more than 1.5 cun, the tip of the needle can enter the subarachnoid space through the posterior atlanto-occipital membrane, epidural space, spinal dura mater and spinal arachnoid mater, and then can pierce the cervical segment of the spinal cord. If the spinal cord injury is mild, headache, dizziness and other symptoms may occur. If the injury is severe, there may be severe headache, vomiting, coma, and quadriplegia, which should be treated in time. ②If the insertion is too deep in the direction of the back of the nose, the tip of the needle can pierce the medulla oblongata through the posterior atlanto-occipital membrane above the tubercula posterius, and then pierce the medulla oblongata. For details of the symptoms of medulla injury, please refer to Fengfu (GV 16) acupoint.

四、天柱

【定位】平哑门，斜方肌外侧缘凹陷中，或哑门旁开 1.3 寸。

【操作】直刺或斜刺 0.5 ～ 1 寸。

【主治】头痛，眩晕，目赤肿痛，目视不明，鼻塞，项强，肩背痛，癫狂痫。

【进针层次】①皮肤；②皮下组织（内有第 3 枕神经的分支）；③斜方肌；④头夹肌；⑤头半棘肌；⑥头后大直肌（图 2–16 ～图 2–21）。

【针刺意外与预防】不宜向内上方深刺，以免刺伤延髓；延髓损伤症状详见风府穴。

4. Tianzhu (BL 10)

【Location】At the level of Yamen (GV 15), and in the depression of lateral border of trapezius m., or 1.3 cun lateral to Yamen (GV 15).

【Method】Puncture perpendicularly or obliquely 0.5-1 cun.

【Indications】Headache, vertigo, pain and swelling in the eyes, blurred vision, nasal obstruction, stiffness in the neck, pain in the back and shoulder, insanity, mania, and epilepsy.

【Stratified anatomy】①Skin; ②Subcutaneous tissue (There are branches of the 3rd occipital n..); ③Trapezius m.; ④Splenius capitis m.; ⑤Semispinalis capitis m.; ⑥Rectus capitis posterior major m. (Fig.2-16 ~ Fig.2-21).

【Cautions】The inward-upward deep insertion is not appropriate, so as not to pierce the medulla oblongata. For details of the symptoms of medulla oblongata injury, please refer to Fengfu (GV 16) acupoint.

五、大椎

【定位】第 7 颈椎棘突下凹陷中，后正中线上。

【操作】微向上斜刺 0.5 ～ 1 寸。

【主治】热病，骨蒸盗汗，感冒，咳嗽，气喘，颈项强痛，肩背痛，小儿惊风，角弓反张，癫狂，瘾疹，黄疸。

【进针层次】①皮肤；②皮下组织（内有第 8 颈神经后支的皮支）；③棘上韧带；④棘间韧带；⑤黄韧带（图 2–16 ～图 2–21）。

【针刺意外与预防】若向上斜刺过深，针尖可通过黄韧带、硬膜外隙、硬脊膜和脊髓蛛网膜进入蛛网膜下隙，进而可刺中脊髓；脊髓损伤症状详见哑门穴。

5. Dazhui (GV 14)

【Location】On the posterior midline, and in the depression below the spinous process of the 7th cervical vertebra.

【Method】Puncture obliquely and slightly upward 0.5-1 cun.

【Indications】Febrile disease, tidal fever and night sweating, common cold, cough, panting, stiffness and pain in the neck, pain in the shoulder and back, infantile convulsions, opisthotonos, insanity and mania, urticaria, and jaundice.

【Stratified anatomy】①Skin; ②Subcutaneous tissue (There are cutaneous branch of the posterior branches of 8th cervical n..); ③Supraspinous lig.; ④Interspinal lig.; ⑤Ligamenta flavum (Fig.2-16 ~ Fig.2-21).

【Cautions】If the oblique-upward insertion is too deep, the tip of the needle can enter the subarachnoid space through the ligamentum flavum, epidural space, spinal dura mater and spinal arachnoid mater, and then can pierce the spinal cord. For details of the symptoms of spinal cord injury, please refer to Yamen (GV 15) acupoint.

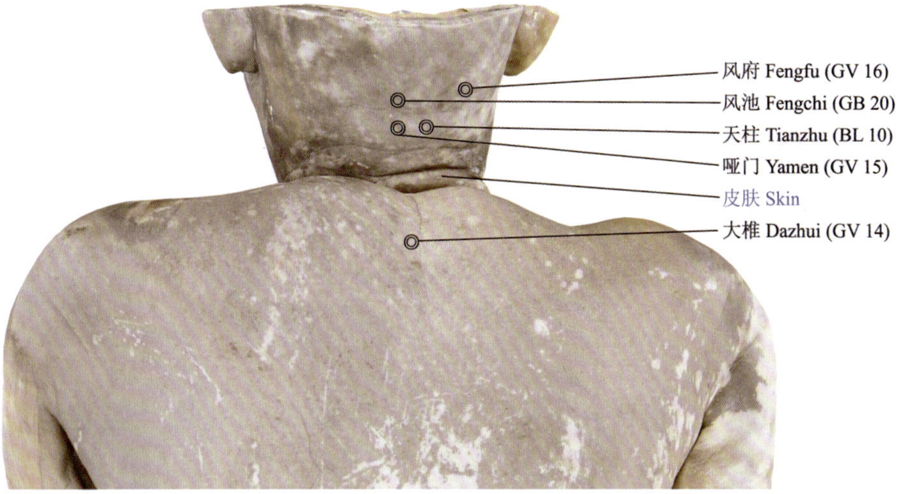

图 2–16　颈后面腧穴层次解剖（1）

Fig.2-16　Layered anatomy of acupoints on the posterior aspect of the neck (1)

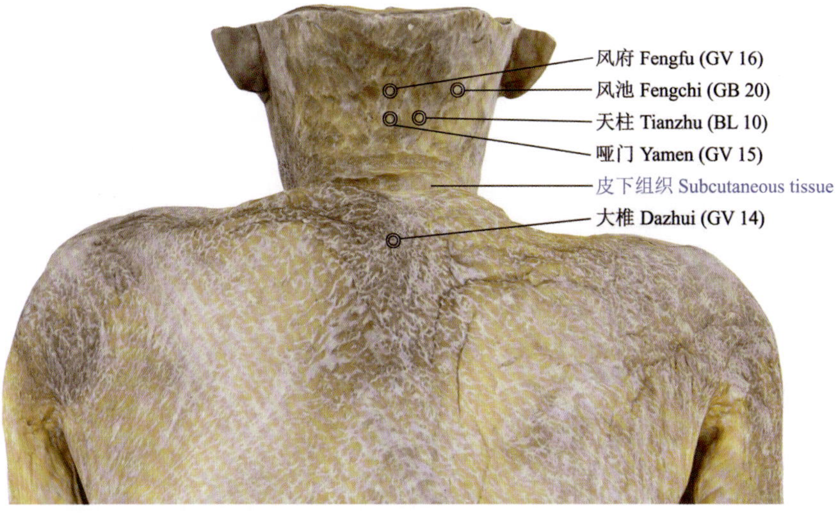

图 2–17　颈后面腧穴层次解剖（2）

Fig.2-17　Layered anatomy of acupoints on the posterior aspect of the neck (2)

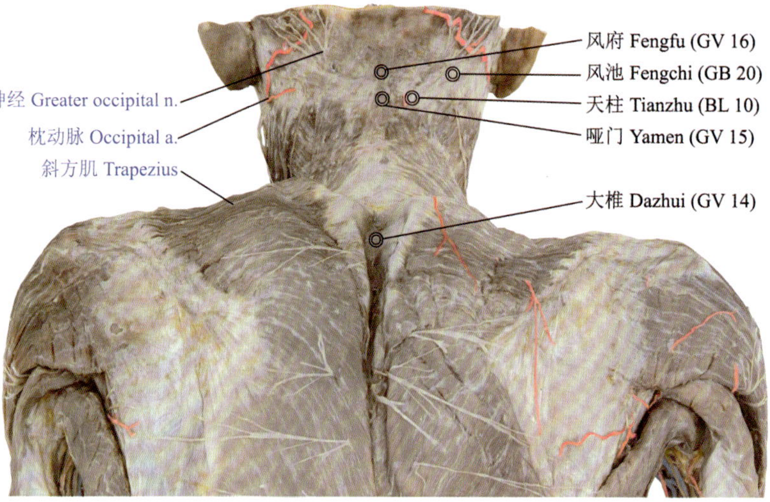

图 2–18　颈后面腧穴层次解剖（3）

Fig.2-18　Layered anatomy of acupoints on the posterior aspect of the neck (3)

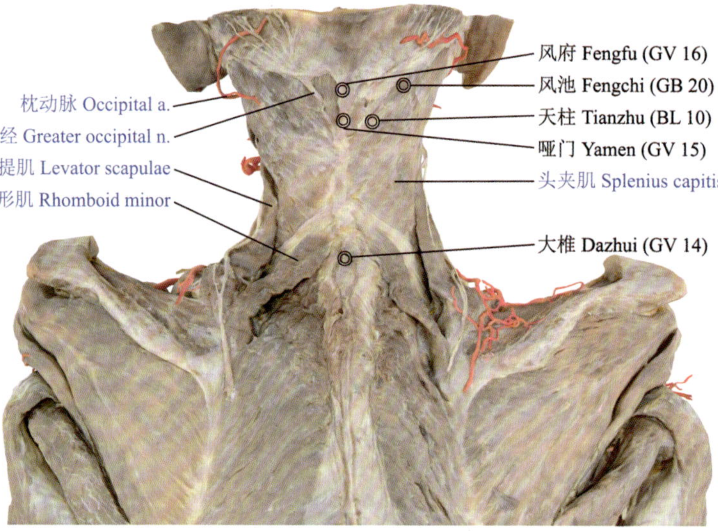

图 2–19　颈后面腧穴层次解剖（4）

Fig.2-19　Layered anatomy of acupoints on the posterior aspect of the neck (4)

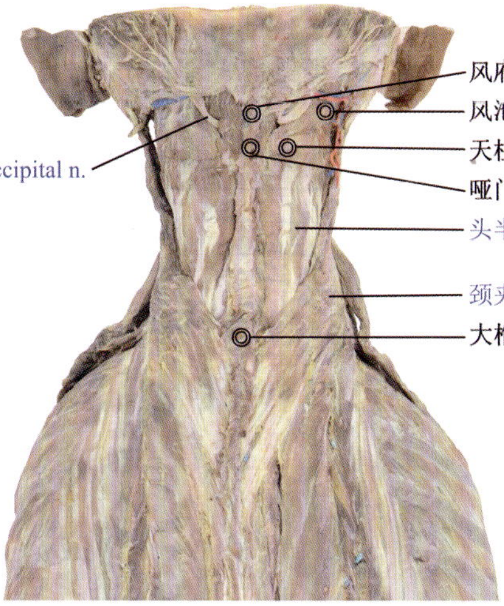

图 2–20 颈后面腧穴层次解剖（5）

Fig.2-20 Layered anatomy of acupoints on the posterior aspect of the neck (5)

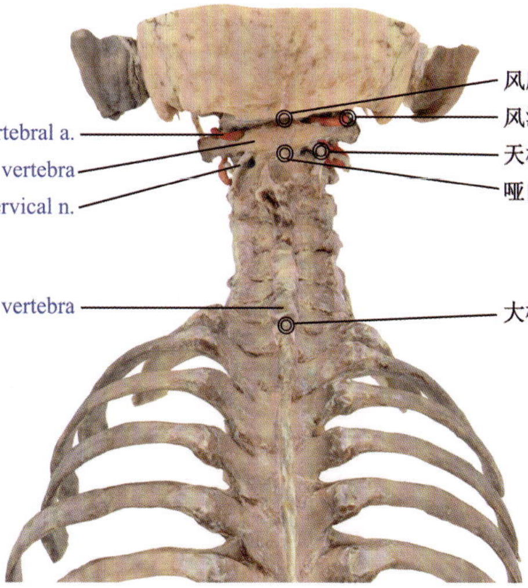

图 2–21 颈后面腧穴层次解剖（6）

Fig.2-21 Layered anatomy of acupoints on the posterior aspect of the neck (6)

第三章　胸背部腧穴层次解剖

Chapter 3　Layered Anatomy of Acupoints on the Chest and Back

第一节　胸前面腧穴

Section 1　Acupoints on the anterior aspect of the chest

一、膻中

【定位】平第 4 肋间隙，前正中线上。

【操作】平刺 0.3 ～ 0.5 寸。

【主治】胸闷，气短，咳喘，胸痛，心悸，心烦，乳少，乳痈，噎膈。

【进针层次】①皮肤；②皮下组织（内有第 4 肋间神经的前皮支，胸廓内动、静脉的穿支）；③左、右胸大肌之间（图 3–1 ～图 3–8）。

1. Danzhong (CV 17)

【Location】On the anterior midline, and at the level of the 4th intercostal space.

【Method】Puncture subcutaneously 0.3-0.5 cun.

【Indications】Stuffy chest, short breath, cough, panting, chest pain, palpitations, vexation, hypogalactia, breast abscess, and dysphagia.

【Stratified anatomy】①Skin; ②Subcutaneous tissue (There are anterior cutaneous branch of the 4th intercostal n., perforating branch of the internal thoracic a. & v..); ③Between the left and right pectoralis major (Fig.3-1 ~ Fig.3-8).

二、俞府

【定位】锁骨下缘，前正中线旁开 2 寸。

【操作】斜刺或平刺 0.5 ～ 0.8 寸。

【主治】咳嗽，气喘，胸痛，呕吐。

【进针层次】①皮肤；②皮下组织（内有锁骨上神经的分支）；③胸大肌；④锁骨与第 1 肋之间（图 3–1 ～图 3–8）。

【针刺意外与预防】①若直刺过深，针尖可刺中锁骨下静脉引起出血；或依次通过胸内筋膜、肋胸膜进入胸膜腔，进而可刺中左肺上叶或右肺上叶，引起气胸。②若针刺左侧俞府穴 1.5 寸以上时，针尖可刺中锁骨下动脉和主动脉弓，引起严重出血，后果甚为严重。

2. Shufu (KI 27)

【Location】At the infraclavicular margin, and 2 cun lateral to the anterior midline.

【Method】Puncture obliquely or subcutaneously 0.5-0.8 cun.

【Indications】Cough, panting, chest pain, and vomiting.

【Stratified anatomy】①Skin; ②Subcutaneous tissue (There are branches of the supraclavicular n..); ③Pectoralis major; ④Between the clavicle and the 1st rib. (Fig.3-1 ~ Fig.3-8).

【Cautions】①If the perpendicular insertion is too deep, the tip of the needle can pierce the subclavian v. and cause bleeding; or enter the pleural cavity through the intrapleural fascia and costal pleura in turn, which can prick the left upper lobe or the right upper lobe of the lung, causing pneumothorax. ②If the depth of insertion at the left Shufu (KI 27) acupoint is more than 1.5 cun, the tip of the needle can prick the subclavian a. and the aortic arch, causing severe bleeding, and the consequences are very serious.

三、中府

【定位】平第 1 肋间隙，锁骨下窝外侧，前正中线旁开 6 寸。

【操作】向外侧斜刺或平刺 0.5 ～ 0.8 寸。

【主治】咳嗽，气喘，胸痛，胸中烦满，肩背痛。

【进针层次】①皮肤；②皮下组织（内有锁骨上神经的分支）；③三角肌和头静脉；④胸大肌；⑤胸小肌（图 3–1 ～图 3–8）。

【针刺意外与预防】若向内侧深刺，针尖可依次通过肋间外肌、肋间内肌、肋间最内肌、胸内筋膜、肋胸膜进入胸膜腔，进而可刺中左肺上叶或右肺上叶，引起气胸。

3. Zhongfu (LU 1)

【Location】At the level of the 1st intercostal space, on the lateral side of the subclavian fossa, and 6 cun lateral to the anterior midline.

【Method】Puncture obliquely outward or subcutaneously 0.5-0.8 cun.

【Indications】Cough, panting, chest pain, irritability and fullness in the chest, and pain in the shoulder and back.

【Stratified anatomy】①Skin; ②Subcutaneous tissue (There are branches of the supraclavicular n..); ③Deltoid m. and cephalic v.; ④Pectoralis major; ⑤Pectoralis minor (Fig.3-1 ~ Fig.3-8).

【Cautions】If the needle is stabbed deep inwards, the tip of the needle can enter the pleural cavity through the extracostal m., intercostal m., intercostales intimi, intrathoracic fascia, and costal pleura, and then can pierce the upper lobe of the left lung or the upper lobe of the right lung, causing pneumothorax.

四、天池

【定位】第 4 肋间隙，前正中线旁开 5 寸。

【操作】平刺或斜刺 0.5 ～ 0.8 寸。

【主治】咳嗽，气喘，胸闷，胸痛，痰多，乳痈，乳少。

【进针层次】①皮肤；②皮下组织（内有第 4 肋间神经的外侧皮支和胸腹壁静脉的属支）；③胸大肌；④胸小肌（图 3–1 ～图 3–8）。

【针刺意外与预防】①若直刺过深，针尖可依次通过肋间外肌、肋间内肌、肋间最内肌、胸内筋膜、肋胸膜进入胸膜腔，进而可刺中肺，引起气胸。②若左侧天池穴直刺过深时，针尖通过肋间隙可刺入心脏，后果甚为严重。

4. Tianchi (PC 1)

【Location】In the 4th intercostal space, and 5 cun lateral to the anterior midline.

【Method】Puncture obliquely or subcutaneously 0.5-0.8 cun.

【Indications】Cough, panting, stuffy chest, chest pain, profuse sputum, acute mastitis, and hypogalactia.

【Stratified anatomy】①Skin; ②Subcutaneous tissue (There are branches of the lateral cutaneous branch of the 4th intercostal n. and tributaries of the thoracoepigastric v..); ③Pectoralis major; ④Pectoralis minor (Fig.3-1 ~ Fig.3-8).

【Cautions】①If the perpendicular insertion is too deep, the tip of the needle can enter the pleural cavity through the extracostal m., intercostal m., intercostales intimi, intrathoracic fascia, and costal pleura, and then can pierce the lungs, causing pneumothorax. ②If the insertion at the left Tianchi (PC 1) acupoint is too deep, the tip of the needle can prick the heart, and the consequences are very serious.

五、期门

【定位】第 6 肋间隙，前正中线旁开 4 寸。

【操作】平刺或斜刺 0.5 ～ 0.8 寸。

【主治】胸胁胀痛，乳痈，呕吐，吞酸，呃逆，腹胀，腹泻，咳嗽，气喘。

【进针层次】①皮肤；②皮下组织（内有第 6 肋间神经的外侧皮支和胸腹壁静脉的属支）；③腹外斜肌（图 3–1 ～图 3–8）。

【针刺意外与预防】①若直刺过深，针尖可通过肋间外肌、肋间内肌、肋间最内肌、胸内筋膜、肋胸膜，刺入肋膈隐窝引起气胸。②若继续深刺，针尖还可通过膈胸膜、膈、壁腹膜进入腹膜腔，进而可刺中肝（右期门穴）或胃（左期门穴）；若大幅度提插、捻转，可引起肝出血或急腹症，后果严重。

5. Qimen (LR 14)

【Location】In the 6th intercostal space, and 4 cun lateral to the anterior midline.

【Method】Puncture subcutaneously or obliquely 0.5-0.8 cun.

【Indications】Distension and pain in the chest and hypochondrium, acute mastitis, vomiting, acid regurgitation, hiccup, abdominal distension, diarrhea, cough, and panting.

【Stratified anatomy】①Skin; ②Subcutaneous tissue (There are lateral cutaneous branch of the 6th intercostal n. and tributaries of thoracoepigastric v..); ③Musculus obliquus externus abdominis (Fig.3-1 ~ Fig.3-8).

【Cautions】①If the perpendicular insertion is too deep, the tip of the needle can enter the costodiaphragmatic recess through the extracostal m., intercostal m., internal intercostal m., intrathoracic fascia, and costal pleura and cause pneumothorax. ②If the insertion is deeper, the tip of the needle can also enter the peritoneal cavity through the diaphragmatic pleura, diaphragm and parietal peritoneum, and then pierce the liver [right Qimen (LR 14) acupoint] or stomach [left Qimen (LR 14) acupoint]. If the manipulation is implemented with strong lifting and thrusting or twirling, it can cause liver bleeding or acute abdomen, and the consequences are serious.

六、日月

【定位】第 7 肋间隙，前正中线旁开 4 寸。

【操作】平刺或斜刺 0.5 ～ 0.8 寸。

【主治】胁肋疼痛，呕吐，吞酸，黄疸，胃脘痛。

【进针层次】①皮肤；②皮下组织（内有第 7 肋间神经的外侧皮支和胸腹壁静脉的属支）；③腹外斜肌（图 3–1 ～图 3–8）。

【针刺意外与预防】若直刺过深，针尖可通过肋间外肌、肋间内肌、肋间最内肌、壁腹膜进入腹膜腔，进而可刺中肝（右期门穴）或横结肠（左期门穴）；若大幅度提插、捻转，可引起肝出血或急腹症，后果严重。

6. Riyue (GB 24)

【Location】In the 7th intercostal space, and 4 cun lateral to the anterior midline.

【Method】Puncture subcutaneously or obliquely 0.5-0.8 cun.

【Indications】Pain in the hypochondrium, vomiting, acid regurgitation, jaundice, and gastric pain.

【Stratified anatomy】①Skin; ②Subcutaneous tissue (There are lateral cutaneous branch of the 7th intercostal n. and tributaries of the thoracoepigastric v..); ③Musculus obliquus externus abdominis (Fig.3-1 ~ Fig.3-8).

【Cautions】If the perpendicular insertion is too deep, the tip of the needle can enter the peritoneal cavity through the extracostal m., intercostal m., intercostales intimi, and parietal peritoneum and then pierce the liver [right Qimen (LR 14) acupoint] or transverse colon [left Qimen (LR 14) acupoint]. If the manipulation is implemented with strong lifting and thrusting or twirling, it can cause liver bleeding or acute abdomen, and the consequences are serious.

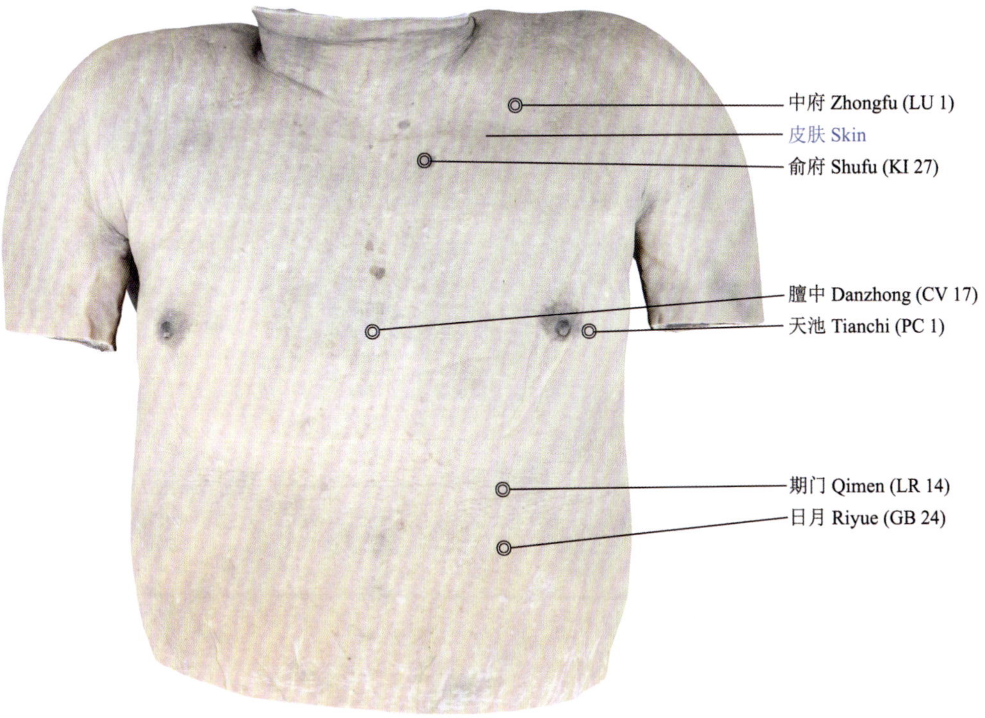
中府 Zhongfu (LU 1)
皮肤 Skin
俞府 Shufu (KI 27)
膻中 Danzhong (CV 17)
天池 Tianchi (PC 1)
期门 Qimen (LR 14)
日月 Riyue (GB 24)

图 3-1 胸前面腧穴层次解剖（1）

Fig.3-1 Layered anatomy of acupoints on the anterior aspect of the chest (1)

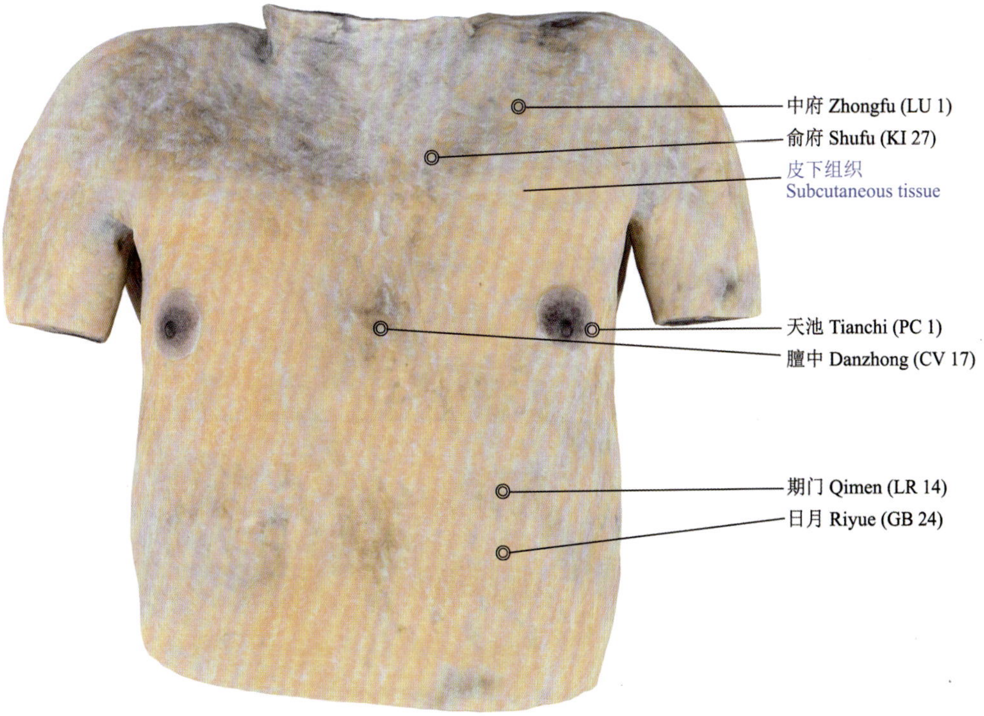
中府 Zhongfu (LU 1)
俞府 Shufu (KI 27)
皮下组织
Subcutaneous tissue
天池 Tianchi (PC 1)
膻中 Danzhong (CV 17)
期门 Qimen (LR 14)
日月 Riyue (GB 24)

图 3-2 胸前面腧穴层次解剖（2）

Fig.3-2 Layered anatomy of acupoints on the anterior aspect of the chest (2)

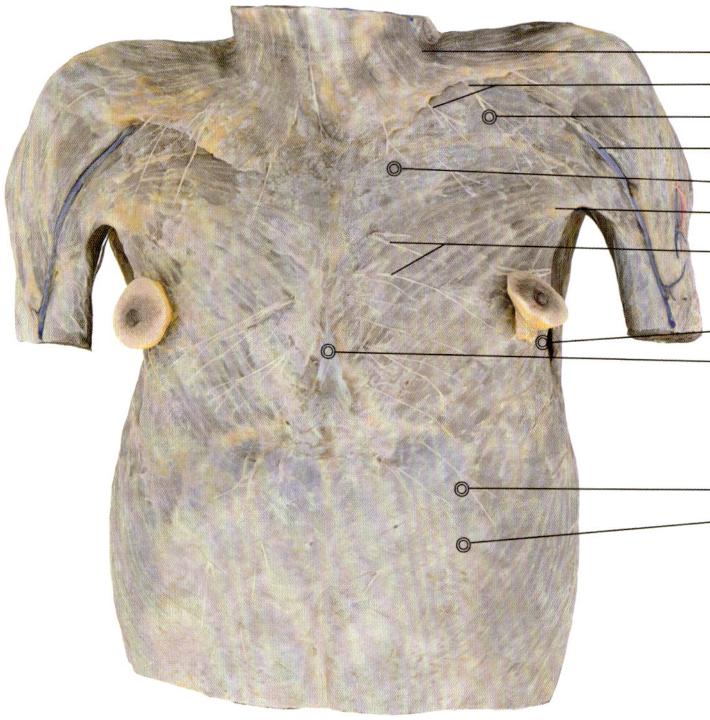
颈阔肌 Platysma
锁骨上神经 Supraclavicular n.
中府 Zhongfu (LU 1)
头静脉 Cephalic v.
俞府 Shufu (KI 27)
深筋膜 Deep fascia
肋间神经内侧皮支 Medial cutaneous branch of intercostal n.
天池 Tianchi (PC 1)
膻中 Danzhong (CV 17)
期门 Qimen (LR 14)
日月 Riyue (GB 24)

图 3–3　胸前面腧穴层次解剖（3）

Fig.3-3　Layered anatomy of acupoints on the anterior aspect of the chest (3)

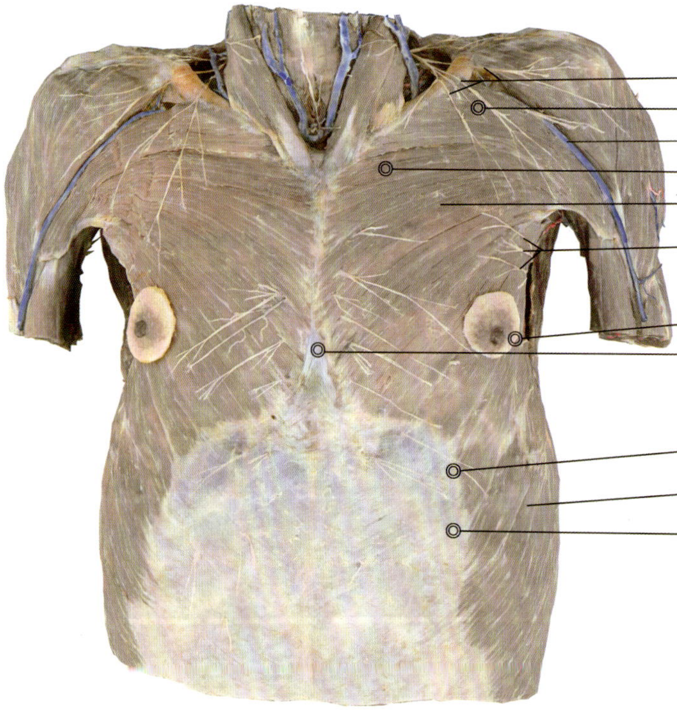
锁骨上神经 Supraclavicular n.
中府 Zhongfu (LU 1)
头静脉 Cephalic v.
俞府 Shufu (KI 27)
胸大肌 Pectoralis major
肋间神经外侧皮支 Lateral cutaneous branch of intercostal n.
天池 Tianchi (PC 1)
膻中 Danzhong (CV 17)
期门 Qimen (LR 14)
腹外斜肌
Musculus obliquus externus abdominis
日月 Riyue (GB 24)

图 3–4　胸前面腧穴层次解剖（4）

Fig.3-4　Layered anatomy of acupoints on the anterior aspect of the chest (4)

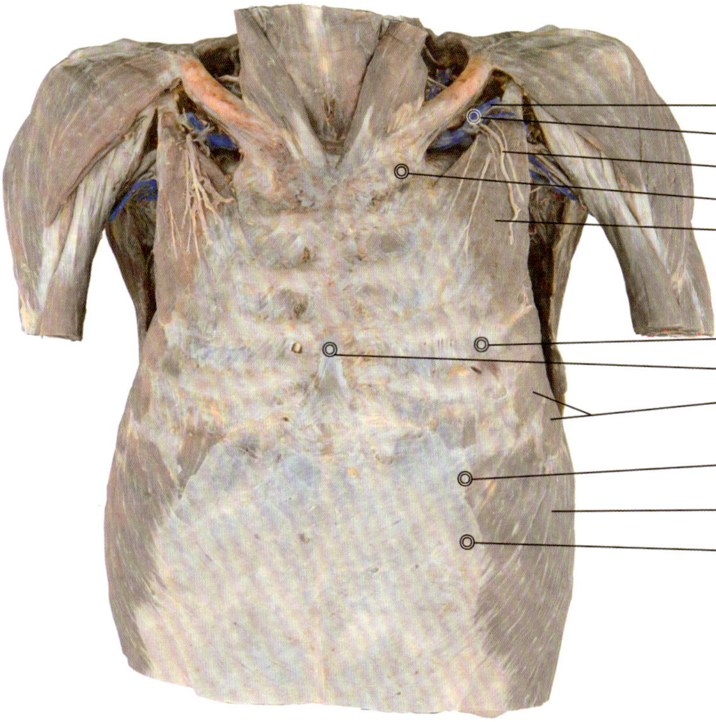
头静脉 Cephalic v.
中府 Zhongfu (LU 1)
胸外侧神经 Lateral pectoral n.
俞府 Shufu (KI 27)
胸小肌 Pectoralis minor
天池 Tianchi (PC 1)
膻中 Danzhong (CV 17)
前锯肌 Serratus anterior
期门 Qimen (LR 14)
腹外斜肌
Musculus obliquus externus abdominis
日月 Riyue (GB 24)

图 3-5 胸前面腧穴层次解剖（5）

Fig.3-5 Layered anatomy of acupoints on the anterior aspect of the chest (5)

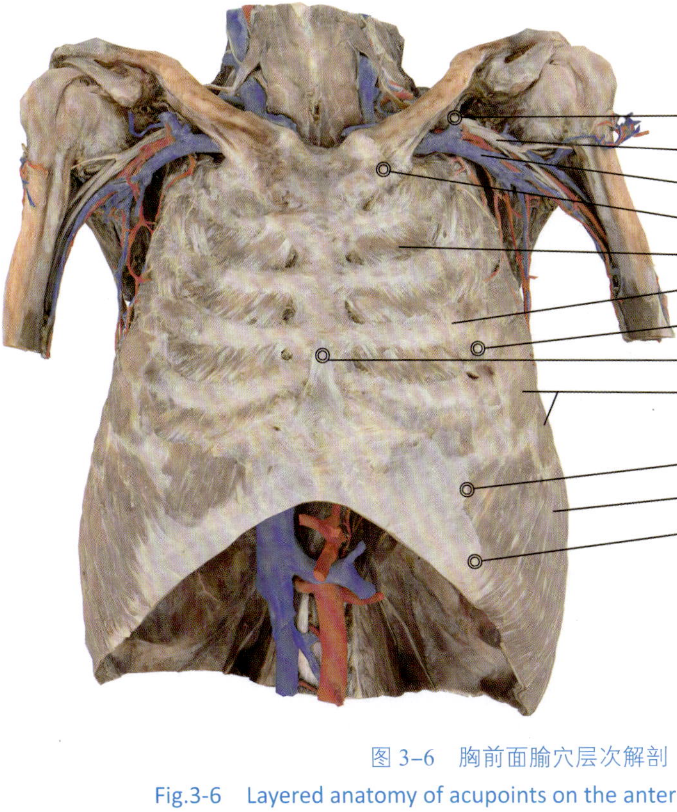
中府 Zhongfu (LU 1)
臂丛 Brachial plexus
腋静脉 Axillary v.
俞府 Shufu (KI 27)
肋间内肌 Intercostales interni
第 4 肋骨 4th rib
天池 Tianchi (PC 1)
膻中 Danzhong (CV 17)
前锯肌 Serratus anterior
期门 Qimen (LR 14)
腹外斜肌 Musculus obliquus externus abdominis
日月 Riyue (GB 24)

图 3-6 胸前面腧穴层次解剖（6）

Fig.3-6 Layered anatomy of acupoints on the anterior aspect of the chest (6)

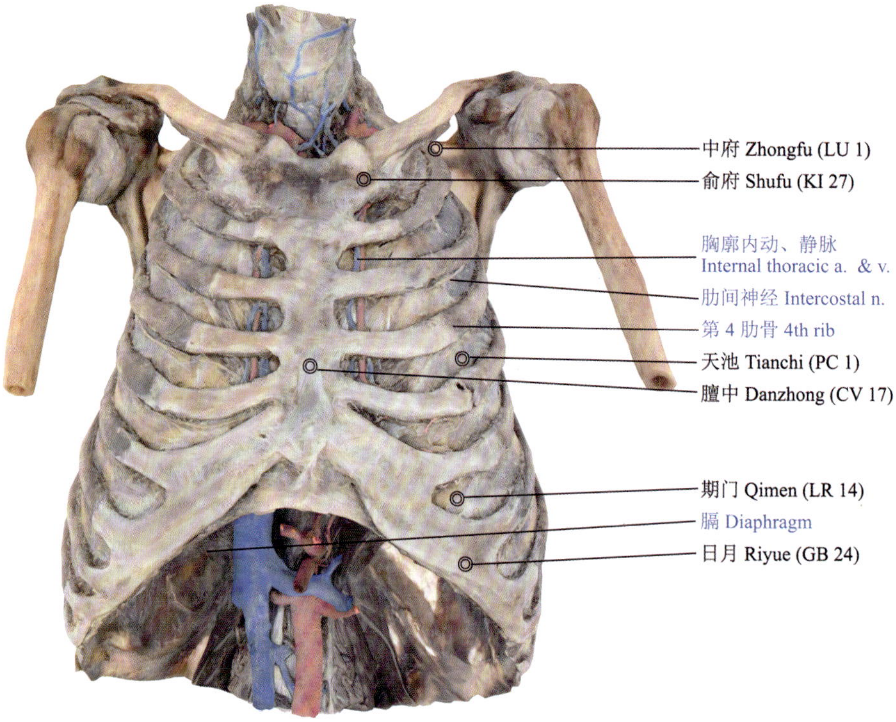
中府 Zhongfu (LU 1)
俞府 Shufu (KI 27)
胸廓内动、静脉
Internal thoracic a. & v.
肋间神经 Intercostal n.
第 4 肋骨 4th rib
天池 Tianchi (PC 1)
膻中 Danzhong (CV 17)
期门 Qimen (LR 14)
膈 Diaphragm
日月 Riyue (GB 24)

图 3–7 胸前面腧穴层次解剖（7）

Fig.3-7 Layered anatomy of acupoints on the anterior aspect of the chest (7)

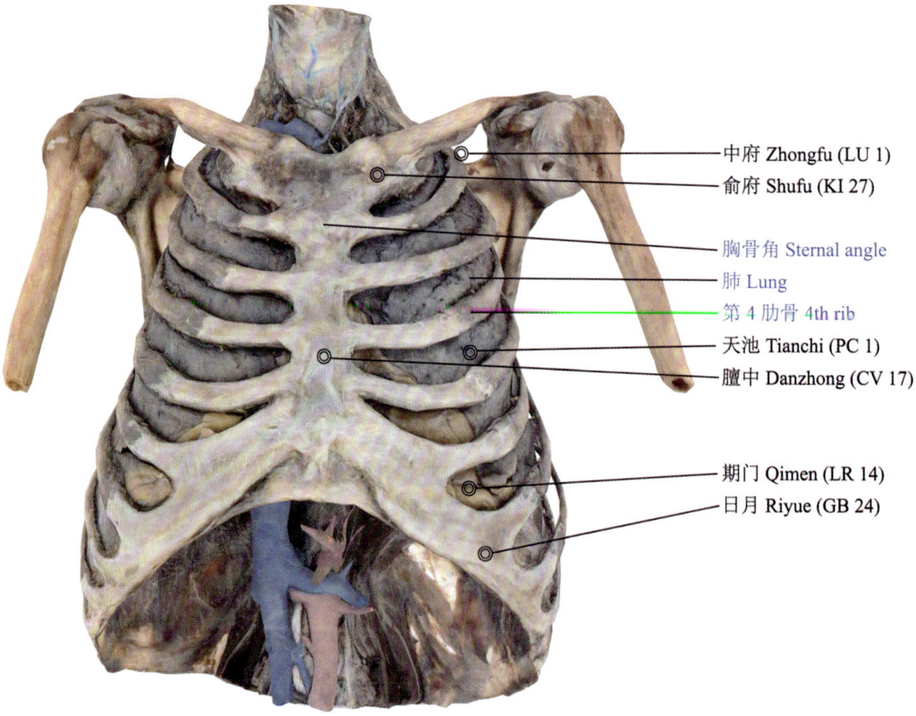
中府 Zhongfu (LU 1)
俞府 Shufu (KI 27)
胸骨角 Sternal angle
肺 Lung
第 4 肋骨 4th rib
天池 Tianchi (PC 1)
膻中 Danzhong (CV 17)
期门 Qimen (LR 14)
日月 Riyue (GB 24)

图 3–8 胸前面腧穴层次解剖（8）

Fig.3-8 Layered anatomy of acupoints on the anterior aspect of the chest (8)

第二节 胸侧面腧穴

Section 2 Acupoints on the lateral aspect of the chest

大包

【定位】第 6 肋间隙，在腋中线上。

【操作】平刺或斜刺 0.5 ～ 0.8 寸。

【主治】咳嗽，气喘，胸闷，胁肋痛，胸胁胀满，全身疼痛，四肢无力。

【进针层次】①皮肤；②皮下组织（内有第 6 肋间神经的外侧皮支，胸长神经，胸外侧动脉的分支和胸外侧静脉的属支）；③前锯肌（图 3–9 ～图 3–16）。

【针刺意外与预防】若直刺过深，针尖可依次通过肋间外肌、肋间内肌、肋间最内肌、胸内筋膜、肋胸膜进入胸膜腔，进而可刺中肺，引起气胸。

Dabao (SP 21)

【Location】On the mid-axillary line, and in the 6th intercostal space.

【Method】Puncture subcutaneously or obliquely 0.5-0.8 cun.

【Indications】Cough, panting, stuffy chest, pain in the hypochondrium, distension in the chest and hypochondrium, pain all over the body, and weakness of limbs.

【Stratified anatomy】①Skin; ②Subcutaneous tissue (There are lateral cutaneous branch of the 6th intercostal n., long thoracic n., branches or tributaries of the lateral thoracic a. & v..); ③Serratus anterior (Fig.3-9 ~ Fig.3-16).

【Cautions】If the perpendicular insertion is too deep, the tip of the needle can enter the pleural cavity through the extracostal m., intracostal m., intercostales intimi, intrathoracic fascia, and costal pleura, and then can prick the lungs and cause pneumothorax.

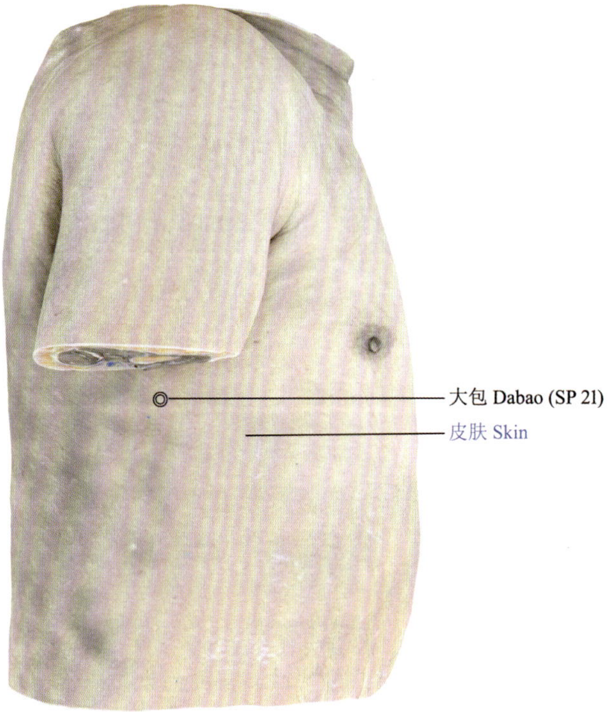

图 3-9　胸侧面腧穴层次解剖（1）
Fig.3-9　Layered anatomy of acupoints on the lateral aspect of the chest (1)

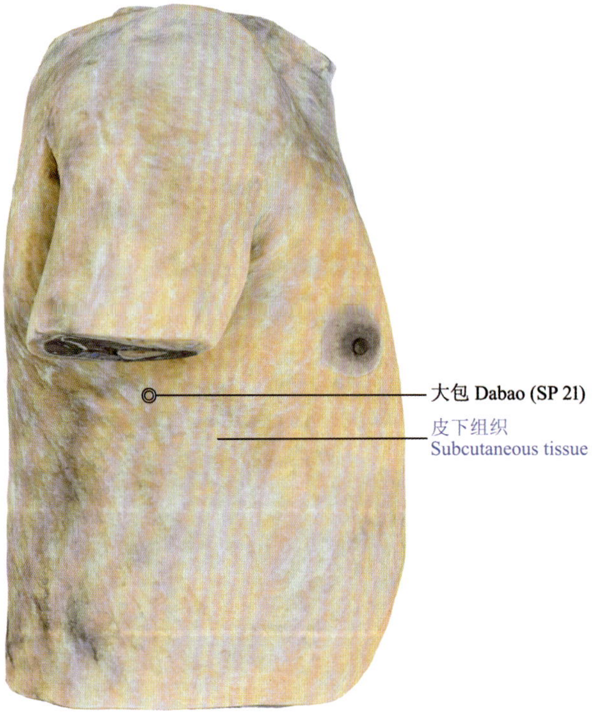

图 3-10　胸侧面腧穴层次解剖（2）
Fig.3-10　Layered anatomy of acupoints on the lateral aspect of the chest (2)

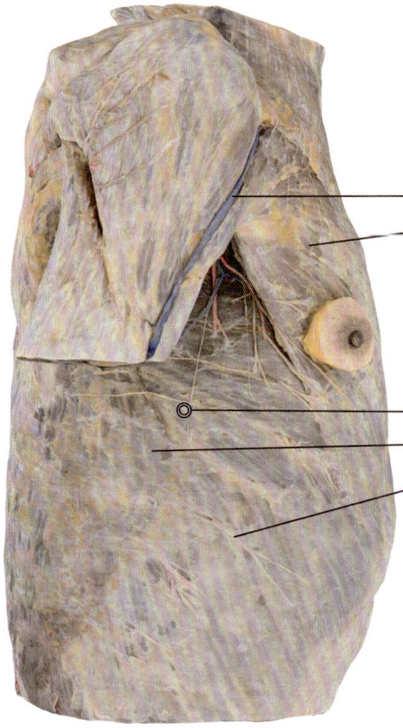
头静脉 Cephalic v.
胸大肌 Pectoralis major
大包 Dabao (SP 21)
深筋膜 Deep fascia
肋间神经外侧皮支 Lateral cutaneous branch of intercostal n.

图 3–11　胸侧面腧穴层次解剖（3）

Fig.3-11　Layered anatomy of acupoints on the lateral aspect of the chest (3)

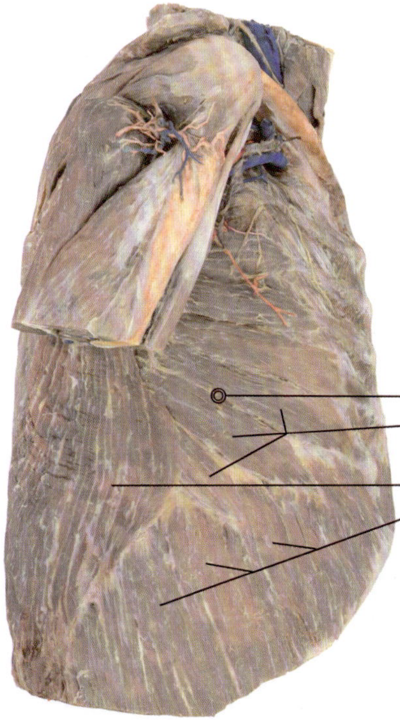
大包 Dabao (SP 21)
前锯肌 Serratus anterior
背阔肌 Latissimus dorsi
腹外斜肌 Musculus obliquus externus abdominis

图 3–12　胸侧面腧穴层次解剖（4）

Fig.3-12　Layered anatomy of acupoints on the lateral aspect of the chest (4)

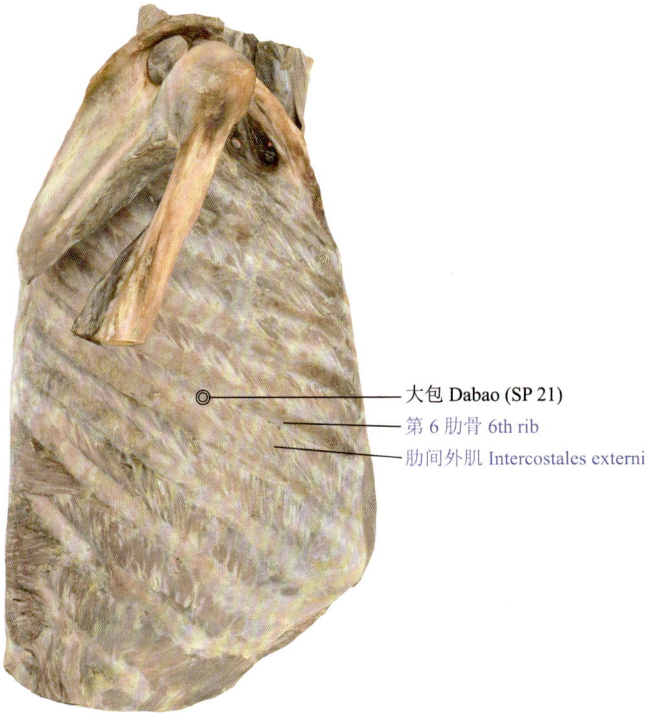
大包 Dabao (SP 21)
第 6 肋骨 6th rib
肋间外肌 Intercostales externi

图 3–13　胸侧面腧穴层次解剖（5）
Fig.3-13　Layered anatomy of acupoints on the lateral aspect of the chest (5)

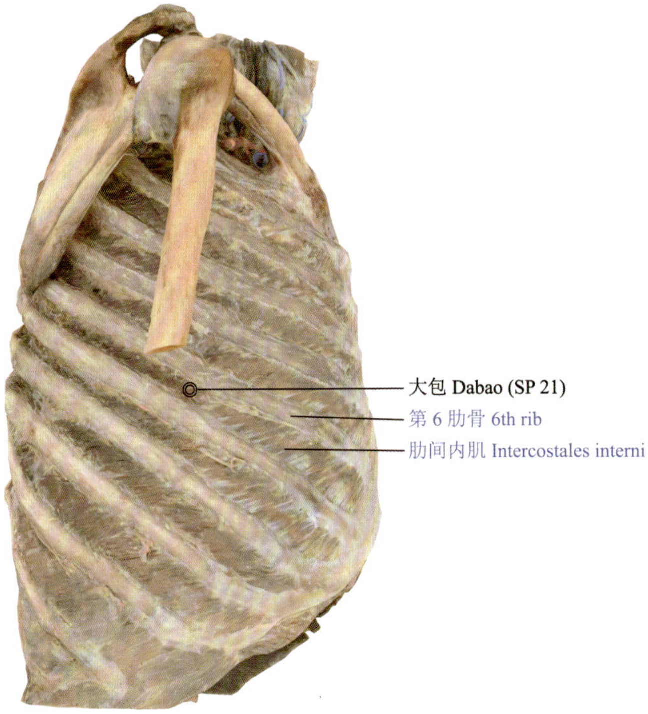
大包 Dabao (SP 21)
第 6 肋骨 6th rib
肋间内肌 Intercostales interni

图 3–14　胸侧面腧穴层次解剖（6）
Fig.3-14　Layered anatomy of acupoints on the lateral aspect of the chest (6)

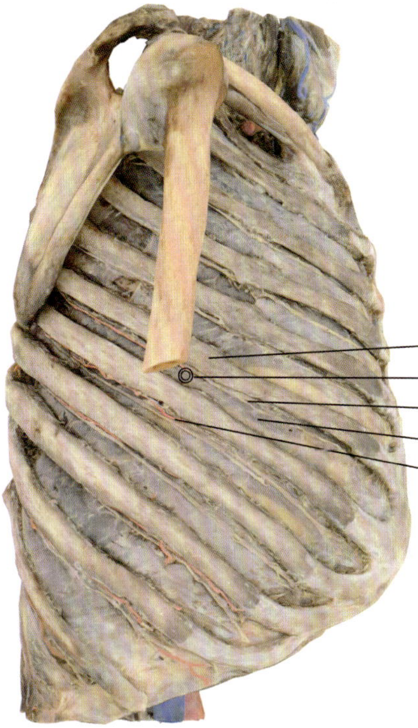
第 6 肋骨 6th rib
大包 Dabao (SP 21)
肋间神经 Intercostal n.
肋间最内肌 Intercostales intimi
肋间后动脉 Post. intercostal a.

图 3-15 胸侧面腧穴层次解剖（7）
Fig.3-15 Layered anatomy of acupoints on the lateral aspect of the chest (7)

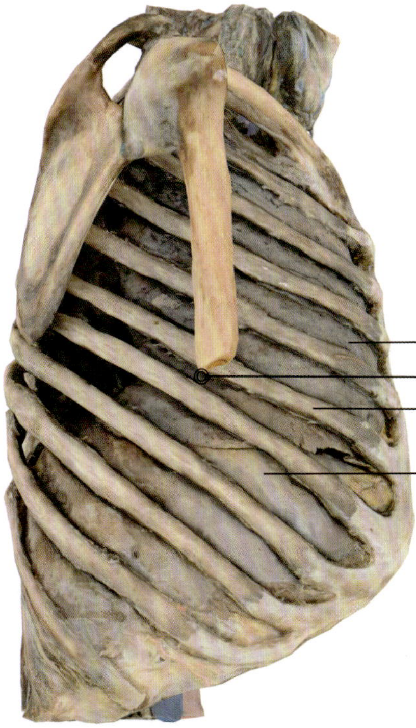
肺 Lung
大包 Dabao (SP 21)
第 6 肋骨 6th rib
膈 Diaphragm

图 3-16 胸侧面腧穴层次解剖（8）
Fig.3-16 Layered anatomy of acupoints on the lateral aspect of the chest (8)

第三节　背部腧穴

Section 3　Acupoints on the back

一、至阳

【定位】第 7 胸椎棘突下凹陷中，后正中线上。

【操作】斜刺 0.5 ～ 1 寸。

【主治】黄疸，身热，胸胁胀痛，心痛，乳痈，咳嗽，气喘，脊背强痛。

【进针层次】①皮肤；②皮下组织（内有第 7 胸神经后支的皮支）；③棘上韧带；④棘间韧带；⑤黄韧带（图 3–17 ～图 3–26）。

【针刺意外与预防】若向上斜刺过深，针尖可通过黄韧带、硬膜外隙、硬脊膜和脊髓蛛网膜进入蛛网膜下隙，进而可刺中脊髓；脊髓损伤症状详见哑门穴。

1. Zhiyang (GV 9)

【Location】On the posterior midline, and in the depression below the spinous process of the 7th thoracic vertebra.

【Method】Puncture obliquely 0.5-1 cun.

【Indications】Jaundice, feverish body, distension and pain in the chest and hypochondrium, angina, acute mastitis, cough, panting, and stiffness and pain in the spine and back.

【Stratified anatomy】①Skin; ②Subcutaneous tissue (There are cutaneous branch of the posterior branches of the 7th thoracic n..); ③Supraspinous lig.; ④Interspinal lig.; ⑤Ligamenta flavum (Fig.3-17 ~ Fig.3-26).

【Cautions】If the oblique-upward insertion is too deep, the tip of the needle can enter the subarachnoid space through the ligamentum flavum, epidural space, dura mater, and spinal arachnoid mater, and then can pierce the spinal cord. For details of the symptoms of spinal cord injury, please refer to Yamen (GV 15) acupoint.

二、风门

【定位】第 2 胸椎棘突下，后正中线旁开 1.5 寸。

【操作】向内侧斜刺 0.5 ～ 0.8 寸。

【主治】感冒，咳嗽，气喘，发热，头痛，项强，肩背痛。

【进针层次】①皮肤；②皮下组织（内有第 2、第 3 胸神经后支的皮支及其伴行的动、静脉）；③斜方肌；④菱形肌；⑤上后锯肌；⑥颈夹肌；⑦胸腰筋膜浅层；⑧竖脊肌（图 3–17 ～图 3–26）。

【针刺意外与预防】若直刺或向外斜刺过深，针尖可通过肋间外肌、肋间内膜、胸内筋膜、肋胸膜进入胸膜腔，进而可刺中肺，引起气胸。

2. Fengmen (BL 12)

【Location】Under the spinous process of the 2nd thoracic vertebra, and 1.5 cun lateral to the posterior midline.

【Method】Puncture obliquely inward 0.5-0.8 cun.

【Indications】Common cold, cough, panting, fever, headache, stiffness in the neck, and pain in the back and shoulder.

【Stratified anatomy】①Skin; ②Subcutaneous tissue (There are cutaneous branch of the posterior branches of the 2nd and 3rd thoracic n. and the accompanying a. & v..); ③Trapezius; ④Rhomboideus; ⑤Serratus posterior superior; ⑥Splenius cervicis; ⑦Superficial layer of the thoracolumbar fascia; ⑧Erector spinae (Fig.3-17 ~ Fig.3-26).

【Cautions】If the perpendicular or oblique-outward insertion is too deep, the tip of the needle can enter the pleural cavity through the extracostal m., intercostal endometrium, intrathoracic fascia, and costal pleura, and then can pierce the lungs and cause pneumothorax.

三、肺俞

【定位】第 3 胸椎棘突下，后正中线旁开 1.5 寸。

【操作】向内侧斜刺 0.5 ～ 0.8 寸。

【主治】咳嗽，气喘，咳血，鼻塞，咽喉肿痛，骨蒸潮热，盗汗，皮肤瘙痒，瘾疹。

【进针层次】①皮肤；②皮下组织（内有第 3、第 4 胸神经后支的皮支及其伴行的动、静脉）；③斜方肌；④菱形肌；⑤上后锯肌；⑥胸腰筋膜浅层；⑦竖脊肌（图 3–17 ～图 3–26）。

【针刺意外与预防】同风门穴。

3. Feishu (BL 13)

【Location】Under the spinous process of the 3rd thoracic vertebra, and 1.5 cun lateral to the posterior midline.

【Method】Puncture obliquely inwards 0.5-0.8 cun.

【Indications】Cough, panting, hemoptysis, nasal obstruction, sore throat, tidal fever, night sweating, pruritus, and urticaria.

【Stratified anatomy】①Skin; ②Subcutaneous tissue (There are cutaneous branch of the posterior branches of the 3rd and 4th thoracic n. and the accompanying a. & v..) ③Trapezius; ④Rhomboideus; ⑤Serratus posterior superior; ⑥Superficial layer of the thoracolumbar fascia; ⑦Erector spinae (Fig.3-17 ~ Fig.3-26).

【Cautions】Same as that of the Fengmen (BL 12) acupoint.

四、膏肓

【定位】第 4 胸椎棘突下，后正中线旁开 3 寸。

【操作】斜刺 0.5 ～ 0.8 寸。

【主治】咳嗽，气喘，盗汗，肺痨，健忘，遗精，完谷不化，虚劳，肩背痛。

【进针层次】①皮肤；②皮下组织（内有第 4、第 5 胸神经后支的皮支及其伴行的动、静脉）；③斜方肌；④菱形肌；⑤胸腰筋膜浅层；⑥竖脊肌（图 3–17 ～图 3–26）。

【针刺意外与预防】同风门穴。

4. Gaohuang (BL 43)

【Location】Under the spinous process of the 4th thoracic vertebra, and 3 cun lateral to the posterior midline.

【Method】Puncture obliquely 0.5-0.8 cun.

【Indications】Cough, panting, night sweating, tuberculosis, forgetfulness, nocturnal emission, diarrhea with undigested food, consumptive diseases, and pain in the back and shoulder.

【Stratified anatomy】①Skin; ②Subcutaneous tissue (There are cutaneous branch of the posterior branches of the 4th and 5th thoracic n. and the accompanying a. & v..); ③Trapezius; ④Rhomboideus; ⑤Superficial layer of the thoracolumbar fascia; ⑥Erector spinae (Fig.3-17 ~ Fig.3-26).

【Cautions】Same as that of the Fengmen (BL 12) acupoint.

五、心俞

【定位】第 5 胸椎棘突下，后正中线旁开 1.5 寸。

【操作】向内侧斜刺 0.5 ～ 0.8 寸。

【主治】心痛，心悸，心烦，失眠，健忘，梦遗，癫狂痫，咳嗽，盗汗。

【进针层次】①皮肤；②皮下组织（内有第 5、第 6 胸神经后支的皮支及其伴行的动、静脉）；③斜方肌；④菱形肌；⑤胸腰筋膜浅层；⑥竖脊肌（图 3–17 ～图 3–26）。

【针刺意外与预防】同风门穴。

5. Xinshu (BL 15)

【Location】Under the spinous process of the 5th thoracic vertebra, and 1.5 cun lateral to the posterior midline.

【Method】Puncture obliquely inwards 0.5-0.8 cun.

【Indications】Angina, palpitations, dysphoria, insomnia, forgetfulness, nocturnal emission, insanity, mania, epilepsy, cough, and night sweating.

【Stratified anatomy】①Skin; ②Subcutaneous tissue (There are cutaneous branch of the posterior branches of the 5th and 6th thoracic n. and the accompanying a. & v..); ③Trapezius; ④Rhomboideus; ⑤Superficial layer of the thoracolumbar fascia; ⑥Erector spinae (Fig.3-17 ~ Fig.3-26).

【Cautions】Same as that of the Fengmen (BL 12) acupoint.

六、膈俞

【定位】第 7 胸椎棘突下，后正中线旁开 1.5 寸。

【操作】向内侧斜刺 0.5 ～ 0.8 寸。

【主治】胃痛，呕吐，呃逆，噎膈，咳嗽，气喘，潮热，盗汗，瘾疹，贫血，瘀血证。

【进针层次】①皮肤；②皮下组织（内有第 7、第 8 胸神经后支的皮支及其伴行的动、静脉）；③斜方肌；④背阔肌；⑤胸腰筋膜浅层；⑥竖脊肌（图 3–17 ～图 3–26）。

【针刺意外与预防】同风门穴。

6. Geshu (BL 17)

【Location】Under the spinous process of the 7th thoracic vertebra, and 1.5 cun lateral to the posterior midline.

【Method】Puncture obliquely inwards 0.5-0.8 cun.

【Indications】Stomachache, vomiting, hiccup, dysphagia, cough, panting, tidal fever, night sweating, urticaria, anemia, and blood stasis syndrome.

【Stratified anatomy】①Skin; ②Subcutaneous tissue (There are cutaneous branch of the posterior branches of the 7th and 8th thoracic n. and the accompanying a. & v..); ③Trapezius; ④Latissimus dorsi; ⑤Superficial layer of the thoracolumbar fascia; ⑥Erector spinae (Fig.3-17 ~ Fig.3-26).

【Cautions】Same as that of the Fengmen (BL 12) acupoint.

七、肝俞

【定位】第 9 胸椎棘突下，后正中线旁开 1.5 寸。

【操作】向内侧斜刺 0.5 ～ 0.8 寸。

【主治】胁痛，黄疸，脊背痛，目赤肿痛，目视不明，夜盲，吐血，衄血，癫狂痫。

【进针层次】①皮肤；②皮下组织（内有第 9、第 10 胸神经后支的皮支及其伴行的动、静脉）；③斜方肌；④背阔肌；⑤胸腰筋膜浅层；⑥竖脊肌（图 3–17 ～图 3–26）。

【针刺意外与预防】同风门穴。

7. Ganshu (BL 18)

【Location】Under the spinous process of the 9th thoracic vertebra, and 1.5 cun lateral to the posterior midline.

【Method】Puncture obliquely inwards 0.5-0.8 cun.

【Indications】Pain in the hypochondrium, jaundice, pain in the back and spine, pain and swelling in the eyes, blurred vision, night blindness, hematemesis, epistaxis, insanity, mania, and epilepsy.

【Stratified anatomy】①Skin; ②Subcutaneous tissue (There are cutaneous branch of the posterior branches of the 9th and 10th thoracic n. and the accompanying a. & v..); ③Trapezius; ④Latissimus dorsi; ⑤Superficial layer of the thoracolumbar fascia; ⑥Erector spinae (Fig.3-17 ~ Fig.3-26).

【Cautions】Same as that of the Fengmen (BL 12) acupoint.

八、胆俞

【定位】第 10 胸椎棘突下，后正中线旁开 1.5 寸。

【操作】向内侧斜刺 0.5 ～ 0.8 寸。

【主治】胁痛，口苦，黄疸，呕吐，噎膈，潮热，盗汗。

【进针层次】①皮肤；②皮下组织（内有第 10、第 11 胸神经后支的皮支及其伴行的动、静脉）；③斜方肌；④背阔肌；⑤下后锯肌腱膜和胸腰筋膜浅层；⑥竖脊肌（图 3–17 ～图 3–26）。

【针刺意外与预防】同风门穴。

8. Danshu (BL 19)

【Location】Under the spinous process of the 10th thoracic vertebra, and 1.5 cun lateral to the posterior midline.

【Method】Puncture obliquely inwards 0.5-0.8 cun.

【Indications】Pain in the hypochondrium, bitter taste in the mouth, jaundice, vomiting, dysphagia, tidal fever and night sweating.

【Stratified anatomy】①Skin; ②Subcutaneous tissue (There are cutaneous branch of the posterior branches of the 10th and 11th thoracic n. and the accompanying a. & v..); ③Trapezius; ④Latissimus dorsi; ⑤Aponeurosis of serratus posterior inferior and superficial layer of the thoracolumbar fascia; ⑥Erector spinae (Fig.3-17 ~ Fig.3-26).

【Cautions】Same as the Fengmen (BL 12) acupoint.

九、脾俞

【定位】第 11 胸椎棘突下，后正中线旁开 1.5 寸。

【操作】向内侧斜刺 0.5 ～ 0.8 寸。

【主治】腹胀，呕吐，泄泻，痢疾，完谷不化，便血，黄疸，水肿，背痛。

【进针层次】①皮肤；②皮下组织（内有第 11、第 12 胸神经后支的皮支及其伴行的动、静脉）；③背阔肌腱膜、下后锯肌腱膜和胸腰筋膜浅层；④竖脊肌（图 3–17 ～图 3–26）。

【针刺意外与预防】①若直刺过深，针尖可依次通过肋间外肌、肋间内肌、肋间最内肌、胸内筋膜、肋胸膜进入胸膜腔，进而可刺中肺，引起气胸。②若向外侧斜刺过深，针尖可经肋间隙进入肋膈隐窝内，进而可刺中肝、肾；若施针时采用大幅度提插、捻转手法，后果严重。

9. Pishu (BL 20)

【Location】Under the spinous process of the 11th thoracic vertebra, and 1.5 cun lateral to the posterior midline.

【Method】Puncture obliquely inwards 0.5-0.8 cun.

【Indications】Abdominal distension, vomiting, diarrhea, dysentery, diarrhea with undigested food, bloody stools, jaundice, edema, and pain in the back.

【Stratified anatomy】①Skin; ②Subcutaneous tissue (There are cutaneous branch of the posterior branches of the 11th and 12th thoracic n. and the accompanying a. & v..); ③Aponeurosis of latissimus dorsi, aponeurosis of serratus posterior inferior and superficial layer of the thoracolumbar fascia; ④Erector spinae (Fig.3-17 ~ Fig.3-26).

【Cautions】①If the perpendicular insertion is too deep, the tip of the needle can enter the pleural cavity through the extracostal m., intercostal m., intercostales intimi, intrathoracic fascia and costal pleura in turn, and then pierce the lungs, causing pneumothorax. ②If the oblique insertion is too deep outward, the tip of the needle can enter the costodiaphragmatic recess through the intercostal space, and then it can pierce the liver and kidney. If the needling is manipulated with strong lifting-thrusting and twisting methods, the consequences will be serious.

十、胃俞

【定位】第 12 胸椎棘突下，后正中线旁开 1.5 寸。

【操作】向内侧斜刺 0.5 ～ 0.8 寸。

【主治】胃痛，呕吐，泄泻，腹胀，完谷不化，背痛。

【进针层次】①皮肤；②皮下组织（内有第 12 胸神经、第 1 腰神经后支的皮支及其伴行的动、静脉）；③背阔肌腱膜、下后锯肌腱膜和胸腰筋膜浅层；④竖脊肌（图 3–17 ～图 3–26）。

【针刺意外与预防】①若直刺过深，针尖可依次通过肋间外肌、肋间内肌、肋间最内肌、胸内筋膜、肋胸膜进入胸膜腔，进而可刺中肺，引起气胸。②若向外侧斜刺过深，针尖可经肋间隙进入肋膈隐窝内，进而可刺中肝、脾、肾；若大幅度提插、捻转手法，后果严重。

10. Weishu (BL 21)

【Location】Under the spinous process of the 12th thoracic vertebra, and 1.5 cun lateral to the posterior midline.

【Method】Puncture obliquely inwards 0.5-0.8 cun.

【Indications】Stomachache, vomiting, diarrhea, abdominal distension, diarrhea with undigested food, and pain in the back.

【Stratified anatomy】①Skin; ②Subcutaneous tissue (There are cutaneous branch of the posterior branches of the 12th thoracic and 1st lumbar n. and the accompanying a. & v..); ③Aponeurosis of latissimus dorsi, aponeurosis of serratus posterior inferior and superficial layer of the thoracolumbar fascia; ④Erector spinae (Fig.3-17 ~ Fig.3-26).

【Cautions】①If the perpendicular insertion is too deep, the tip of the needle can enter the pleural cavity through the extracostal m., intercostal m., intercostales intimi, intrathoracic fascia and costal pleura in turn, and then pierce the lungs, causing pneumothorax. ②If the oblique insertion is too deep outward, the tip of the needle can enter the costodiaphragmatic recess through the intercostal space, and then it can pierce the liver, spleen, and kidney. If the needling is manipulated with strong lifting-thrusting and twisting methods, the consequences will be serious.

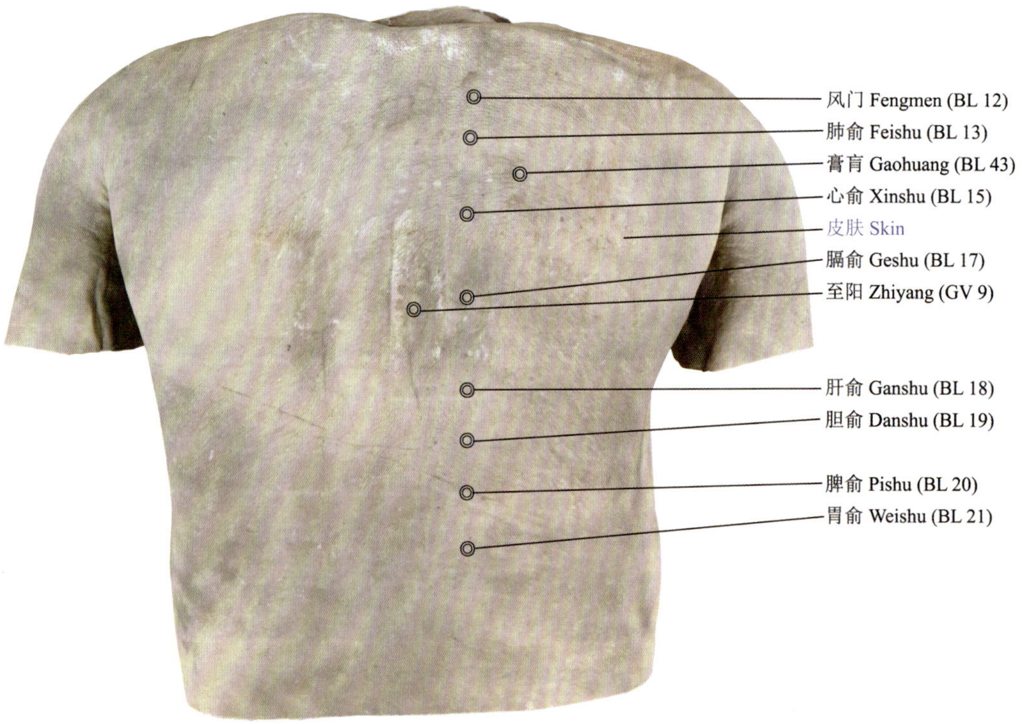
风门 Fengmen (BL 12)
肺俞 Feishu (BL 13)
膏肓 Gaohuang (BL 43)
心俞 Xinshu (BL 15)
皮肤 Skin
膈俞 Geshu (BL 17)
至阳 Zhiyang (GV 9)
肝俞 Ganshu (BL 18)
胆俞 Danshu (BL 19)
脾俞 Pishu (BL 20)
胃俞 Weishu (BL 21)

图 3-17　背部腧穴层次解剖（1）
Fig.3-17　Layered anatomy of acupoints on the back (1)

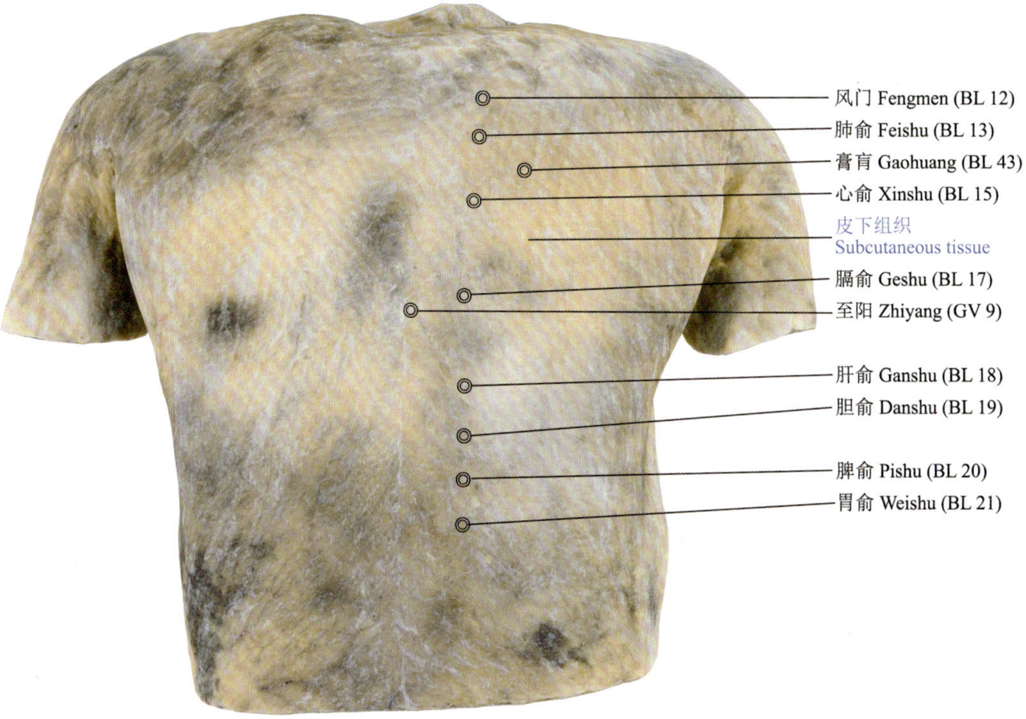
风门 Fengmen (BL 12)
肺俞 Feishu (BL 13)
膏肓 Gaohuang (BL 43)
心俞 Xinshu (BL 15)
皮下组织
Subcutaneous tissue
膈俞 Geshu (BL 17)
至阳 Zhiyang (GV 9)
肝俞 Ganshu (BL 18)
胆俞 Danshu (BL 19)
脾俞 Pishu (BL 20)
胃俞 Weishu (BL 21)

图 3–18　背部腧穴层次解剖（2）

Fig.3-18　Layered anatomy of acupoints on the back (2)

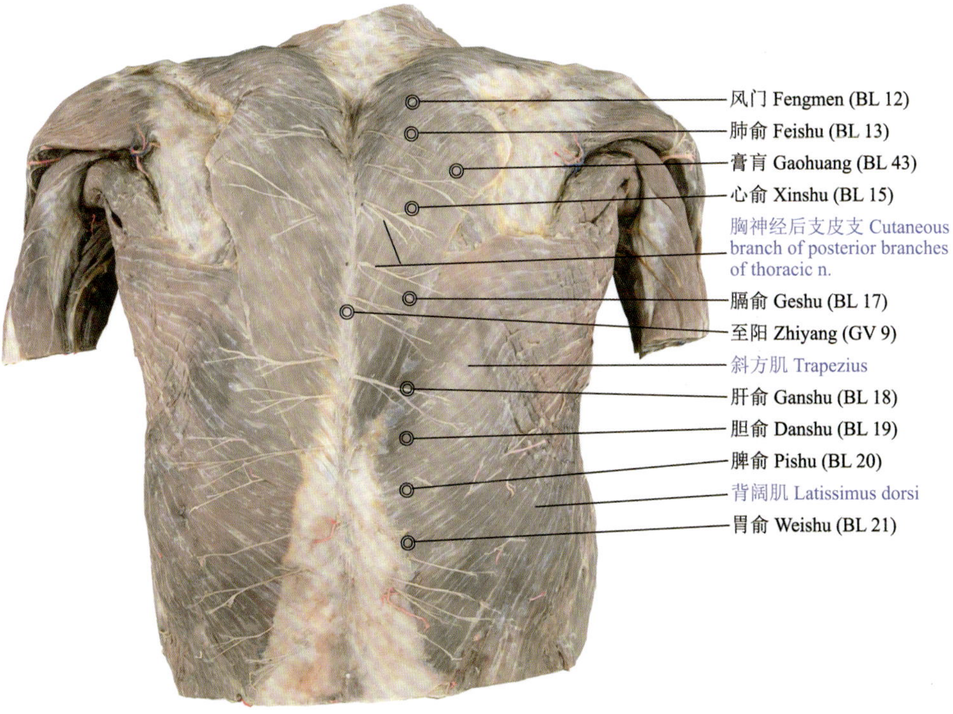
风门 Fengmen (BL 12)
肺俞 Feishu (BL 13)
膏肓 Gaohuang (BL 43)
心俞 Xinshu (BL 15)
胸神经后支皮支 Cutaneous branch of posterior branches of thoracic n.
膈俞 Geshu (BL 17)
至阳 Zhiyang (GV 9)
斜方肌 Trapezius
肝俞 Ganshu (BL 18)
胆俞 Danshu (BL 19)
脾俞 Pishu (BL 20)
背阔肌 Latissimus dorsi
胃俞 Weishu (BL 21)

图 3–19　背部腧穴层次解剖（3）

Fig.3-19　Layered anatomy of acupoints on the back (3)

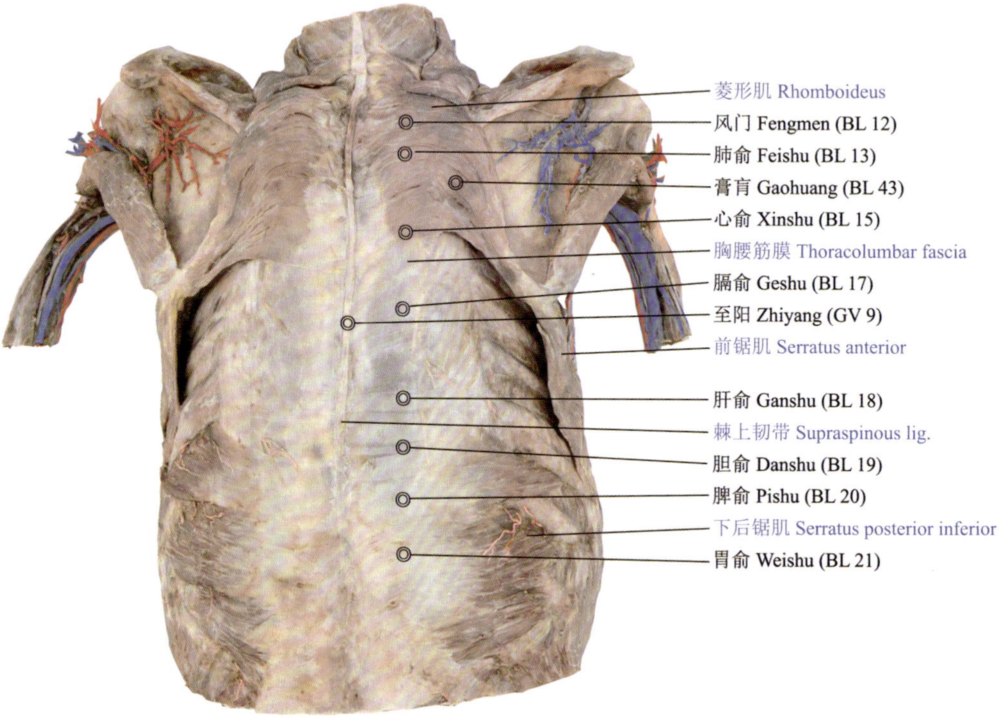
菱形肌 Rhomboideus
风门 Fengmen (BL 12)
肺俞 Feishu (BL 13)
膏肓 Gaohuang (BL 43)
心俞 Xinshu (BL 15)
胸腰筋膜 Thoracolumbar fascia
膈俞 Geshu (BL 17)
至阳 Zhiyang (GV 9)
前锯肌 Serratus anterior
肝俞 Ganshu (BL 18)
棘上韧带 Supraspinous lig.
胆俞 Danshu (BL 19)
脾俞 Pishu (BL 20)
下后锯肌 Serratus posterior inferior
胃俞 Weishu (BL 21)

图 3–20　背部腧穴层次解剖（4）

Fig.3-20　Layered anatomy of acupoints on the back (4)

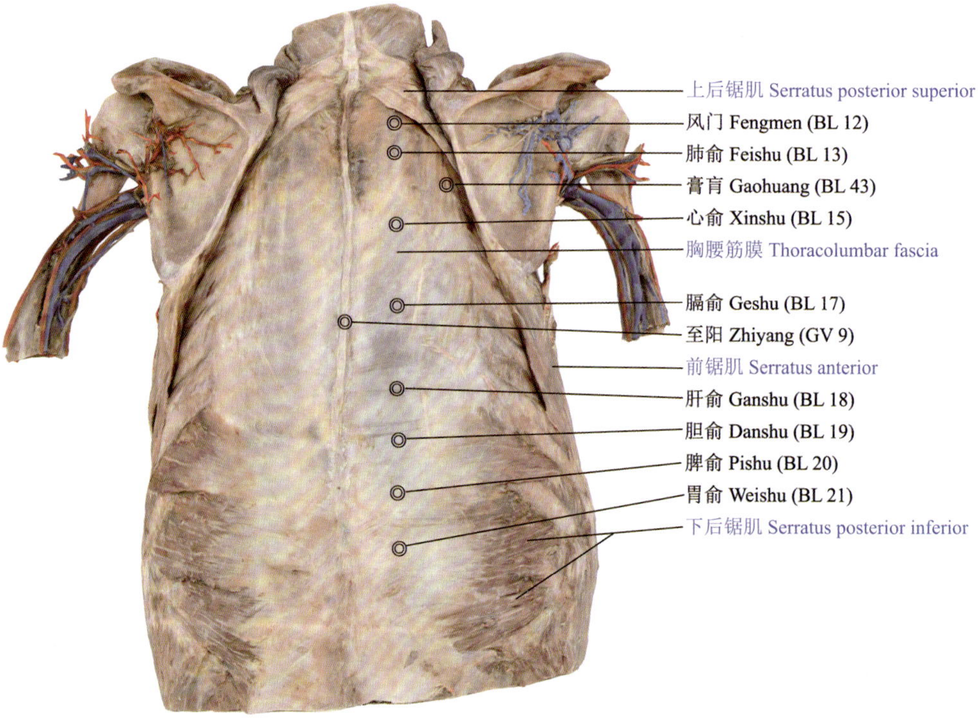
上后锯肌 Serratus posterior superior
风门 Fengmen (BL 12)
肺俞 Feishu (BL 13)
膏肓 Gaohuang (BL 43)
心俞 Xinshu (BL 15)
胸腰筋膜 Thoracolumbar fascia
膈俞 Geshu (BL 17)
至阳 Zhiyang (GV 9)
前锯肌 Serratus anterior
肝俞 Ganshu (BL 18)
胆俞 Danshu (BL 19)
脾俞 Pishu (BL 20)
胃俞 Weishu (BL 21)
下后锯肌 Serratus posterior inferior

图 3–21　背部腧穴层次解剖（5）

Fig.3-21　Layered anatomy of acupoints on the back (5)

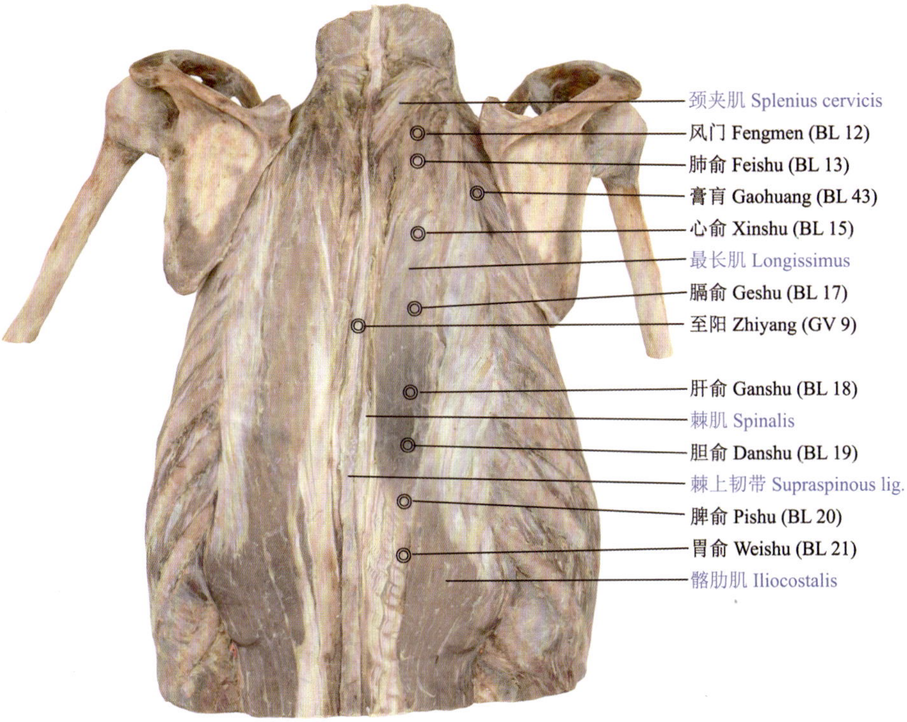
颈夹肌 Splenius cervicis
风门 Fengmen (BL 12)
肺俞 Feishu (BL 13)
膏肓 Gaohuang (BL 43)
心俞 Xinshu (BL 15)
最长肌 Longissimus
膈俞 Geshu (BL 17)
至阳 Zhiyang (GV 9)
肝俞 Ganshu (BL 18)
棘肌 Spinalis
胆俞 Danshu (BL 19)
棘上韧带 Supraspinous lig.
脾俞 Pishu (BL 20)
胃俞 Weishu (BL 21)
髂肋肌 Iliocostalis

图 3–22 背部腧穴层次解剖（6）

Fig.3-22 Layered anatomy of acupoints on the back (6)

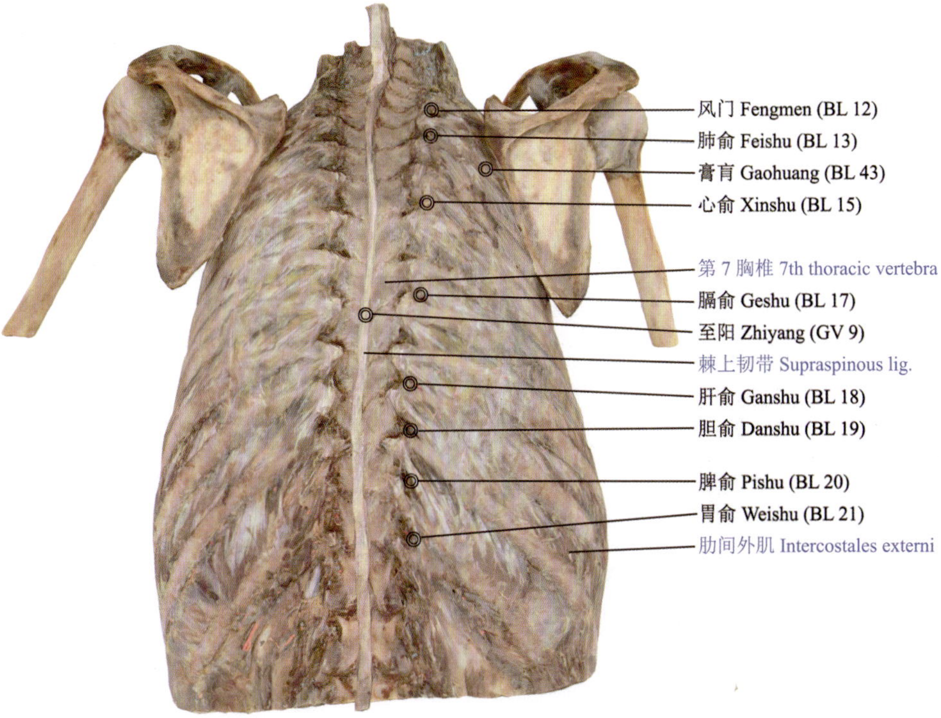
风门 Fengmen (BL 12)
肺俞 Feishu (BL 13)
膏肓 Gaohuang (BL 43)
心俞 Xinshu (BL 15)
第 7 胸椎 7th thoracic vertebra
膈俞 Geshu (BL 17)
至阳 Zhiyang (GV 9)
棘上韧带 Supraspinous lig.
肝俞 Ganshu (BL 18)
胆俞 Danshu (BL 19)
脾俞 Pishu (BL 20)
胃俞 Weishu (BL 21)
肋间外肌 Intercostales externi

图 3–23 背部腧穴层次解剖（7）

Fig.3-23 Layered anatomy of acupoints on the back (7)

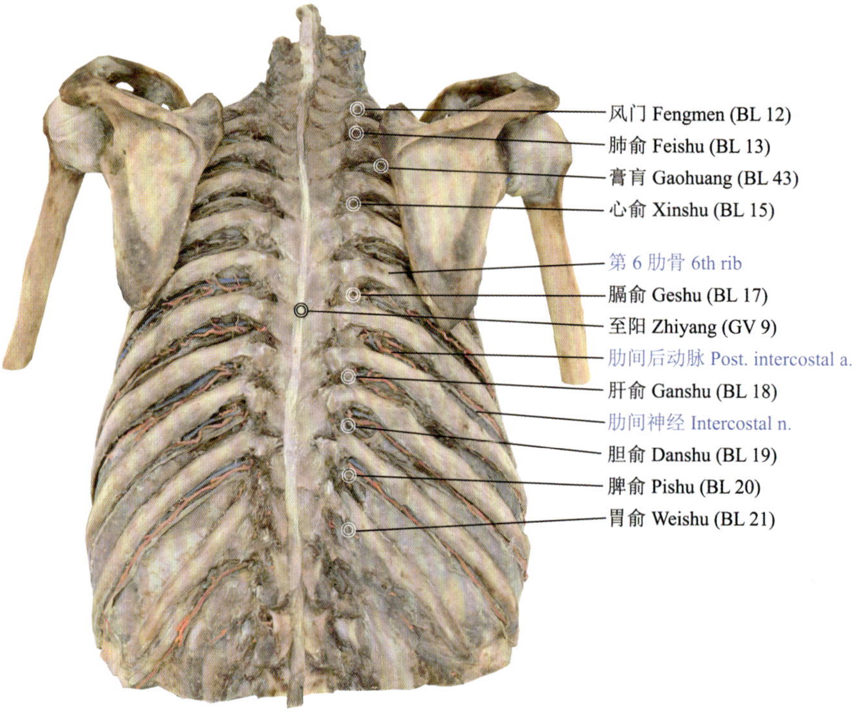
风门 Fengmen (BL 12)
肺俞 Feishu (BL 13)
膏肓 Gaohuang (BL 43)
心俞 Xinshu (BL 15)
第 6 肋骨 6th rib
膈俞 Geshu (BL 17)
至阳 Zhiyang (GV 9)
肋间后动脉 Post. intercostal a.
肝俞 Ganshu (BL 18)
肋间神经 Intercostal n.
胆俞 Danshu (BL 19)
脾俞 Pishu (BL 20)
胃俞 Weishu (BL 21)

图 3-24　背部腧穴层次解剖（8）
Fig.3-24　Layered anatomy of acupoints on the back (8)

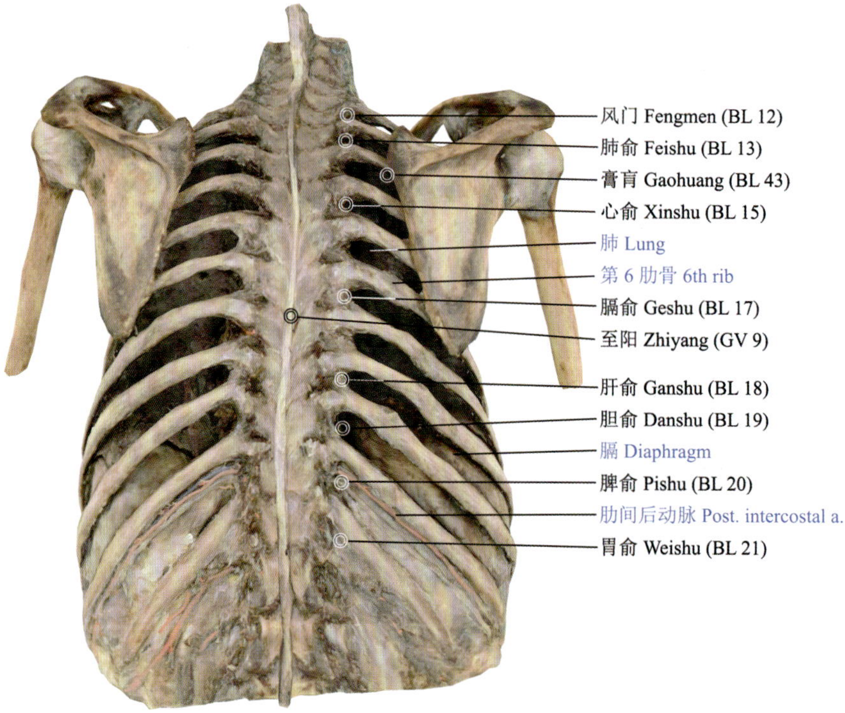
风门 Fengmen (BL 12)
肺俞 Feishu (BL 13)
膏肓 Gaohuang (BL 43)
心俞 Xinshu (BL 15)
肺 Lung
第 6 肋骨 6th rib
膈俞 Geshu (BL 17)
至阳 Zhiyang (GV 9)
肝俞 Ganshu (BL 18)
胆俞 Danshu (BL 19)
膈 Diaphragm
脾俞 Pishu (BL 20)
肋间后动脉 Post. intercostal a.
胃俞 Weishu (BL 21)

图 3-25　背部腧穴层次解剖（9）
Fig.3-25　Layered anatomy of acupoints on the back (9)

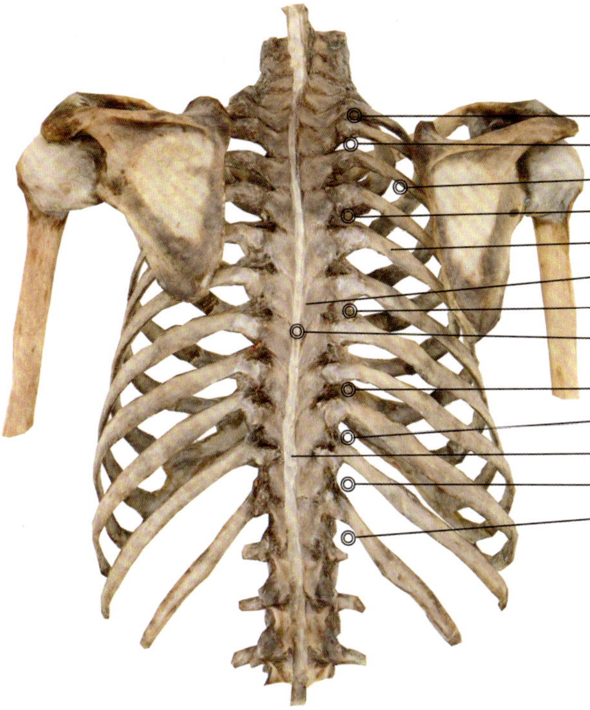

图 3–26　背部腧穴层次解剖（10）

Fig.3-26　Layered anatomy of acupoints on the back (10)

第四章　腹腰部腧穴层次解剖

Chapter 4　Layered Anatomy of Acupoints on the Abdomen and Waist

第一节　腹前面腧穴

Section 1　Acupoints on the anterior aspect of the abdomen

一、鸠尾

【定位】胸剑结合下 1 寸，前正中线上。

【操作】向下斜刺 0.3 ～ 0.6 寸。

【主治】胸闷，心痛，心悸，胃痛，噎膈，癫狂痫。

【进针层次】①皮肤；②皮下组织（内有第 6 肋间神经的前皮支和胸腹壁静脉的属支）；③腹白线（图 4–1 ～图 4–8）。

【针刺意外与预防】①若向下或两侧斜刺过深，针尖可越过剑突，通过腹直肌、壁腹膜而进入腹膜腔，进而可刺中肝或胃；若大幅度提插和捻转，可引起肝出血或急腹症，后果严重。②若向上斜刺过深，针尖可穿过膈进入胸腔，再进入纵隔，刺中心包和心脏，轻者仅有心前区的疼痛，重者可有胸闷、心慌、心悸，甚至休克、心包腔出血和心脏骤停。③若向左上或右上斜刺过深，针尖可刺入两肺的内下角，引起气胸。

1. Jiuwei (CV 15)

【Location】1 cun under the xiphoid process, and on the anterior midline.

【Method】Puncture obliquely downward 0.3-0.6 cun.

【Indications】Stuffy chest, angina, palpitations, stomachache, dysphagia, insanity, mania, and epilepsy.

【Stratified anatomy】①Skin; ②Subcutaneous tissue (There are anterior cutaneous branch of the 6th intercostal n. and tributaries of the thoracoepigastric v..); ③Linea alba (Fig.4-1 ~ Fig.4-8).

【Cautions】①If the oblique insertion is too deep downward or toward both sides, the tip of the needle can cross the xiphoid process and enter the peritoneal cavity through the rectus abdominis and parietal peritoneum, and then pierce the liver or stomach. If the needling is manipulated with strong lifting-thrusting and twisting methods, it can cause liver bleeding or acute abdomen, and the consequences will be serious. ②If the upward-oblique insertion is too deep, the tip of the needle can pass through the diaphragm into the chest, and then enter the mediastinum, pierce the pericardium and heart. In mild cases, there may only pain in the anterior mediastinum, and in severe cases, there may be chest tightness, panic, palpitations, and even shock, pericardium bleeding and cardiac arrest. ③If the oblique insertion is too deep toward the upper left or upper right, the tip of the needle can pierce the inner and inferior corners of the two lungs, causing pneumothorax.

二、中脘

【定位】脐中上 4 寸，前正中线上。

【操作】直刺 1 ～ 1.5 寸。

【主治】胃痛，腹痛，腹胀，呕吐，完谷不化，肠鸣，泄泻，便秘，咳喘，痰多，失眠，癫痫。

【进针层次】①皮肤；②皮下组织（内有第 8 肋间神经的前皮支和胸腹壁静脉的属支）；③腹白线（图 4–1 ～图 4–8）。

【针刺意外与预防】若直刺过深，针尖可通过腹横筋膜、腹膜外筋膜、壁腹膜而进入腹膜腔，可刺中胃、横结肠、肝或脾（肝脾肿大时）；若大幅度提插和捻转，可引起肝脾出血或急腹症，后果严重。

2. Zhongwan (CV 12)

【Location】4 cun above the umbilicus, and on the anterior midline.

【Method】Puncture perpendicularly 1-1.5cun.

【Indications】Stomachache, abdominal pain, abdominal distension, vomiting, diarrhea with undigested food, borborygmus, diarrhea, constipation, asthma, profuse sputum, insomnia, and epilepsy.

【Stratified anatomy】①Skin; ②Subcutaneous tissue (There are anterior cutaneous branch of the 8th intercostal n. and tributaries of the thoracoepigastric v..); ③Linea alba (Fig.4-1 ~ Fig.4-8).

【Cautions】If the perpendicular insertion is too deep, the tip of the needle can enter the peritoneal cavity through the transabdominal fascia, extraperitoneal fascia, and parietal peritoneum, which can prick the stomach, transverse colon, liver or spleen (when the liver and spleen are enlarged). If the needling is manipulated with strong lifting-thrusting and twisting methods, it can cause liver and spleen bleeding or acute abdomen, and the consequences will be serious.

三、梁门

【定位】脐中上 4 寸，前正中线旁开 2 寸。

【操作】直刺 0.5 ～ 1 寸。

【主治】胃痛，呕吐，食欲不振，腹胀，泄泻。

【进针层次】①皮肤；②皮下组织（内有第 8 肋间神经的前皮支和胸腹壁静脉的属支）；③腹直肌鞘前层；④腹直肌（图 4–1 ～图 4–8）。

【针刺意外与预防】若直刺过深，针尖可过通过腹直肌鞘后层、腹横筋膜、腹膜外筋膜和壁腹膜而进入腹膜腔，进而可刺中小肠、胃或横结肠；若大幅度提插和捻转，可引起急腹症，后果严重。

3. Liangmen (ST 21)

【Location】4 cun above the umbilicus, and 2 cun lateral to the anterior midline.

【Method】Puncture perpendicularly 0.5-1.0 cun.

【Indications】Stomachache, vomiting, poor appetite, abdominal distension, and diarrhea.

【Stratified anatomy】①Skin; ②Subcutaneous tissue (There are anterior cutaneous branch of the 8th intercostal n. and tributaries of the thoracoepigastric v..); ③Anterior wall of sheath of rectus abdominis. ④Rectus abdominis (Fig.4-1 ~ Fig.4-8).

【Cautions】If the perpendicular insertion is too deep, the tip of the needle can enter the peritoneal cavity through the posterior layer of the sheath of rectus abdominis, transversalis fascia, extraperitoneal fascia and the parietal peritoneum, and then can pierce the small intestine, stomach or transverse colon. If the needling is manipulated with strong lifting-thrusting and twisting methods, it can cause acute abdomen, and the consequences will be serious.

四、下脘

【定位】脐中上 2 寸，前正中线上。

【操作】直刺 1 ～ 1.5 寸。

【主治】腹胀，痞块，完谷不化，腹痛，呕吐，泄泻，虚肿，消瘦。

【进针层次】①皮肤；②皮下组织（内有第 9 肋间神经的前皮支和胸腹壁静脉的属支）；③腹白线（图 4–1 ~图 4–8）。

【针刺意外与预防】若直刺过深，针尖可通过腹横筋膜、腹膜外筋膜、壁腹膜而进入腹膜腔，进而可刺中小肠、胃或横结肠；若大幅度提插和捻转，可引起急腹症，后果严重。

4. Xiawan (CV 10)

【Location】2 cun above the umbilicus, and on the anterior midline.

【Method】Puncture perpendicularly 1-1.5 cun.

【Indications】Abdominal distension, abdominal mass, diarrhea with undigested food, abdominal pain, vomiting, diarrhea, puffiness and emaciation.

【Stratified anatomy】①Skin; ②Subcutaneous tissue (There are anterior cutaneous branch of the 9th intercostal n. and tributaries of the thoracoepigastric v..); ③Linea alba (Fig.4-1 ~ Fig.4-8).

【Cautions】If the perpendicular insertion is too deep, the tip of the needle can enter the peritoneal cavity through the transabdominal fascia, extraperitoneal fascia and parietal peritoneum, and then pierce the small intestines, stomach or transverse colons. If the needling is manipulated with strong lifting-thrusting and twisting methods, it can cause acute abdomen, and the consequences will be serious.

五、神阙

【定位】脐中央。

【操作】禁刺；可灸或敷贴。

【主治】腹痛，泄泻，水肿，脱肛，小便不利，中风脱证，虚劳。

【进针层次】①皮肤；②皮下组织（内有第 10 肋间神经的前皮支和胸腹壁静脉的属支）；③腹白线（图 4–1 ～图 4–8）。

5. Shenque (CV 8)

【Location】At the centre of the navel.

【Method】No needling. Moxibustion or acupoint application therapy can be used.

【Indications】Abdominal pain, diarrhea, edema, prolapse of the anus, difficulty in urinating, wind-stroke collapse pattern, and deficiency-consumption.

【Stratified anatomy】①Skin; ②Subcutaneous tissue (There are anterior cutaneous branch of the 10th intercostal n. and tributaries of the thoracoepigastric v..); ③Linea alba (Fig.4-1 ~ Fig.4-8).

六、天枢

【定位】脐中旁开 2 寸。

【操作】直刺 1～ 1.5 寸。

【主治】腹胀，肠鸣，腹痛，便秘，泄泻，痢疾，痞块，痛经，月经不调。

【进针层次】①皮肤；②皮下组织（内有第 10 肋间神经的前皮支和腹壁浅动、静脉）；③腹直肌鞘前层；④腹直肌（图 4–1 ～图 4–8）。

【针刺意外与预防】若直刺过深，针尖可通过腹直肌鞘后层、腹横筋膜、腹膜外筋膜和壁腹膜而进入腹膜腔，可刺中大网膜、空肠或回肠；若大幅度提插和捻转，可引起急腹症，后果严重。

6. Tianshu (ST 25)

【Location】2 cun lateral to the navel.

【Method】Puncture perpendicularly l-1.5 cun.

【Indications】Abdominal distension, borborygmus, abdominal pain, constipation, diarrhea, dysentery, abdominal mass, dysmenorrhea, and irregular menstruation.

【Stratified anatomy】①Skin; ②Subcutaneous tissue (There are anterior cutaneous branch of the 10th intercostal n. and superficial epigastric a. & v..); ③Anterior layer of the rectus abdominis sheath; ④Rectus abdominis (Fig.4-1 ~ Fig.4-8).

【Cautions】If the perpendicular insertion is too deep, the tip of the needle can enter the abdominal cavity through the posterior layer of the rectus abdominis sheath, transabdominal fascia, fascia extraperitonealis and parietal peritoneum, and can pierce the greater omentum, jejunum or ileum. If the needling is manipulated with strong lifting-thrusting and twisting methods, it can cause acute abdomen, and the consequences will be serious.

七、大横

【定位】脐中旁开 4 寸。

【操作】直刺 0.5 ～ 1 寸。

【主治】腹痛，便秘，泄泻，痢疾。

【进针层次】①皮肤；②皮下组织（内有第 10 肋间神经的前皮支和腹壁浅动、静脉）；③腹外斜肌；④腹内斜肌；⑤腹横肌（图 4–1 ～图 4–8）。

【针刺意外与预防】若直刺过深，针尖可通过腹横筋膜、腹膜外筋膜和壁腹膜而进入腹膜腔，进而可刺中升结肠（右侧大横穴）、降结肠（左侧大横穴）、空肠或回肠；若大幅度提插和捻转，可引起急腹症，后果严重。

7. Daheng (SP 15)

【Location】4 cun lateral to the navel.

【Method】Puncture perpendicularly 0.5-1 cun.

【Indications】Abdominal pain, constipation, diarrhea, and dysentery.

【Stratified anatomy】①Skin; ②Subcutaneous tissue (There are anterior cutaneous branch of the 10th intercostal n. and superficial epigastric a. & v..); ③Musculus obliquus externus abdominis; ④Musculus obliquus internus abdominis; ⑤Transversus abdominis (Fig.4-1 ~ Fig.4-8).

【Cautions】If the perpendicular insertion is too deep, the tip of the needle can enter the peritoneal cavity through the transversalis fascia, extraperitoneal fascia and parietal peritoneum, and then it can prick the ascending colon [right Daheng (SP 15) acupoint], descending colon [left Daheng (SP 15) acupoint], jejunum or ileum. If the needling is manipulated with strong lifting-thrusting and twisting methods, it can cause acute abdomen, and the consequences will be serious.

八、气海

【定位】脐中下 1.5 寸，前正中线上。

【操作】直刺 1 ～ 2 寸。

【主治】少腹疼痛，便秘，泻痢，疝气，癃闭，淋证，遗尿，遗精，阳痿，闭经，痛经，崩漏，带下，阴挺，中风脱证，虚劳（图 4–1 ～图 4–8）。

【进针层次】①皮肤；②皮下组织（内有第 11 肋间神经的前皮支和腹壁浅动、静脉）；③腹白线。

【针刺意外与预防】若直刺过深，针尖可穿过白线、腹横筋膜、腹膜外筋膜和壁腹膜刺入腹膜腔，进而可刺中空肠或回肠；若大幅度提插和捻转，可引起急腹症，后果严重。

8. Qihai (CV 6)

【Location】1.5 cun below the navel, and on the anterior midline.

【Method】Puncture perpendicularly 1-2 cun.

【Indications】Pain in the lower abdomen, constipation, diarrhea, hernia, retention of urine, stranguria, enuresis, nocturnal emission, impotence, amenorrhea, dysmenorrhea, metrorrhagia and metrostaxis, leukorrhea, prolapse of uterus, collapse syndrome due to apoplexy, and deficiency-consumption.

【Stratified anatomy】①Skin; ②Subcutaneous tissue (There are anterior cutaneous branch of the 11th intercostal n. and superficial epigastric a. & v..); ③Linea alba (Fig.4-1 ~ Fig.4-8).

【Cautions】If the perpendicular insertion is too deep, the tip of the needle can enter the peritoneal cavity through the linea alba, transversalis fascia, extraperitoneal fascia and parietal peritoneum, and then can pierce the jejunum or ileum. If the needling is manipulated with strong lifting-thrusting and twisting methods, it can cause acute abdomen, and the consequences will be serious.

九、关元

【定位】脐中下 3 寸，前正中线上。

【操作】直刺 1 ～ 2 寸。

【主治】遗精，阳痿，早泄，痛经，闭经，不孕，带下，尿频，癃闭，中风脱证，虚劳，眩晕，少腹疼痛，疝气，腹泻。

【进针层次】①皮肤；②皮下组织（内有肋下神经前皮支和腹壁浅动、静脉）；③腹白线（图 4–1 ～图 4–8）。

【针刺意外与预防】若直刺过深，针尖可穿过白线、腹横筋膜、腹膜外筋膜和壁腹膜刺入腹膜腔，进而可刺中空肠、回肠或膀胱（膀胱充盈、尿潴留或小儿）；若大幅度提插和捻转，可引起尿液、肠内容物等流入腹膜腔，引起急腹症，后果严重。故针刺此穴时，宜先排空膀胱。

9. Guanyuan (CV 4)

【Location】3 cun below the navel, and on the anterior midline.

【Method】Puncture perpendicularly 1-2 cun.

【Indications】Nocturnal emission, impotence, premature ejaculation, dysmenorrhea, amenorrhea, sterility, leukorrhea, frequent urination, retention of urine, collapse syndrome due to apoplexy, deficiency-consumption, vertigo, pain in the lower abdomen, hernia, and diarrhea.

【Stratified anatomy】①Skin; ②Subcutaneous tissue (There are anterior cutaneous branch of the subcostal n. and superficial epigastric a. & v..); ③Linea alba (Fig.4-1 ~ Fig.4-8).

【Cautions】If the perpendicular insertion is too deep, the tip of the needle can enter the peritoneal cavity through the linea alba, transversalis fascia, extraperitoneal fascia and parietal peritoneum, and then pierce the jejunum, ileum or bladder (bladder filling, urinary retention or children). If the needling is manipulated with strong lifting-thrusting and twisting methods, it can cause urine, intestinal contents, etc. to flow into the peritoneal cavity, causing acute abdomen with serious consequences. Therefore, when pricking this acupoint, it is appropriate to empty the bladder first.

十、中极

【定位】脐中下 4 寸，前正中线上。

【操作】直刺 1 ～ 1.5 寸。

【主治】癃闭，遗尿，尿频，遗精，阳痿，痛经，闭经，带下，崩漏，水肿，疝气。

【进针层次】①皮肤；②皮下组织（内有髂腹下神经前皮支和腹壁浅动、静脉）；③腹白线（图 4–1 ～图 4–8）。

【针刺意外与预防】同关元穴。

10. Zhongji (CV 3)

【Location】4 cun below the navel, and on the anterior midline.

【Method】Puncture perpendicularly 1-1.5 cun.

【Indications】Retention of urine, enuresis, frequent urination, nocturnal emission, impotence, dysmenorrhea, amenorrhea, leukorrhea, metrorrhagia and metrostaxis, edema, and hernia.

【Stratified anatomy】①Skin; ②Subcutaneous tissue (There are anterior cutaneous branch of iliohypogastric n. and superficial epigastric a. & v..); ③Linea alba (Fig.4-1 ~ Fig.4-8).

【Cautions】Same as that of Guanyuan (CV 4) acupoint.

十一、大赫

【定位】脐中下 4 寸，前正中线旁开 0.5 寸。

【操作】直刺 1 ～ 1.5 寸。

【主治】遗精，阳痿，阴挺，带下。

【进针层次】①皮肤；②皮下组织（内有髂腹下神经前皮支和腹壁浅动、静脉）；③腹直肌鞘前层；④腹直肌（图 4–1 ～图 4–8）。

【针刺意外与预防】同关元穴。

11. Dahe (KI 12)

【Location】4 cun below the navel, 0.5 cun lateral to the anterior midline.

【Method】Puncture perpendicularly 1-1.5cun.

【Indications】Nocturnal emission, impotence, prolapse of uterus, and leukorrhea.

【Stratified anatomy】①Skin; ②Subcutaneous tissue (There are anterior cutaneous branch of iliohypogastric n. and superficial epigastric a. & v..); ③Anterior layer of the rectus abdominis sheath; ④Rectus abdominis (Fig.4-1 ~ Fig.4-8).

【Cautions】Same as that of Guanyuan (CV 4) acupoint.

十二、归来

【定位】脐中下 4 寸，前正中线旁开 2 寸。

【操作】直刺 1 ～ 1.5 寸。

【主治】腹痛，疝气，闭经，月经不调，阴挺，带下。

【进针层次】①皮肤；②皮下组织（内有肋下神经的前皮支和腹壁浅动、静脉）；③腹直肌鞘前层；④腹直肌外侧缘（图 4–1 ～图 4–8）。

【针刺意外与预防】若直刺过深，针尖可穿过腹直肌鞘后层、腹横筋膜、腹膜外筋膜和壁腹膜刺入腹膜腔，进而可刺中小肠；若大幅度提插和捻转，可引起急腹症，后果严重。

12. Guilai (ST 29)

【Location】4 cun below the navel, and 2cun lateral to the anterior midline.

【Method】Puncture perpendicularly 1-1.5 cun.

【Indications】Abdominal pain, hernia, amenorrhea, irregular menstruation, prolapse of uterus, and leukorrhea.

【Stratified anatomy】①Skin; ②Subcutaneous tissue (There are anterior cutaneous branch of the subcostal n. and superficial epigastric a. & v..); ③Anterior layer of the rectus abdominis sheath; ④Lateral border of rectus abdominis (Fig.4-1 ~ Fig.4-8).

【Cautions】If the perpendicular insertion is too deep, the tip of the needle can enter the peritoneal cavity through the posterior layer of the rectus abdominis sheath, transversalis fascia, extraperitoneal fascia and parietal peritoneum, and then pierce the small intestines. If the needling is manipulated with strong lifting-thrusting and twisting methods, it can cause acute abdomen, and the consequences will be serious.

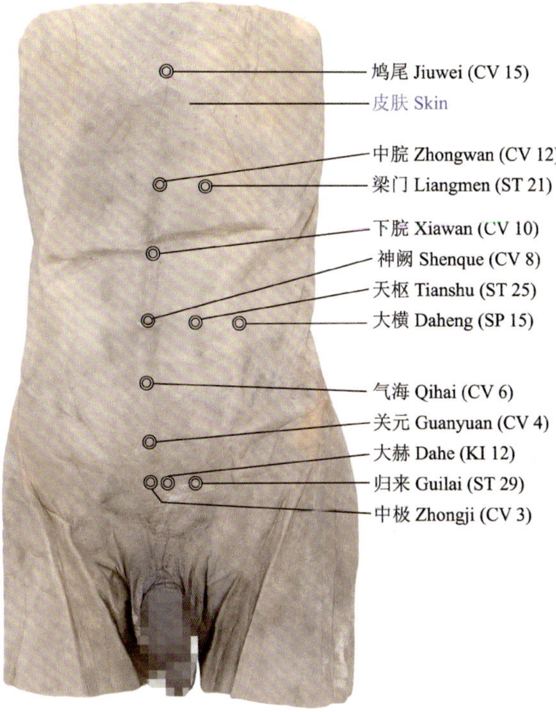

图 4–1 腹前面腧穴层次解剖（1）

Fig.4-1 Layered anatomy of acupoints on the anterior aspect of the abdomen (1)

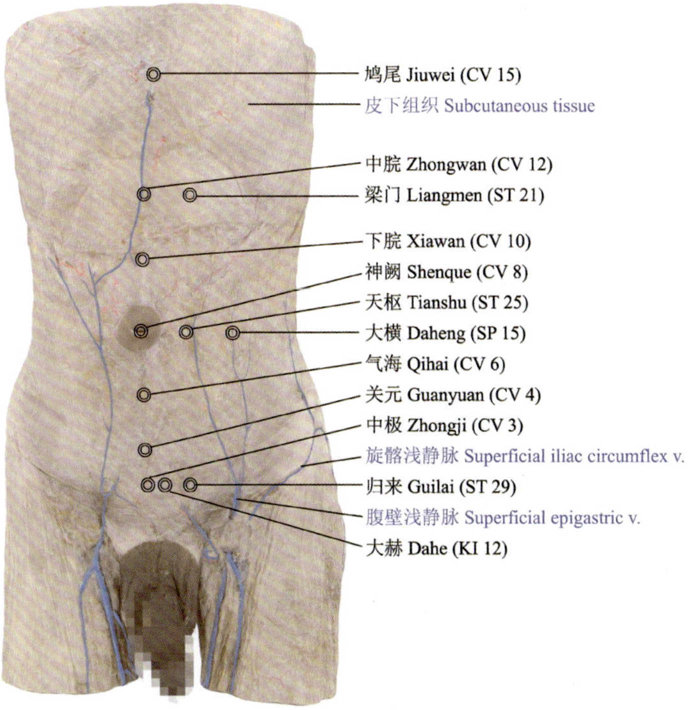

图 4–2 腹前面腧穴层次解剖（2）

Fig.4-2 Layered anatomy of acupoints on the anterior aspect of the abdomen (2)

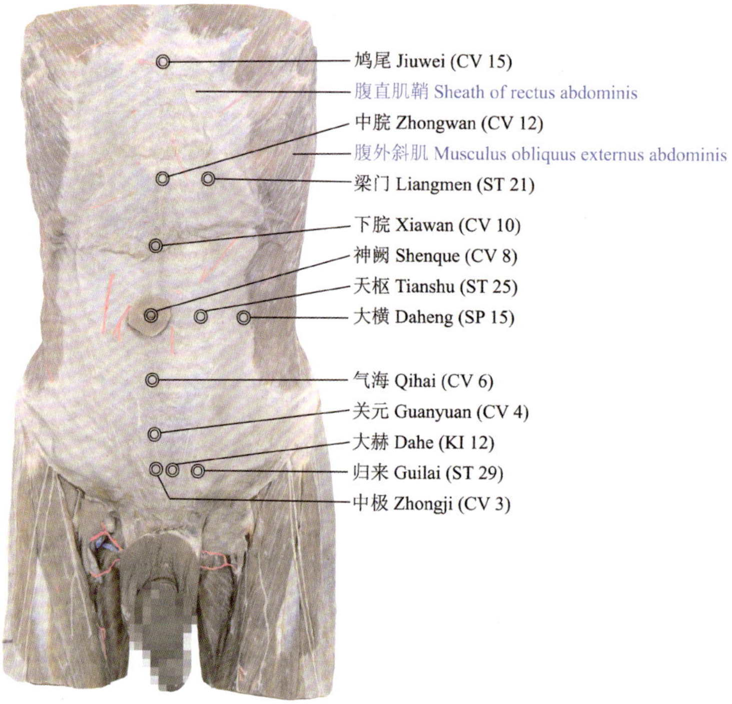
鸠尾 Jiuwei (CV 15)
腹直肌鞘 Sheath of rectus abdominis
中脘 Zhongwan (CV 12)
腹外斜肌 Musculus obliquus externus abdominis
梁门 Liangmen (ST 21)
下脘 Xiawan (CV 10)
神阙 Shenque (CV 8)
天枢 Tianshu (ST 25)
大横 Daheng (SP 15)
气海 Qihai (CV 6)
关元 Guanyuan (CV 4)
大赫 Dahe (KI 12)
归来 Guilai (ST 29)
中极 Zhongji (CV 3)

图 4–3　腹前面腧穴层次解剖（3）

Fig.4-3　Layered anatomy of acupoints on the anterior aspect of the abdomen (3)

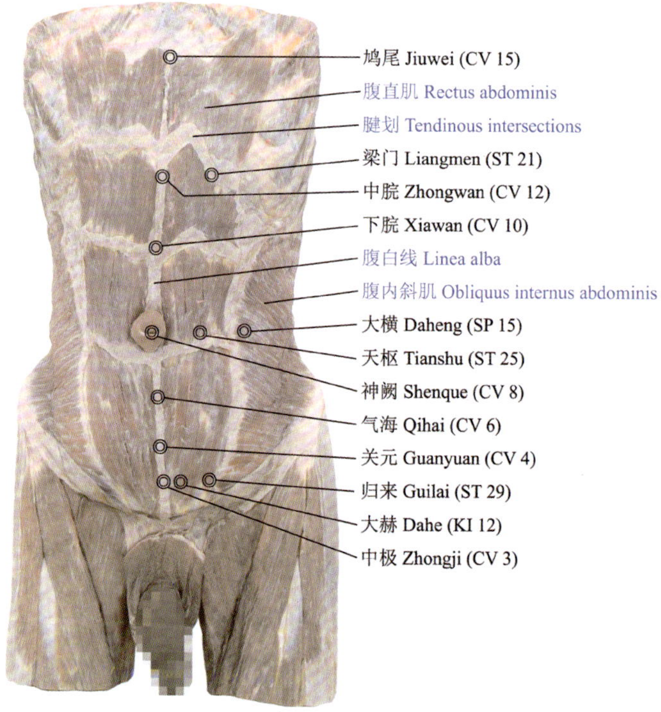
鸠尾 Jiuwei (CV 15)
腹直肌 Rectus abdominis
腱划 Tendinous intersections
梁门 Liangmen (ST 21)
中脘 Zhongwan (CV 12)
下脘 Xiawan (CV 10)
腹白线 Linea alba
腹内斜肌 Obliquus internus abdominis
大横 Daheng (SP 15)
天枢 Tianshu (ST 25)
神阙 Shenque (CV 8)
气海 Qihai (CV 6)
关元 Guanyuan (CV 4)
归来 Guilai (ST 29)
大赫 Dahe (KI 12)
中极 Zhongji (CV 3)

图 4–4　腹前面腧穴层次解剖（4）

Fig.4-4　Layered anatomy of acupoints on the anterior aspect of the abdomen (4)

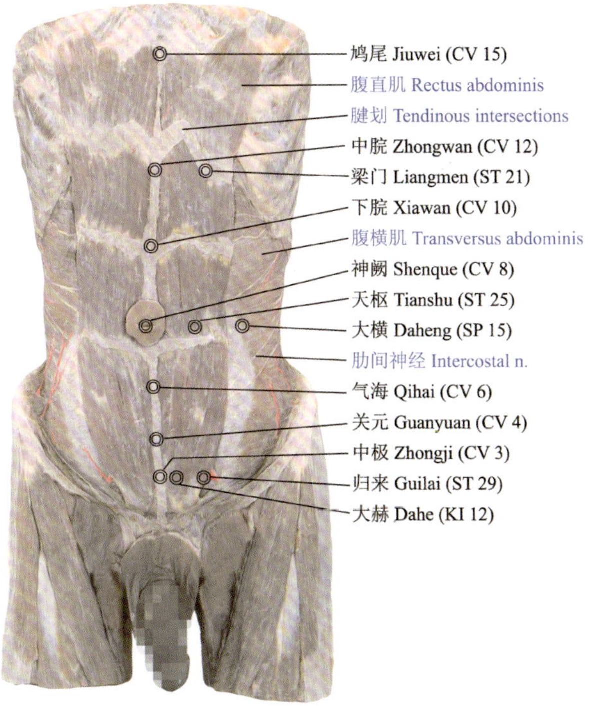
鸠尾 Jiuwei (CV 15)
腹直肌 Rectus abdominis
腱划 Tendinous intersections
中脘 Zhongwan (CV 12)
梁门 Liangmen (ST 21)
下脘 Xiawan (CV 10)
腹横肌 Transversus abdominis
神阙 Shenque (CV 8)
天枢 Tianshu (ST 25)
大横 Daheng (SP 15)
肋间神经 Intercostal n.
气海 Qihai (CV 6)
关元 Guanyuan (CV 4)
中极 Zhongji (CV 3)
归来 Guilai (ST 29)
大赫 Dahe (KI 12)

图 4–5　腹前面腧穴层次解剖（5）

Fig.4-5　Layered anatomy of acupoints on the anterior aspect of the abdomen (5)

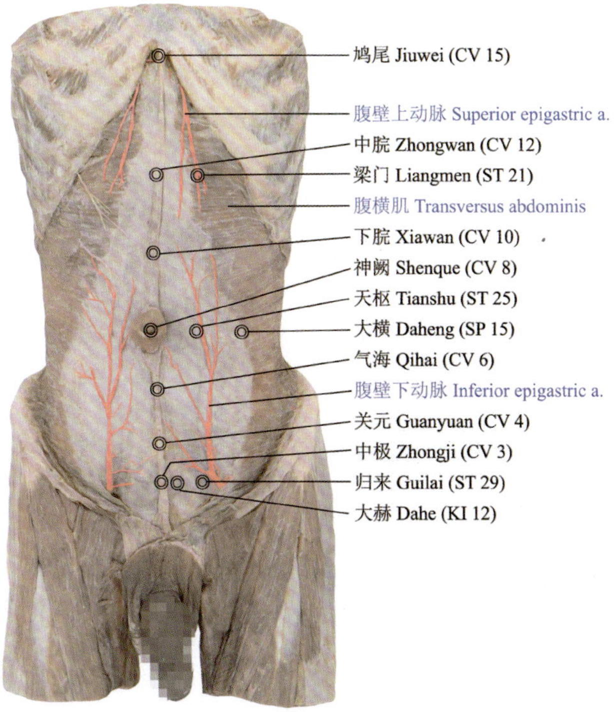
鸠尾 Jiuwei (CV 15)
腹壁上动脉 Superior epigastric a.
中脘 Zhongwan (CV 12)
梁门 Liangmen (ST 21)
腹横肌 Transversus abdominis
下脘 Xiawan (CV 10)
神阙 Shenque (CV 8)
天枢 Tianshu (ST 25)
大横 Daheng (SP 15)
气海 Qihai (CV 6)
腹壁下动脉 Inferior epigastric a.
关元 Guanyuan (CV 4)
中极 Zhongji (CV 3)
归来 Guilai (ST 29)
大赫 Dahe (KI 12)

图 4–6　腹前面腧穴层次解剖（6）

Fig.4-6　Layered anatomy of acupoints on the anterior aspect of the abdomen (6)

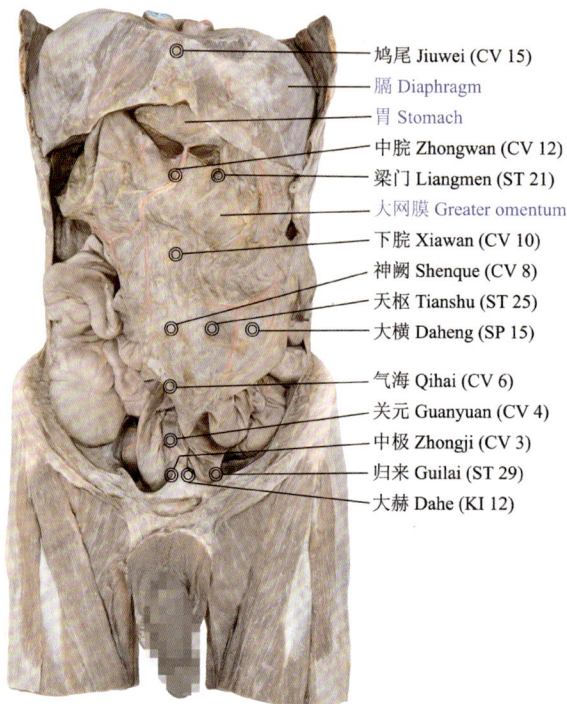

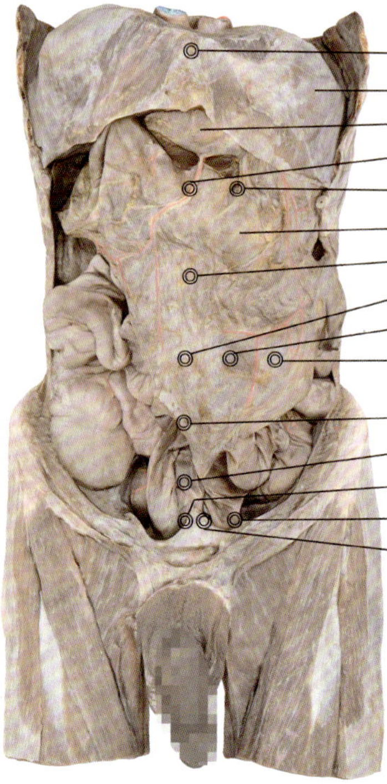
鸠尾 Jiuwei (CV 15)
膈 Diaphragm
胃 Stomach
中脘 Zhongwan (CV 12)
梁门 Liangmen (ST 21)
大网膜 Greater omentum
下脘 Xiawan (CV 10)
神阙 Shenque (CV 8)
天枢 Tianshu (ST 25)
大横 Daheng (SP 15)
气海 Qihai (CV 6)
关元 Guanyuan (CV 4)
中极 Zhongji (CV 3)
归来 Guilai (ST 29)
大赫 Dahe (KI 12)

图 4–7　腹前面腧穴层次解剖（7）

Fig.4-7　Layered anatomy of acupoints on the anterior aspect of the abdomen (7)

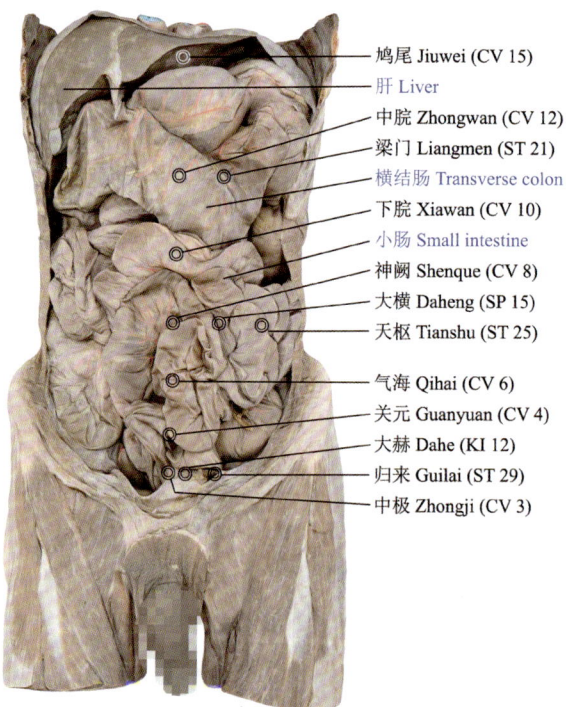

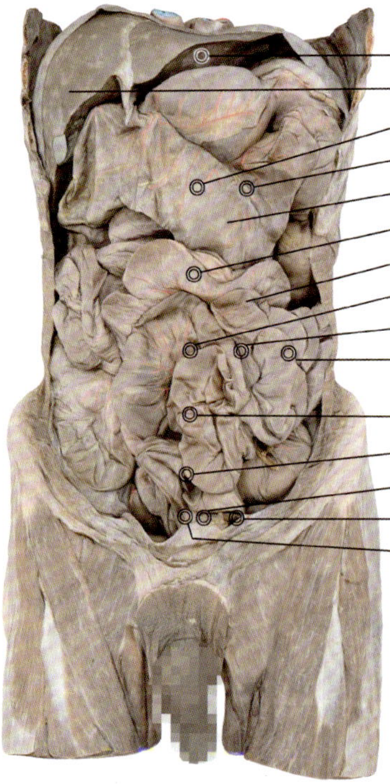
鸠尾 Jiuwei (CV 15)
肝 Liver
中脘 Zhongwan (CV 12)
梁门 Liangmen (ST 21)
横结肠 Transverse colon
下脘 Xiawan (CV 10)
小肠 Small intestine
神阙 Shenque (CV 8)
大横 Daheng (SP 15)
天枢 Tianshu (ST 25)
气海 Qihai (CV 6)
关元 Guanyuan (CV 4)
大赫 Dahe (KI 12)
归来 Guilai (ST 29)
中极 Zhongji (CV 3)

图 4–8　腹前面腧穴层次解剖（8）

Fig.4-8　Layered anatomy of acupoints on the anterior aspect of the abdomen (8)

第二节　腹外侧面腧穴

Section 2　Acupoints on the lateral aspect of the abdomen

一、章门

【定位】第 11 肋骨游离端的下际。

【操作】直刺 0.5 ～ 1 寸。

【主治】腹痛，腹胀，肠鸣，腹泻，呕吐，便秘，神疲乏力，胁痛，黄疸，小儿疳疾，痞块。

【进针层次】①皮肤；②皮下组织（内有第 10 肋间神经的前皮支和胸腹壁静脉的属支）；③腹外斜肌；④腹内斜肌；⑤腹横肌（图 4–9 ～图 4–15）。

【针刺意外与预防】若直刺过深，针尖可通过腹横筋膜、腹膜外筋膜、壁腹膜进入腹膜腔，进而可刺中肝（右章门穴）或小肠；若大幅度提插、捻转，可引起肝出血或急腹症，后果严重。

1. Zhangmen (LR 13)

【Location】Below the free end of the 11th rib.

【Method】Puncture perpendicularly 0.5-1.0 cun.

【Indications】Abdominal pain, abdominal distension, borborygmus, diarrhea, vomiting, constipation, mental weariness, pain in the hypochondrium, jaundice, infantile malnutritional stagnation, and abdominal mass.

【Stratified anatomy】①Skin; ②Subcutaneous tissue (There are anterior cutaneous branch of the 10th intercostal n. and tributaries of the thoracoepigastric v..); ③Musculus obliquus externus abdominis; ④Musculus obliquus internus abdominis; ⑤Transversus abdominis (Fig.4-9 ~ Fig.4-15).

【Cautions】If the perpendicular insertion is too deep, the tip of the needle can enter the peritoneal cavity through the transversalis fascia, extraperitoneal fascia and parietal peritoneum, and then can pierce the liver [right Zhangmen (LR 13) acupoint] or small intestine. If the needling is manipulated with strong lifting-thrusting and twisting methods, it can cause liver bleeding or acute abdomen, and the consequences will be serious.

二、京门

【定位】第 12 肋骨游离端的下际。

【操作】直刺 0.5 ～ 1 寸。

【主治】小便不利，水肿，腹胀，肠鸣，腹泻，腰痛，胁痛。

【进针层次】①皮肤；②皮下组织（内有第 11 肋间神经前皮支和胸腹壁静脉的属支）；③腹外斜肌；④腹内斜肌；⑤腹横肌（图 4–9 ～图 4–15）。

【针刺意外与预防】若直刺过深，针尖可通过腹横筋膜、腹膜外筋膜、壁腹膜进入腹膜腔，进而可刺中肝或升结肠（右京门穴）、降结肠（左京门穴）；若大幅度提插、捻转，可引起肝出血或急腹症，后果严重。

2. Jingmen (GB 25)

【Location】Below the free end of the 12th rib.

【Method】Puncture perpendicularly 0. 5-1.0 cun.

【Indications】Dysuria, edema, abdominal distension, borborygmus, diarrhea, lumbago, and pain in the hypochondrium.

【Stratified anatomy】①Skin; ②Subcutaneous tissue (There are anterior cutaneous branch of the 11th intercostal n. and tributaries of the thoracoepigastric v..); ③Musculus obliquus externus abdominis; ④Musculus obliquus internus abdominis; ⑤Transversus abdominis (Fig.4-9 ~ Fig.4-15).

【Cautions】If the perpendicular insertion is too deep, the needle tip can enter the peritoneal cavity through the transversalis fascia, extraperitoneal fascia and parietal peritoneum, and then can pierce the liver or ascending colon [right Jingmen (GB 25) acupoint] and descending colon [left Jingmen (GB 25) acupoint]. If the needling is manipulated with strong lifting-thrusting and twisting methods, it can cause liver bleeding or acute abdomen, and the consequences will be serious.

三、带脉

【定位】第 11 肋骨游离端垂线与脐水平线的交点上。

【操作】直刺 0.8 ～ 1.2 寸。

【主治】月经不调，带下，腰痛，胁痛，疝气。

【进针层次】①皮肤；②皮下组织（内有第 11 肋间神经前皮支和胸腹壁静脉的属支）；③腹外斜肌；④腹内斜肌；⑤腹横肌（图 4–9 ～图 4–15）。

【针刺意外与预防】若直刺过深，针尖可通过腹横筋膜、腹膜外筋膜、壁腹膜进入腹膜腔，进而可刺中升结肠（右带脉穴）、降结肠（左带脉穴）；若大幅度提插、捻转，可引起急腹症，后果严重。

3. Daimai (GB 26)

【Location】At the intersection point between the vertical line from the free end of the 11th rib and the umbilical horizontal line.

【Method】Puncture perpendicularly 0.8-1.2 cun.

【Indications】Irregular menstruation, leukorrhea, lumbago, pain in the hypochondrium, and hernia.

【Stratified anatomy】①Skin; ②Subcutaneous tissue (There are branches of the 11th intercostal n. and tributaries of the thoracoepigastric v..); ③Musculus obliquus externus abdominis; ④Musculus obliquus internus abdominis; ⑤Transversus abdominis (Fig.4-9 ~ Fig.4-15).

【Cautions】If the perpendicular insertion is too deep, the tip of the needle can enter the peritoneal cavity through the transversalis fascia, extraperitoneal fascia and parietal peritoneum, and then can pierce the ascending colon [right Daimai (GB 26) acupoint] and the descending colon [left Daimai (GB 26) acupoint]. If the needling is manipulated with strong lifting-thrusting and twisting methods, it can cause acute abdomen, and the consequences will be serious.

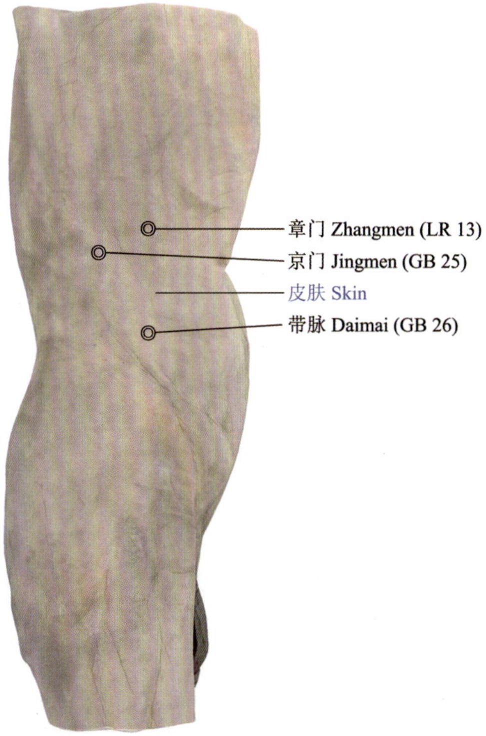

图 4–9　腹外侧面腧穴层次解剖（1）
Fig.4-9　Layered anatomy of acupoints on the lateral aspect of the abdomen (1)

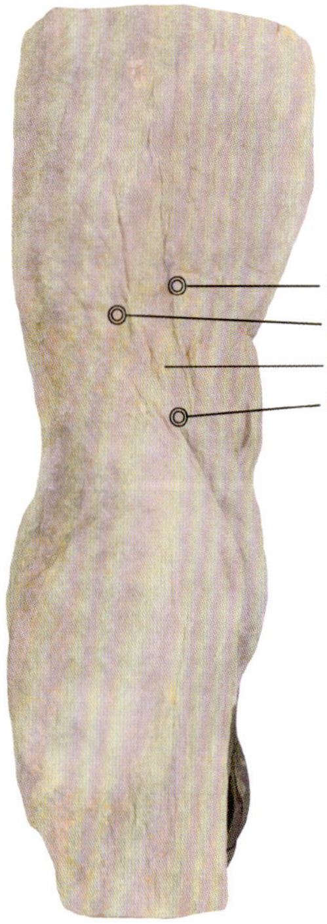

图 4-10　腹外侧面腧穴层次解剖（2）

Fig.4-10　Layered anatomy of acupoints on the lateral aspect of the abdomen (2)

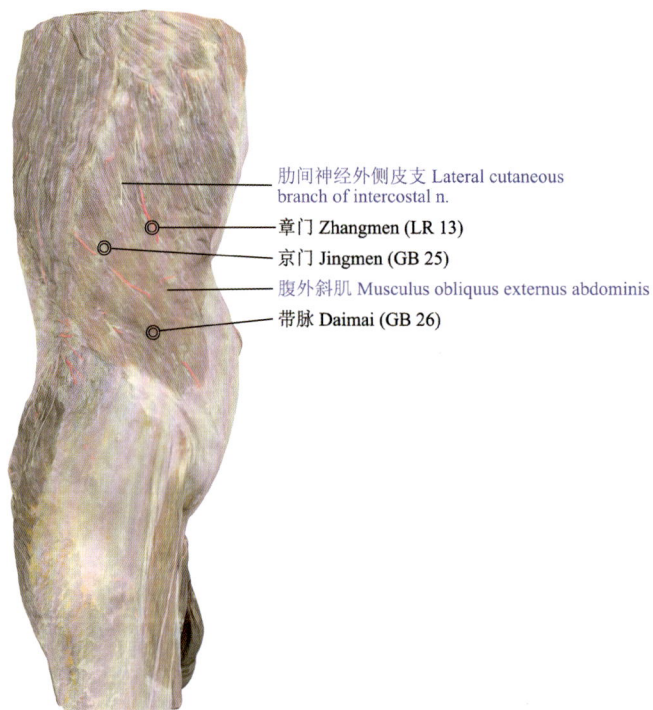

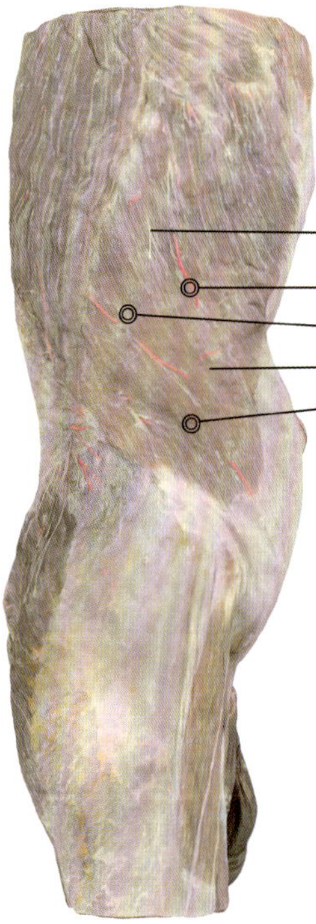

图 4-11　腹外侧面腧穴层次解剖（3）

Fig.4-11　Layered anatomy of acupoints on the lateral aspect of the abdomen (3)

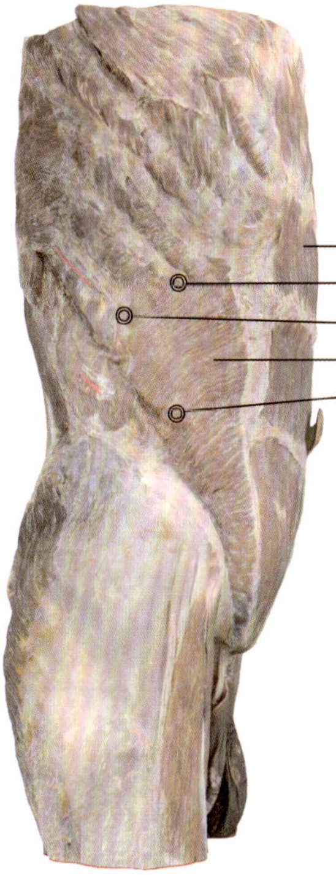
腹直肌 Rectus abdominis
章门 Zhangmen (LR 13)
京门 Jingmen (GB 25)
腹内斜肌 Musculus obliquus internus abdominis
带脉 Daimai (GB 26)

图 4–12　腹外侧面腧穴层次解剖（4）
Fig.4-12　Layered anatomy of acupoints on the lateral aspect of the abdomen (4)

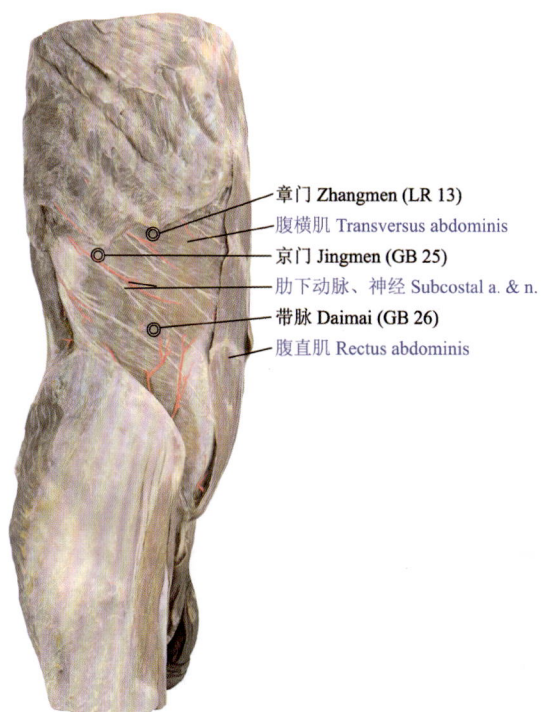

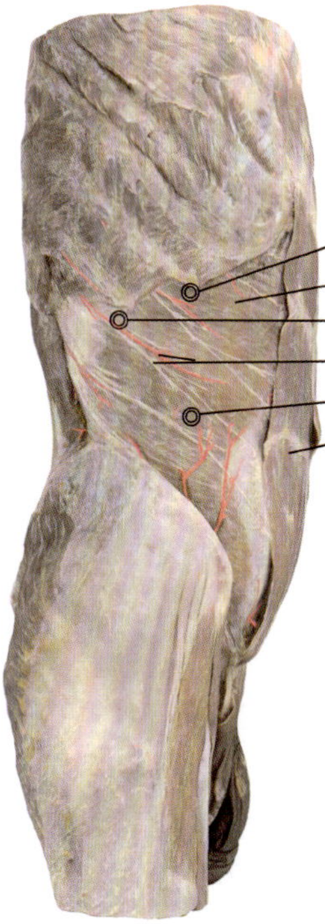
章门 Zhangmen (LR 13)
腹横肌 Transversus abdominis
京门 Jingmen (GB 25)
肋下动脉、神经 Subcostal a. & n.
带脉 Daimai (GB 26)
腹直肌 Rectus abdominis

图 4–13　腹外侧面腧穴层次解剖（5）
Fig.4-13　Layered anatomy of acupoints on the lateral aspect of the abdomen (5)

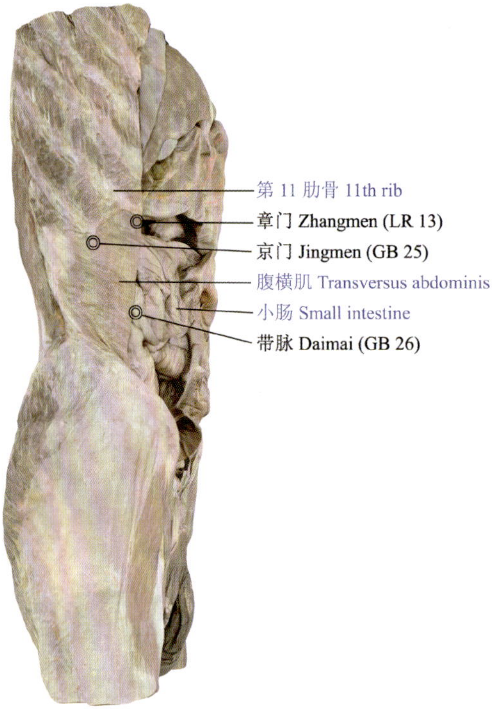
第 11 肋骨 11th rib
章门 Zhangmen (LR 13)
京门 Jingmen (GB 25)
腹横肌 Transversus abdominis
小肠 Small intestine
带脉 Daimai (GB 26)

图 4–14　腹外侧面腧穴层次解剖（6）

Fig.4-14　Layered anatomy of acupoints on the lateral aspect of the abdomen (6)

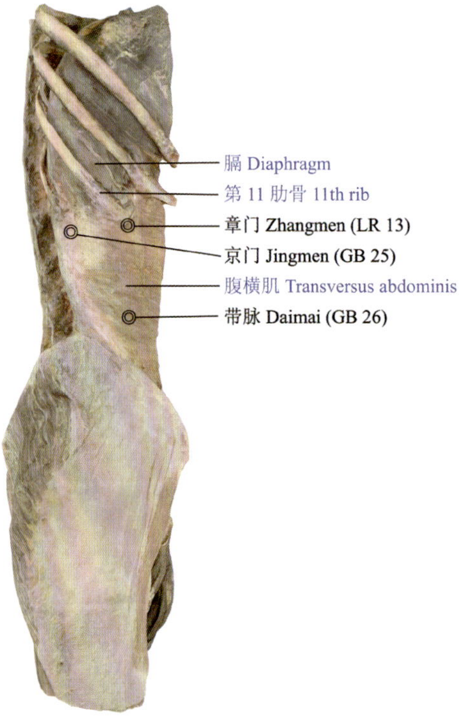
膈 Diaphragm
第 11 肋骨 11th rib
章门 Zhangmen (LR 13)
京门 Jingmen (GB 25)
腹横肌 Transversus abdominis
带脉 Daimai (GB 26)

图 4–15　腹外侧面腧穴层次解剖（7）

Fig.4-15　Layered anatomy of acupoints on the lateral aspect of the abdomen (7)

第三节　腰骶部腧穴

Section 3　Acupoints on the lumbosacral regions

一、命门

【定位】第 2 腰椎棘突下凹陷中，后正中线上。

【操作】直刺 0.5 ～ 1 寸。

【主治】虚损腰痛，下肢痿痹，遗精，阳痿，早泄，月经不调，带下，遗尿，尿频，泄泻，小儿惊风。

【进针层次】①皮肤；②皮下组织（内有第 2 腰神经后支的皮支）；③棘上韧带；④棘间韧带；⑤黄韧带（图 4–16 ～图 4–23）。

【针刺意外与预防】若直刺过深，针尖可通过黄韧带、硬膜外隙、硬脊膜、脊髓蛛网膜，进入蛛网膜下隙。此处椎管内无脊髓，只有马尾神经，若刺中马尾神经，可出现下肢的强烈触电感。

1. Mingmen (GV 4)

【Location】In the depression below the spinous process of the 2nd lumbar vertebra, and on the posterior midline.

【Method】Puncture perpendicularly 0.5-1 cun.

【Indications】Low back pain due to deficiency, flaccidity and impediment of lower limbs, nocturnal emission, impotence, premature ejaculation, irregular menstruation, leukorrhea, enuresis, frequent urination, diarrhea, and infantile convulsions.

【Stratified anatomy】①Skin; ②Subcutaneous tissue (There are cutaneous branch of the posterior branches of the 2nd lumbar n..); ③Supraspinous lig.; ④Interspinal lig.; ⑤Ligamenta flavum (Fig.4-16 ~ Fig.4-23).

【Cautions】If the perpendicular insertion is too deep, the tip of the needle can enter the subarachnoid gap through the ligamentum flavum, epidural space, dura mater and spinal arachnoid mater. There is no spinal cord in the spinal canal, only a cauda equina. If the cauda equina is pierced, an intense electrical sensation can appear in the lower limbs.

二、肾俞

【定位】第 2 腰椎棘突下，后正中线旁开 1.5 寸。

【操作】直刺 0.8 ～ 1 寸。

【主治】头晕，目昏，耳鸣，耳聋，腰痛，遗精，阳痿，早泄，月经不调，带下，遗尿，水肿，小便不利，完谷不化，咳喘少气。

【进针层次】①皮肤；②皮下组织（内有第 2、第 3 腰神经后支的皮支及伴行动、静脉）；③背阔肌腱膜和胸腰筋膜浅层；④竖脊肌（图 4–16 ～图 4–23）。

【针刺意外与预防】若向外斜刺过深，可刺中肾，出现腰痛和尿血。

2. Shenshu (BL 23)

【Location】Below the spinous process of the 2nd lumbar vertebra, and 1.5 cun lateral to the posterior midline.

【Method】Puncture perpendicularly 0.8-1 cun.

【Indications】Dizziness, blurred vision, tinnitus, deafness, lumbago, nocturnal emission, impotence, premature ejaculation, irregular menstruation, leukorrhea, enuresis, edema, dysuria, diarrhea with undigested food, asthma and weak breathing.

【Stratified anatomy】①Skin; ②Subcutaneous tissue (There are cutaneous branch of the posterior branches of the 2nd and 3rd lumbar n. and the accompanying a. & v..); ③Tendinous membrane of latissimus dorsi and superficial layer of the thoracolumbar fascia; ④Erector spinae (Fig.4-16 ~ Fig.4-23).

【Cautions】If the oblique insertion is too deep and outward, it can pierce the kidney, and low back pain and hematuria will occur.

三、志室

【定位】第 2 腰椎棘突下，后正中线旁开 3 寸。

【操作】直刺 0.8 ～ 1 寸。

【主治】遗精，阳痿，月经不调，水肿，小便不利，腰脊强痛。

【进针层次】①皮肤；②皮下组织（内有第 1、第 2 腰神经后支的皮支及伴行动、静脉）；③背阔肌腱膜和胸腰筋膜浅层；④竖脊肌；⑤腰方肌（图 4–16 ～图 4–22）。

【针刺意外与预防】若直刺过深，可刺中肾，出现腰痛和尿血。

3. Zhishi (BL 52)

【Location】Below the spinous process of the 2nd lumbar vertebra, and 3 cun lateral to the posterior midline.

【Method】Puncture perpendicularly 0.8-1 cun.

【Indications】Nocturnal emission, impotence, irregular menstruation, edema, dysuria, and stiffness and pain in the loins and spine.

【Stratified anatomy】①Skin; ②Subcutaneous tissue (There are cutaneous branch of the posterior branches of the 1st and 2nd lumbar n. and the accompanying a. & v..); ③Tendinous membrane of latissimus dorsi and superficial layer of the thoracolumbar fascia; ④Erector spinae; ⑤Quadratus lumborum (Fig.4-16 ~ Fig.4-22).

【Cautions】If the perpendicular insertion is too deep, it can pierce the kidney, and low back pain and hematuria will occur.

四、腰阳关

【定位】第 4 腰椎棘突下凹陷中，后正中线上。

【操作】直刺 0.5 ～ 1 寸。

【主治】腰骶疼痛，下肢痿痹，遗精，阳痿，月经不调，带下，便血。

【进针层次】①皮肤；②皮下组织（内有第 4 腰神经后支的皮支及伴行的动、静脉）；③棘上韧带；④棘间韧带；⑤黄韧带（图 4–16 ～图 4–23）。

【针刺意外与预防】同命门穴。

4. Yaoyangguan (GV 3)

【Location】Below the spinous process of the 4th lumbar vertebra, and on the posterior midline.

【Method】Puncture perpendicularly 0.5-1 cun.

【Indications】Lumbosacral pain, flaccidity and impediment of lower limbs, nocturnal emission, impotence, irregular menstruation, leukorrhea, and bloody stools.

【Stratified anatomy】①Skin; ②Subcutaneous tissue (There are cutaneous branch of the posterior branches of the 4th lumbar n. and the accompanying a. & v..); ③Supraspinous lig.; ④Interspinal lig.; ⑤Ligamenta flavum (Fig.4-16 ~ Fig.4-23).

【Cautions】Same as that of the Mingmen (GV 4) acupoint.

五、大肠俞

【定位】第 4 腰椎棘突下，后正中线旁开 1.5 寸。

【操作】直刺 0.8 ～ 1 寸。

【主治】腰痛，腹痛，腹胀，肠鸣，泄泻，便秘，痢疾，脱肛，痔疾。

【进针层次】①皮肤；②皮下组织（内有第 3、第 4 腰神经后支的皮支及伴行动、静脉）；③背阔肌腱膜和胸腰筋膜浅层；④竖脊肌（图 4–16 ～图 4–23）。

【针刺意外与预防】若直刺过深，针尖可通过腰方筋膜、腹膜外筋膜、壁腹膜进入腹膜腔，进而可刺中小肠；若大幅度提插、捻转，可引起急腹症，后果严重。

5. Dachangshu (BL 25)

【Location】Below the spinous process of the 4th lumbar vertebra, and 1.5 cun lateral to the posterior midline.

【Method】Puncture perpendicularly 0.8-1 cun.

【Indications】Lumbago, abdominal pain, abdominal distension, borborygmus, diarrhea, constipation, dysentery, prolapse of the rectum, and hemorrhoids.

【Stratified anatomy】①Skin; ②Subcutaneous tissue (There are cutaneous branch of the posterior branches of the 3rd and 4th lumbar n. and the accompanying a. & v..); ③Tendinous membrane of latissimus dorsi and superficial layer of the thoracolumbar fascia; ④Erector spinae. (Fig.4-16 ~ Fig.4-23).

【Cautions】If the perpendicular insertion is too deep, the tip of the needle can enter the peritoneal cavity through the thoracolumbar fascia, extraperitoneal fascia and parietal peritoneum, and then can pierce the small intestines. If the needling is manipulated with strong lifting-thrusting and twisting methods, it can cause acute abdomen, and the consequences will be serious.

六、关元俞

【定位】第 5 腰椎棘突下，后正中线旁开 1.5 寸。

【操作】直刺 0.8 ～ 1 寸。

【主治】腰痛，腹痛，腹胀，肠鸣，泄泻，小便不利，遗尿。

【进针层次】①皮肤；②皮下组织（内有第 5 腰神经和第 1 骶神经后支的皮支及伴行动、静脉）；③背阔肌腱膜和胸腰筋膜浅层；④竖脊肌（图 4–16 ～图 4–23）。

6. Guanyuanshu (BL 26)

【Location】Below the spinous process of the 5th lumbar vertebra, and 1.5 cun lateral to the posterior midline.

【Method】Puncture perpendicularly 0.8-1 cun.

【Indications】Lumbago, abdominal pain, abdominal distension, borborygmus, diarrhea, difficulty in urinating and enuresis.

【Stratified anatomy】①Skin; ②Subcutaneous tissue (There are cutaneous branch of the posterior branches of the 5th lumbar n. and 1st sacral n. and the accompanying a. & v..); ③Tendinous membrane of latissimus dorsi and superficial layer of the thoracolumbar fascia; ④Erector spinae (Fig.4-16 ~ Fig.4-23).

七、膀胱俞

【定位】平第 2 骶后孔，骶正中嵴旁开 1.5 寸。

【操作】直刺 0.8 ～ 1 寸。

【主治】小便不利，尿频，遗尿，遗精，腹痛，泄泻，便秘，腰骶痛。

【进针层次】①皮肤；②皮下组织（内有第 1、第 2 骶神经后支的皮支及伴行动、静脉）；③臀大肌；④背阔肌腱膜和胸腰筋膜浅层；⑤竖脊肌（图 4–16 ～图 4–23）。

7. Pangguangshu (BL 28)

【Location】At the level of the 2nd posterior sacral foramen, and 1.5 cun lateral to the sacral median crest.

【Method】Puncture perpendicularly 0.8-1 cun.

【Indications】Dysuria, frequent urination, enuresis, nocturnal emission, abdominal pain, diarrhea, constipation, and lumbosacral pain.

【Stratified anatomy】①Skin; ②Subcutaneous tissue (There are cutaneous branch of the posterior branches of the 1st and 2nd sacral n. and the accompanying a. & v..); ③Gluteus maximus; ④Tendinous membrane of latissimus dorsi and superficial layer of the thoracolumbar fascia; ⑤Erector spinae (Fig.4-16 ~ Fig.4-23).

八、次髎

【定位】正对第 2 骶后孔。

【操作】直刺 0.8 ～ 1 寸。

【主治】月经不调，痛经，带下，遗精，阳痿，疝气，小便不利，癃闭，腰骶痛，下肢痿痹。

【进针层次】①皮肤；②皮下组织（内有臀中皮神经的分支）；③背阔肌腱膜和胸腰筋膜浅层；④竖脊肌；⑤第 2 骶后孔（图 4–16 ～图 4–23）。

【针刺意外与预防】若深刺过度，针尖可穿过骶后孔，达骶前孔，可刺中第 2 骶神经本干，可产生强烈的触电感。

8. Ciliao (BL 32)

【Location】In the 2nd posterior sacral foramen.

【Method】Puncture perpendicularly 0.8-1 cun.

【Indications】Irregular menstruation, dysmenorrhea, leukorrhea, nocturnal emission, impotence, hernia, dysuria, retention of urine, lumbosacral pain, and flaccidity and impediment of lower limbs.

【Stratified anatomy】①Skin; ②Subcutaneous tissue (There are branches of the intermediate gluteal n..); ③Tendinous membrane of latissimus dorsi and superficial layer of the thoracolumbar fascia; ④Erector spinae; ⑤The 2nd posterior sacral foramina (Fig.4-16 ~ Fig.4-23).

【Cautions】If the insertion is too deep, the tip of the needle can pass through the posterior sacral hole, reach the anterior sacral hole, and can pierce the second sacral n. trunk, which can produce an intense electrical sensation.

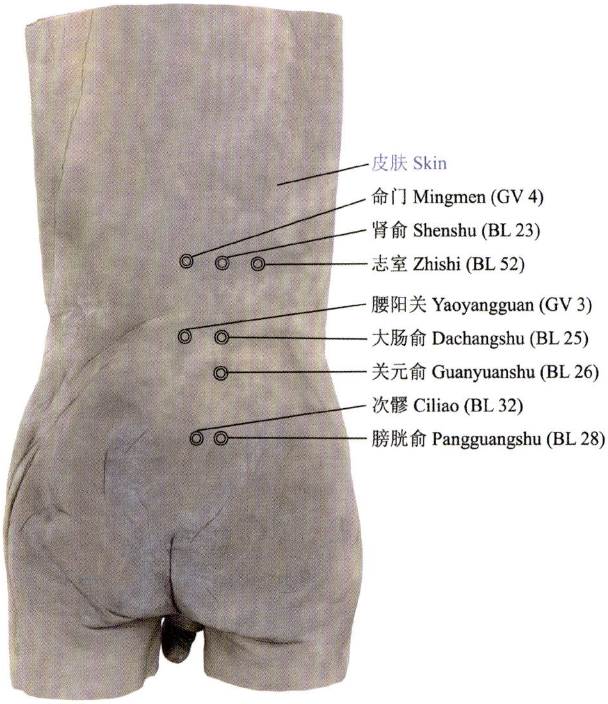
皮肤 Skin
命门 Mingmen (GV 4)
肾俞 Shenshu (BL 23)
志室 Zhishi (BL 52)
腰阳关 Yaoyangguan (GV 3)
大肠俞 Dachangshu (BL 25)
关元俞 Guanyuanshu (BL 26)
次髎 Ciliao (BL 32)
膀胱俞 Pangguangshu (BL 28)

图 4–16　腰骶部腧穴层次解剖（1）
Fig.4-16　Layered anatomy of acupoints on the lumbosacral regions (1)

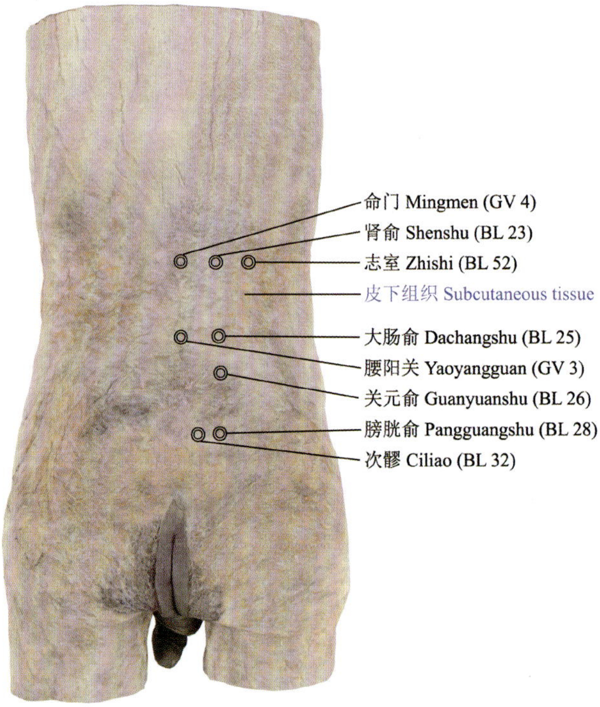
命门 Mingmen (GV 4)
肾俞 Shenshu (BL 23)
志室 Zhishi (BL 52)
皮下组织 Subcutaneous tissue
大肠俞 Dachangshu (BL 25)
腰阳关 Yaoyangguan (GV 3)
关元俞 Guanyuanshu (BL 26)
膀胱俞 Pangguangshu (BL 28)
次髎 Ciliao (BL 32)

图 4–17　腰骶部腧穴层次解剖（2）
Fig.4-17　Layered anatomy of acupoints on the lumbosacral regions (2)

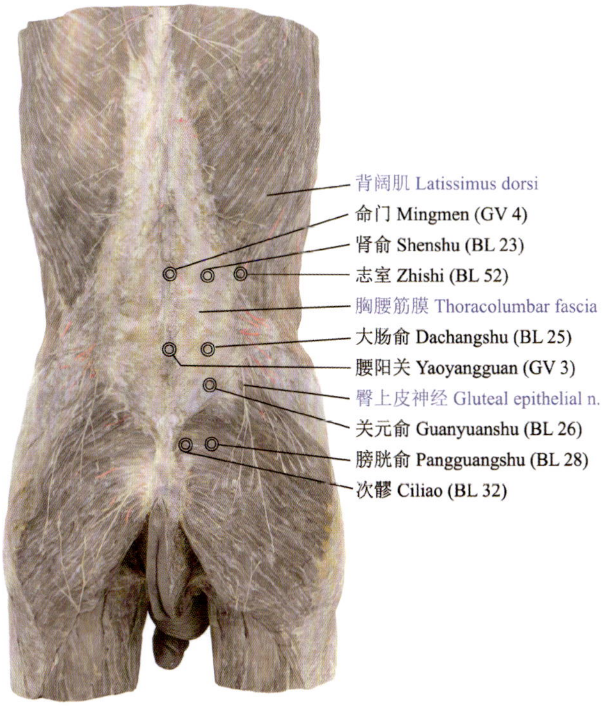
背阔肌 Latissimus dorsi
命门 Mingmen (GV 4)
肾俞 Shenshu (BL 23)
志室 Zhishi (BL 52)
胸腰筋膜 Thoracolumbar fascia
大肠俞 Dachangshu (BL 25)
腰阳关 Yaoyangguan (GV 3)
臀上皮神经 Gluteal epithelial n.
关元俞 Guanyuanshu (BL 26)
膀胱俞 Pangguangshu (BL 28)
次髎 Ciliao (BL 32)

图 4–18　腰骶部腧穴层次解剖（3）
Fig.4-18　Layered anatomy of acupoints on the lumbosacral regions (3)

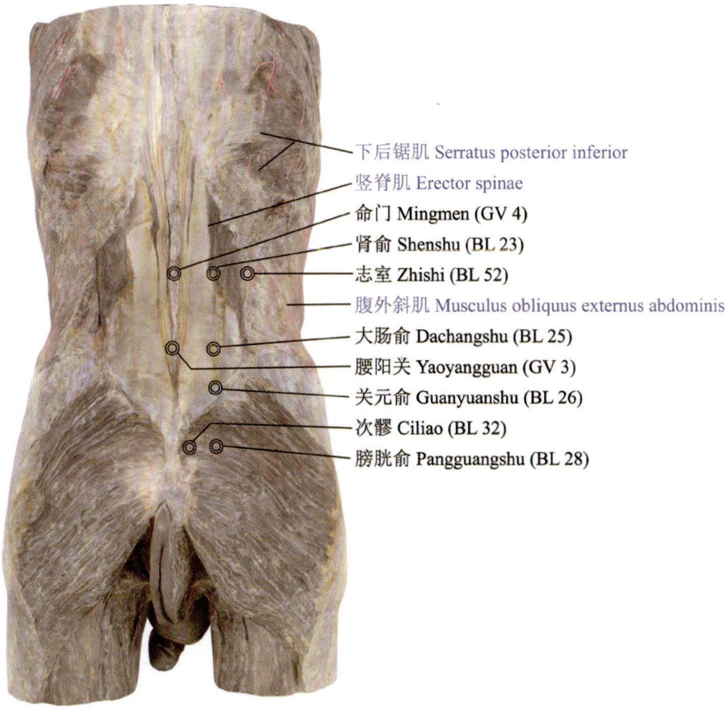
下后锯肌 Serratus posterior inferior
竖脊肌 Erector spinae
命门 Mingmen (GV 4)
肾俞 Shenshu (BL 23)
志室 Zhishi (BL 52)
腹外斜肌 Musculus obliquus externus abdominis
大肠俞 Dachangshu (BL 25)
腰阳关 Yaoyangguan (GV 3)
关元俞 Guanyuanshu (BL 26)
次髎 Ciliao (BL 32)
膀胱俞 Pangguangshu (BL 28)

图 4–19　腰骶部腧穴层次解剖（4）
Fig.4-19　Layered anatomy of acupoints on the lumbosacral regions (4)

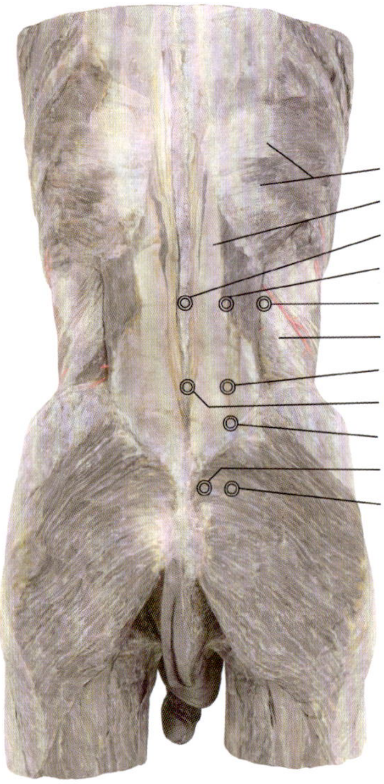

图 4–20　腰骶部腧穴层次解剖（5）

Fig.4-20　Layered anatomy of acupoints on the lumbosacral regions (5)

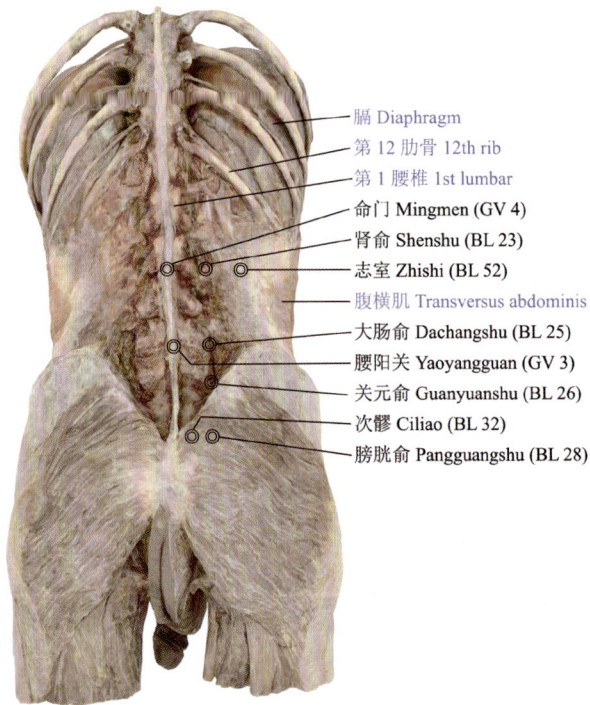

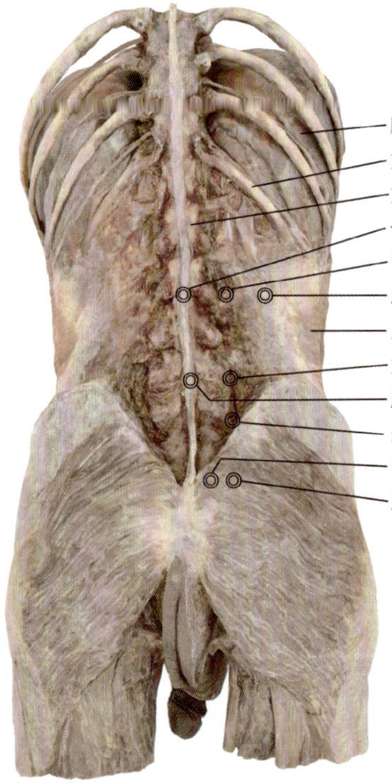

图 4–21　腰骶部腧穴层次解剖（6）

Fig.4-21　Layered anatomy of acupoints on the lumbosacral regions (6)

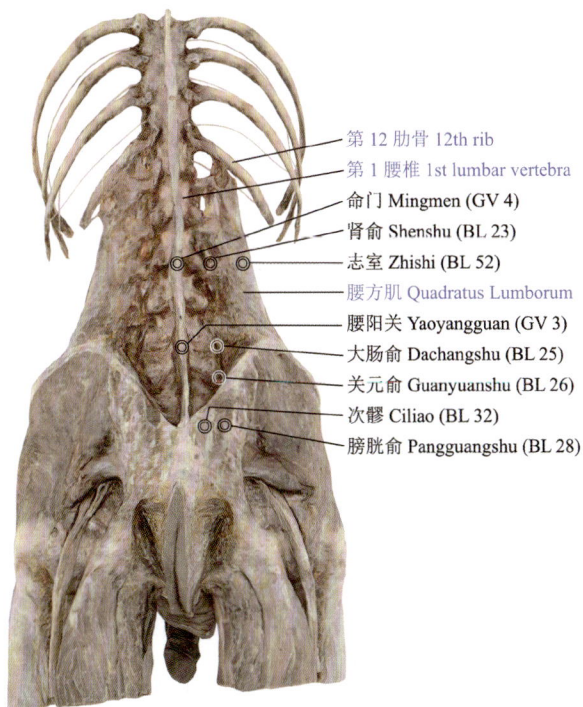

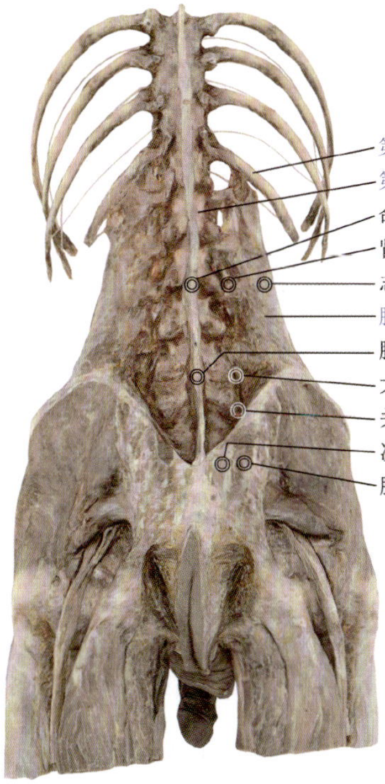
第 12 肋骨 12th rib
第 1 腰椎 1st lumbar vertebra
命门 Mingmen (GV 4)
肾俞 Shenshu (BL 23)
志室 Zhishi (BL 52)
腰方肌 Quadratus Lumborum
腰阳关 Yaoyangguan (GV 3)
大肠俞 Dachangshu (BL 25)
关元俞 Guanyuanshu (BL 26)
次髎 Ciliao (BL 32)
膀胱俞 Pangguangshu (BL 28)

图 4–22　腰骶部腧穴层次解剖（7）

Fig.4-22　Layered anatomy of acupoints on the lumbosacral regions (7)

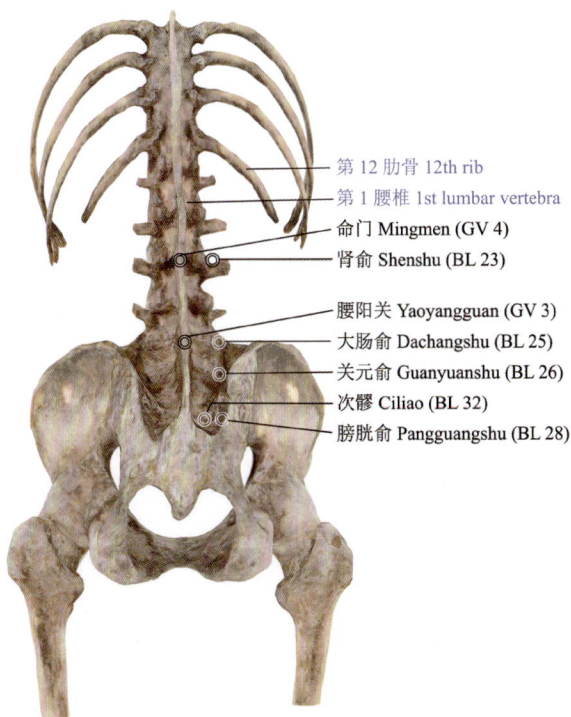

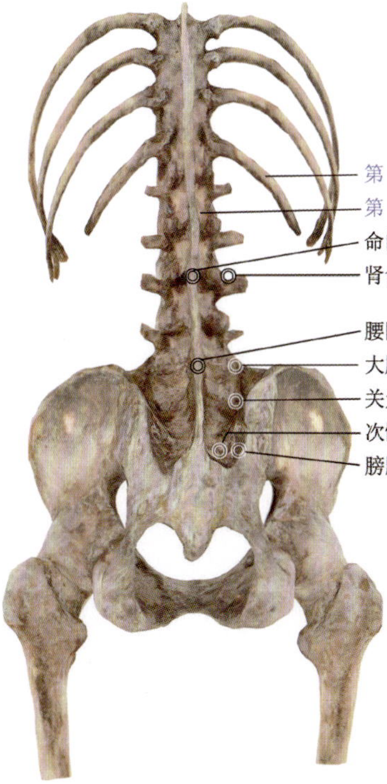
第 12 肋骨 12th rib
第 1 腰椎 1st lumbar vertebra
命门 Mingmen (GV 4)
肾俞 Shenshu (BL 23)
腰阳关 Yaoyangguan (GV 3)
大肠俞 Dachangshu (BL 25)
关元俞 Guanyuanshu (BL 26)
次髎 Ciliao (BL 32)
膀胱俞 Pangguangshu (BL 28)

图 4–23　腰骶部腧穴层次解剖（8）

Fig.4-23　Layered anatomy of acupoints on the lumbosacral regions (8)

第五章　上肢腧穴层次解剖

Chapter 5　Layered Anatomy of Acupoints on the Upper Limb

第一节　肩臂后面腧穴

Section 1　Acupoints on the posterior aspect of the shoulder and arm

一、肩井

【定位】第 7 颈椎棘突与肩峰最外侧点连线的中点。

【操作】直刺 0.3 ～ 0.5 寸。

【主治】颈项强痛，上肢不遂，乳汁不下，乳痈，瘰疬。

【进针层次】①皮肤；②皮下组织（内有锁骨上神经的分支、颈浅动脉的分支和颈浅静脉的属支）；③斜方肌；④颈横动、静脉浅支；⑤前锯肌（图 5–1 ～图 5–6）。

【针刺意外与预防】若朝前下方针刺过深，针尖可穿过第 1 肋间隙进入胸膜腔，进而刺中肺上叶，引起气胸。

1. Jianjing (GB 21)

【Location】At the midpoint of the line joining the spinous process of the 7th cervical vertebra and the outermost point of the acromion.

【Method】Puncture perpendicularly 0.3-0.5 cun.

【Indications】Stiffness and pain in the neck, paralysis of upper limbs, insufficient lactation, acute mastitis, and scrofula.

【Stratified anatomy】①Skin; ②Subcutaneous tissue (There are branches of the supraclavicular n., branches or tributaries of the superficial cervical a. & v..); ③Trapezius; ④Superficial branches of the transverse cervical a. & v.; ⑤Serratus anterior (Fig.5-1 ~ Fig.5-6).

【Cautions】If the insertion is too deep forward and downward, the tip of the needle can enter the pleural cavity through the first intercostal space, and then pierce the upper lobe of the lung, causing pneumothorax.

二、天宗

【定位】肩胛冈中点与肩胛骨下角连线的上 1/3 与下 2/3 交点处。

【操作】直刺或向四周斜刺 0.5 ～ 1 寸。

【主治】肩胛疼痛，乳痈，气喘。

【进针层次】①皮肤；②皮下组织（内有第 3 ～ 5 胸神经后支的皮支）；③斜方肌；④冈下肌（图 5–1 ～图 5–6）。

【针刺意外与预防】该穴的深面为冈下窝的骨面。70 岁以上的老年人冈下窝的骨质薄弱，甚至中央有孔；在这种情况下，若针刺过深时，针尖可穿过冈下窝，再经肩胛下肌、前锯肌、肋间隙进入胸膜腔，进而刺中肺，引起气胸。

2. Tianzong (SI 11)

【Location】At the intersection of the upper 1/3 and lower 2/3 of the line connecting the midpoint of the mesoscapula and the inferior angle of scapula.

【Method】Puncture perpendicularly or obliquely around 0.5-1 cun.

【Indications】Scapulalgia, acute mastitis, and panting.

【Stratified anatomy】①Skin; ②Subcutaneous tissue (There are cutaneous branches of the posterior branches of the 3rd, 4th, 5th thoracic n..); ③Trapezius; ④Infraspinatus (Fig.5-1 ~ Fig.5-6).

【Cautions】The deep side of the acupoint is the bone surface of the fossa infraspinata. The bone of the fossa infraspinata is weak in the elderly over the age of 70, and even there are pores in the centre. In this case, if the piercing is too deep, the tip of the needle can pass through the fossa infraspinata, and then enter the pleural cavity through the subscapularis, serratus anterior and intercostal space, and then pierce the lungs, causing pneumothorax.

三、肩髎

【定位】肩峰外侧缘后端与肱骨大结节之间的凹陷中；或肩髃穴后 1 寸处。

【操作】直刺 0.8 ～ 1.2 寸。

【主治】肩臂痛，肩重不能举，中风瘫痪，瘾疹。

【进针层次】①皮肤；②皮下组织（内有锁骨上神经的分支）；③三角肌；④小圆肌；⑤腋神经和旋肱后动、静脉；⑥大圆肌；⑦背阔肌腱（图 5–1 ～图 5–6）。

【针刺意外与预防】若直刺过深，针尖可进入腋窝，进而可刺中腋窝内的腋动、静脉；若大幅度提插捻转，可引造成大的血肿。

3. Jianliao (TE 14)

【Location】In the depression between the rear end of the outer edge of the acromion and the greater tubercle of the humerus, or 1 cun posteror to the Jianyu (LI 15) acupoint.

【Method】Puncture perpendicularly 0.8-1.2 cun.

【Indications】Pain in the shoulder and arm, heavy shoulders with failing to lift, hemiplegia due to apoplexy, and urticaria.

【Stratified anatomy】①Skin; ②Subcutaneous tissue (There are branches of the supraclavicular n..); ③Deltoid m.; ④Teres minor; ⑤Axillary n., posterior circumflex humeral a. & v.; ⑥Teres major; ⑦Tendon of latissimus dorsi (Fig.5-1 ~ Fig.5-6).

【Cautions】If the piercing is too deep, the tip of the needle can enter the armpit, and then it can pierce the axillary a. & v. in the armpit. If the needling is manipulated with an intense lifting-thrusting and twirling methods, it can cause large hematoma.

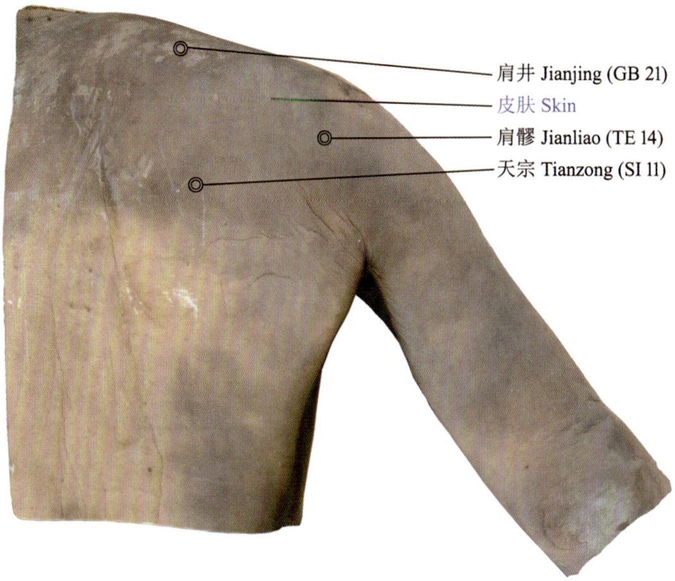

图 5-1　肩臂后面腧穴层次解剖（1）
Fig.5-1　Layered anatomy of acupoints on the posterior aspect of the shoulder and arm (1)

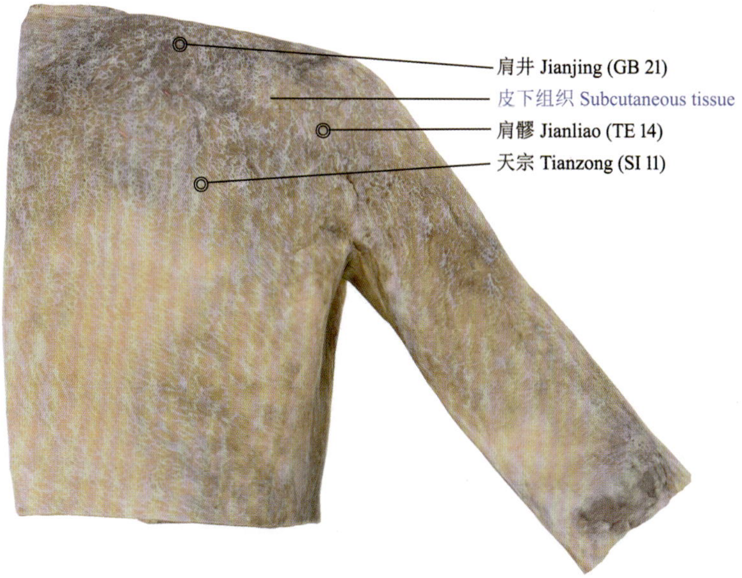

图 5-2　肩臂后面腧穴层次解剖（2）
Fig.5-2　Layered anatomy of acupoints on the posterior aspect of the shoulder and arm (2)

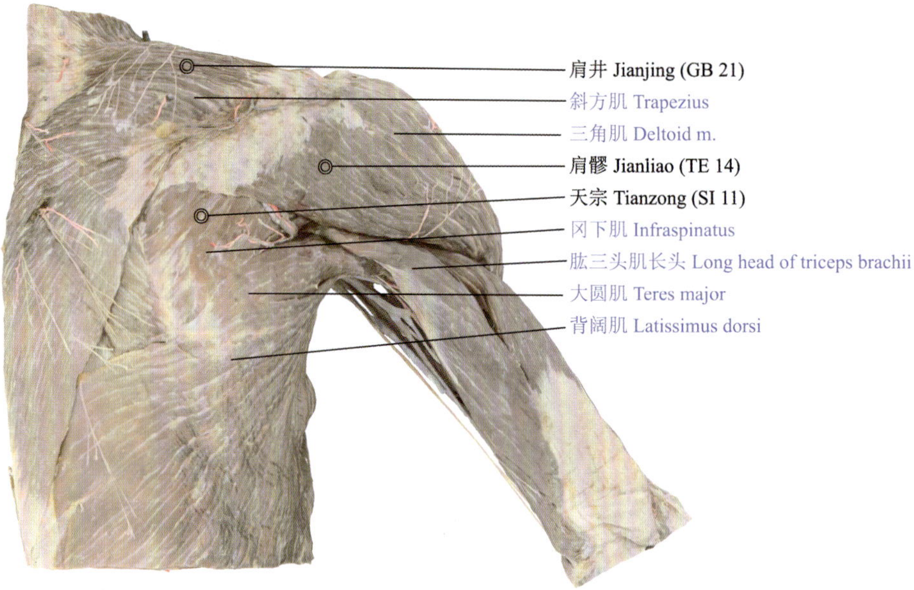
肩井 Jianjing (GB 21)
斜方肌 Trapezius
三角肌 Deltoid m.
肩髎 Jianliao (TE 14)
天宗 Tianzong (SI 11)
冈下肌 Infraspinatus
肱三头肌长头 Long head of triceps brachii
大圆肌 Teres major
背阔肌 Latissimus dorsi

图 5-3　肩臂后面腧穴层次解剖（3）

Fig.5-3　Layered anatomy of acupoints on the posterior aspect of the shoulder and arm (3)

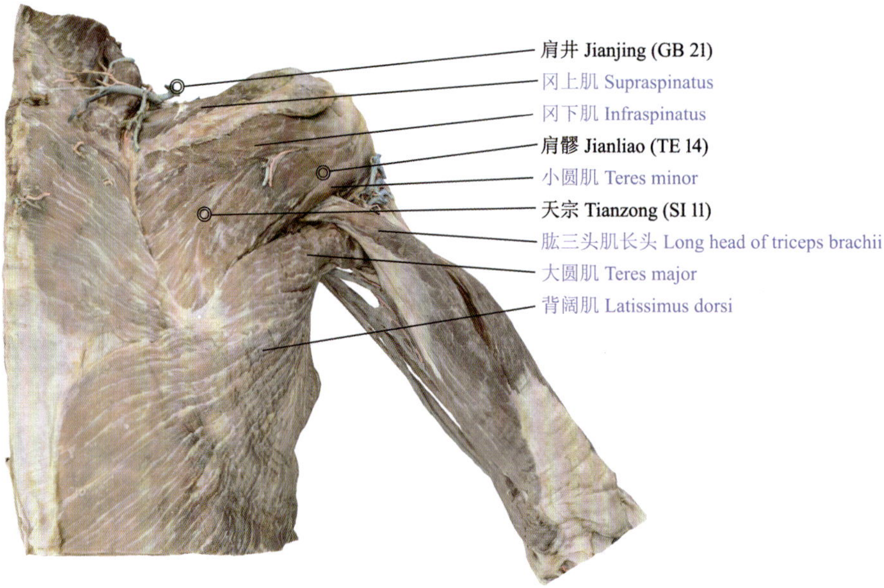
肩井 Jianjing (GB 21)
冈上肌 Supraspinatus
冈下肌 Infraspinatus
肩髎 Jianliao (TE 14)
小圆肌 Teres minor
天宗 Tianzong (SI 11)
肱三头肌长头 Long head of triceps brachii
大圆肌 Teres major
背阔肌 Latissimus dorsi

图 5-4　肩臂后面腧穴层次解剖（4）

Fig.5-4　Layered anatomy of acupoints on the posterior aspect of the shoulder and arm (4)

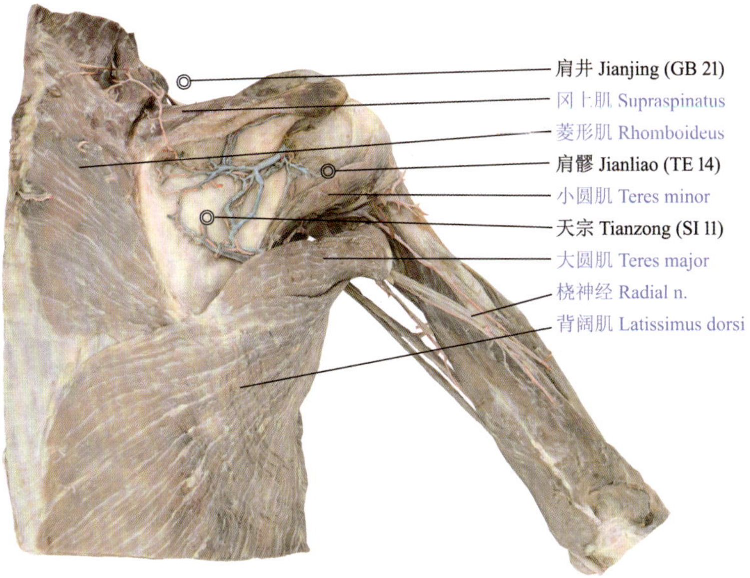
肩井 Jianjing (GB 21)
冈上肌 Supraspinatus
菱形肌 Rhomboideus
肩髎 Jianliao (TE 14)
小圆肌 Teres minor
天宗 Tianzong (SI 11)
大圆肌 Teres major
桡神经 Radial n.
背阔肌 Latissimus dorsi

图 5–5　肩臂后面腧穴层次解剖（5）

Fig.5-5　Layered anatomy of acupoints on the posterior aspect of the shoulder and arm (5)

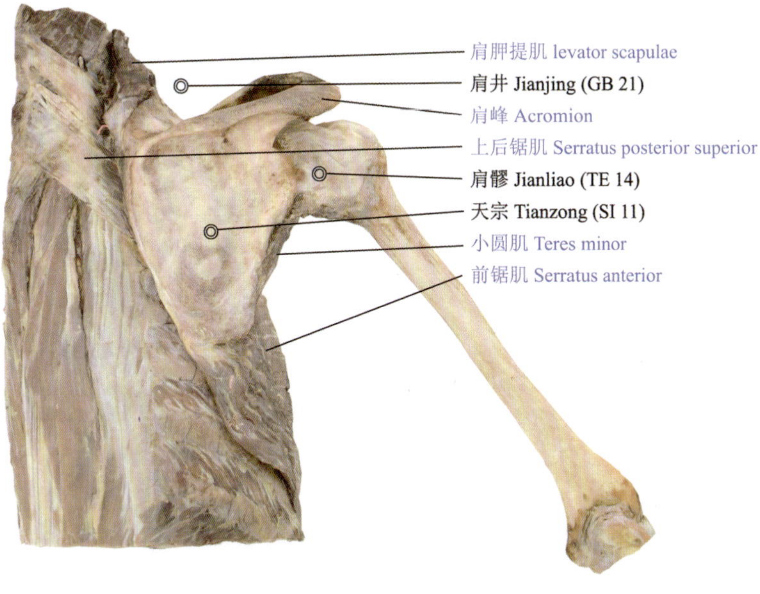
肩胛提肌 levator scapulae
肩井 Jianjing (GB 21)
肩峰 Acromion
上后锯肌 Serratus posterior superior
肩髎 Jianliao (TE 14)
天宗 Tianzong (SI 11)
小圆肌 Teres minor
前锯肌 Serratus anterior

图 5–6　肩臂后面腧穴层次解剖（6）

Fig.5-6　Layered anatomy of acupoints on the posterior aspect of the shoulder and arm (6)

第二节　肩臂外侧面腧穴

Section 2　Acupoints on the lateral aspect of the shoulder and arm

一、肩髃

【定位】当肩峰外侧缘前端与肱骨大结节之间的凹陷中。

【操作】直刺或向下斜刺 0.8 ～ 1.5 寸。

【主治】上肢不遂，肩痛不举，瘾疹。

【进针层次】①皮肤；②皮下组织（内有锁骨上神经的分支）；③三角肌；④三角肌下囊；⑤冈上肌腱（图 5–7 ～图 5–12）。

1. Jianyu (LI 15)

【Location】In the depression between the anterolateral border of the acromion and the greater tubercle of humerus.

【Method】Puncture perpendicularly or obliquely downward 0.8-1.5 cun.

【Indications】Paralysis of upper limbs, heavy shoulders with failing to lift, and urticaria.

【Stratified anatomy】①Skin; ②Subcutaneous tissue (There are branches of the supraclavicular n..); ③Deltoid m.; ④Subdeltoid bursa; ⑤Supraspinatus tendon (Fig.5-7 ~ Fig.5-12).

二、臂臑

【定位】曲池穴与肩髃穴连线上，曲池穴上 7 寸处，相当于三角肌下端。

【操作】直刺或向上斜刺 0.8 ～ 1.5 寸。

【主治】肩臂痛，瘰疬，目疾。

【进针层次】①皮肤；②皮下组织（内有臂外侧上皮神经的分支）；③三角肌（图 5–7 ～图 5–12）。

2. Binao (LI 14)

【Location】On the line connecting Quchi (LI 11) and Jianyu (LI 15), 7 cun above Quchi (LI 11), and equivalent to the lower border of deltoid m..

【Method】Puncture perpendicularly or obliquely upwards 0.8-1.5 cun.

【Indications】Pain in the shoulder and arm, scrofula, and diseases in the eyes.

【Stratified anatomy】①Skin; ②Subcutaneous tissue (There are branches of the superior lateral brachial cutaneous n..); ③Deltoid m. (Fig.5-7 ~ Fig.5-12).

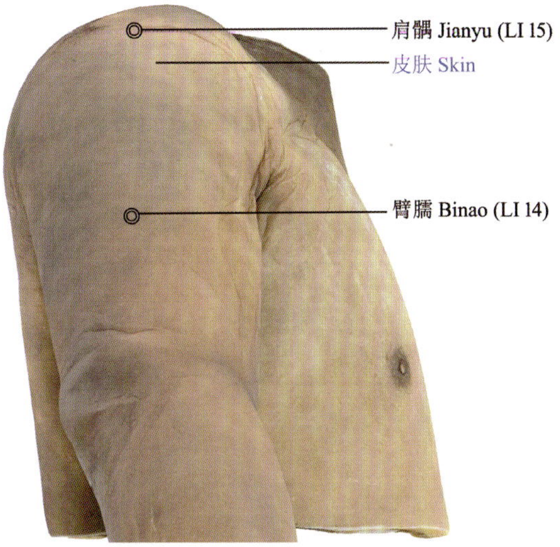

图 5-7　肩臂外侧面腧穴层次解剖（1）
Fig.5-7　Layered anatomy of acupoints on the lateral aspect of the shoulder and arm (1)

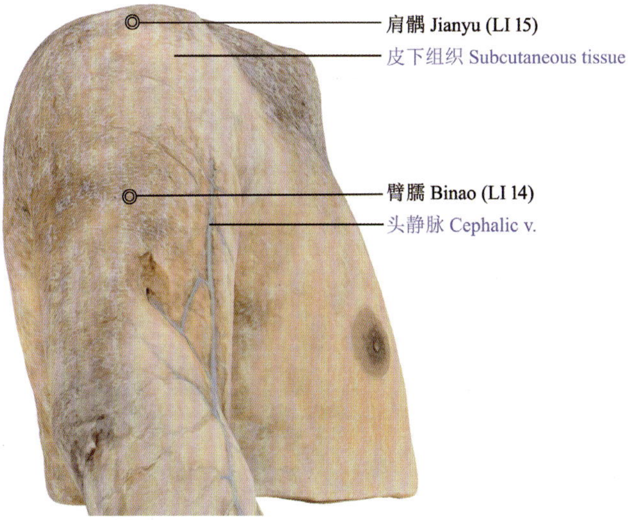

图 5-8　肩臂外侧面腧穴层次解剖（2）
Fig.5-8　Layered anatomy of acupoints on the lateral aspect of the shoulder and arm (2)

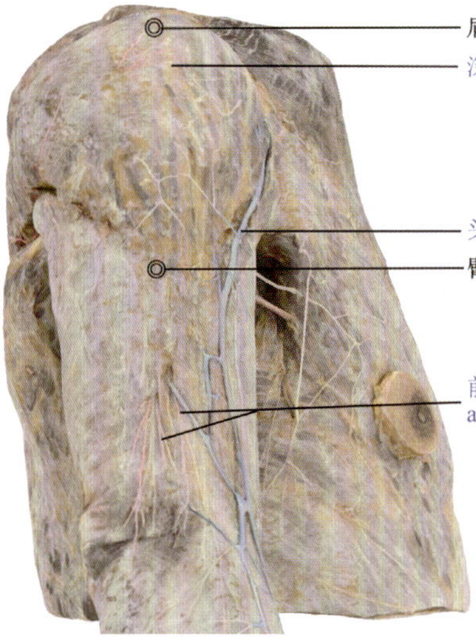
肩髃 Jianyu (LI 15)
深筋膜 Deep fascia
头静脉 Cephalic v.
臂臑 Binao (LI 14)
前臂后皮神经 Posterior antebrachial cutaneous n.

图 5–9　肩臂外侧面腧穴层次解剖（3）

Fig.5-9　Layered anatomy of acupoints on the lateral aspect of the shoulder and arm (3)

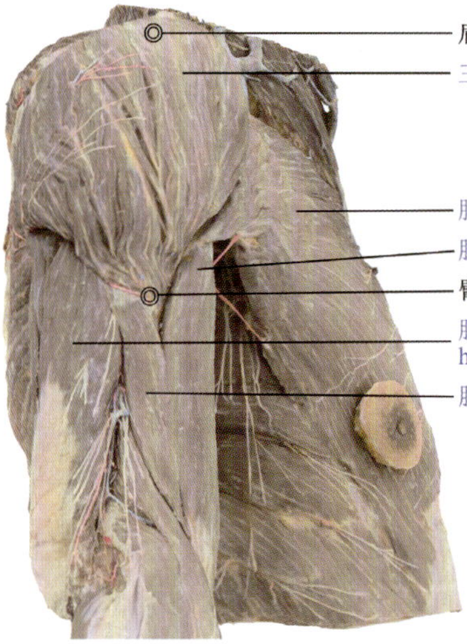
肩髃 Jianyu (LI 15)
三角肌 Deltoid m.
胸大肌 Pectoralis major
肱二头肌 Biceps brachii
臂臑 Binao (LI 14)
肱三头肌外侧头 Lateral head of triceps brachii
肱肌 Brachialis

图 5–10　肩臂外侧面腧穴层次解剖（4）

Fig.5-10　Layered anatomy of acupoints on the lateral aspect of the shoulder and arm (4)

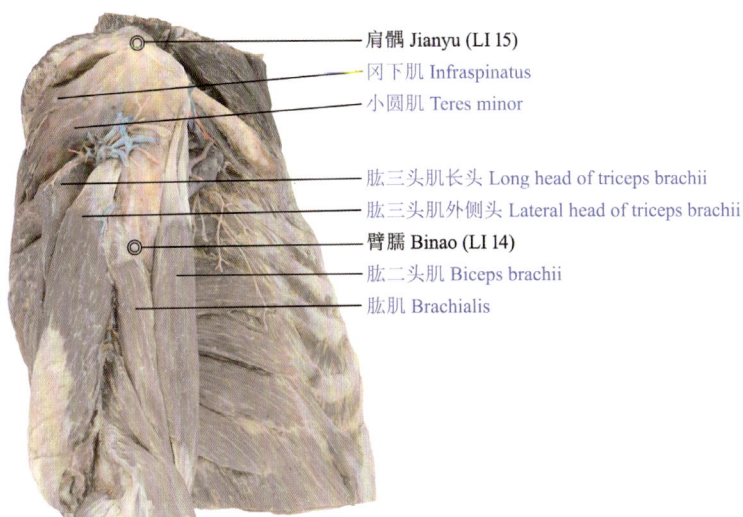

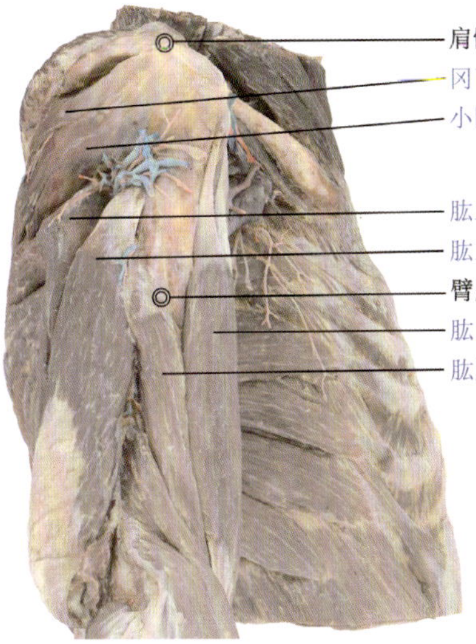
肩髃 Jianyu (LI 15)
冈下肌 Infraspinatus
小圆肌 Teres minor
肱三头肌长头 Long head of triceps brachii
肱三头肌外侧头 Lateral head of triceps brachii
臂臑 Binao (LI 14)
肱二头肌 Biceps brachii
肱肌 Brachialis

图 5-11　肩臂外侧面腧穴层次解剖（5）

Fig.5-11　Layered anatomy of acupoints on the lateral aspect of the shoulder and arm (5)

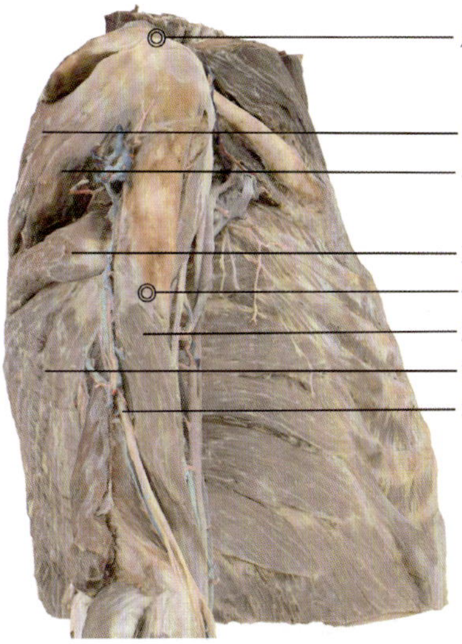
肩髃 Jianyu (LI 15)
冈下肌 Infraspinatus
小圆肌 Teres minor
大圆肌 Teres major
臂臑 Binao (LI 14)
肱肌 Brachialis
背阔肌 Latissimus dorsi
桡神经 Radial n.

图 5-12　肩臂外侧面腧穴层次解剖（6）

Fig.5-12　Layered anatomy of acupoints on the lateral aspect of the shoulder and arm (6)

第三节　肩臂前面腧穴

Section 3　Acupoints on the anterior aspect of the shoulder and arm

一、极泉

【定位】腋窝中央，腋动脉搏动处。

【操作】臂外展，避开腋动脉，直刺或斜刺 0.5 ～ 0.8 寸。

【主治】心痛，心悸，胸闷，气短，胁肋疼痛，肩臂疼痛，上肢不遂，腋臭。

【进针层次】①皮肤；②皮下组织（内有肋间臂神经的分支）；③臂丛和腋动、静脉；④背阔肌腱；⑤大圆肌（图 5–13 ～图 5–18）。

【针刺意外与预防】进针时，医者押手扪住搏动的腋动脉，在指尖引导下，刺手于腋动脉的后缘处进针。针刺入腋窝后，不宜大幅度提插，否则有可能刺破腋血管，造成大的血肿。

1. Jiquan (HT 1)

【Location】In the centre of the axilla, and on the throbbing point of the axillary a..

【Method】Ask the patient to abduct his arms, avoid the axillary a., and puncture perpendicularly or obliquely 0.5-0.8 cun.

【Indications】Angina, palpitations, stuffy chest, short breath, pain in the hypochondrium, pain in the shoulder and arm, paralysis of upper limbs, and osmidrosis.

【Stratified anatomy】①Skin; ②Subcutaneous tissue (There are branches of the intercostobrachial n..) ③Brachial plexus, axillary a. & v.; ④Tendon of latissimus dorsi; ⑤Teres major (Fig.5-13 ~ Fig.5-18).

【Cautions】When the needle is inserted, the acupuncturist presses the pulsating axillary a. with his pressing hand, and under the guidance of the fingertips, he inserts the needle at the posterior edge of the axillary a. with his needling hand. After the needle is pierced into the armpit, it should not be inserted drastically with lifting-thrusting and twirling methods, otherwise it may pierce the axillary blood vessels, causing large hematoma.

二、曲池

【定位】屈肘，肱骨外上髁与肘横纹桡侧端连线的中点。

【操作】直刺 0.8 ～ 1.2 寸。

【主治】热病，咽喉肿痛，齿痛，目赤肿痛，头痛，眩晕，上肢不遂，手臂肿痛，瘰疬，瘾疹，腹痛，吐泻，癫狂。

【进针层次】①皮肤；②皮下组织（内有前臂后皮神经的分支）；③桡侧腕长、短伸肌；④肱桡肌；⑤桡神经及桡侧副动、静脉前支；⑥肱肌（图 5–13 ～图 5–18）。

2. Quchi (LI 11)

【Location】With the patient's elbow flexed, the acupoint is located at the midpoint of the line connecting the lateral epicondyle of the humerus and the radial end of the transverse crease of the elbow.

【Method】Puncture perpendicularly 0.8-1.2 cun.

【Indications】Febrile disease, sore throat, toothache, pain and swelling in the eyes, headache, vertigo, paralysis of upper limbs, swelling and pain of the hand and arm, scrofula, urticaria, abdominal pain, vomiting, diarrhea, insanity and mania.

【Stratified anatomy】①Skin; ②Subcutaneous tissue (There are branches of the posterior antebrachial cutaneous n..); ③Extensor carpiradialis longus and brevis; ④Brachioradialis m.; ⑤Radial n. and anterior branch of the radial collateral a. & v.; ⑥Brachialis m. (Fig.5-13 ~ Fig.5-18).

三、尺泽

【定位】肘横纹上，肱二头肌腱桡侧缘凹陷中。

【操作】直刺 0.5 ～ 0.8 寸，或点刺出血。

【主治】咳嗽，气喘，咳血，咽喉肿痛，肘臂挛痛，吐泻，小儿惊风。

【进针层次】①皮肤；②皮下组织（内有前臂外侧皮神经的分支）；③肱桡肌；④桡神经及桡侧副动、静脉的前支；⑤肱肌（图 5–13 ～图 5–18）。

3. Chize (LU 5)

【Location】On the transverse crease of the elbow, and in the depression of the radial edge of the tendon of biceps brachii.

【Method】Puncture perpendicularly 0.5-0.8 cun, or prick with a three-edged needle to cause bleeding.

【Indications】Cough, panting, hemoptysis, sore throat, spasmodic pain of the elbow and arm, vomiting, diarrhea, and infantile convulsions.

【Stratified anatomy】①Skin; ②Subcutaneous tissue (There are branches of the lateral antebrachial cutaneous n..); ③Brachioradialis m.; ④Radial n. and anterior branch of the radial collateral a. & v.; ⑤Brachialis m. (Fig.5-13 ~ Fig.5-18).

四、曲泽

【定位】肘横纹上，肱二头肌腱尺侧缘凹陷中。

【操作】避开肱动脉，直刺 1 ～ 1.5 寸，或点刺出血。

【主治】心痛，心悸，善惊，胃痛，呕吐，泄泻，热病，中暑，肘臂挛痛。

【进针层次】①皮肤；②皮下组织（内有前臂内侧皮神经的分支）；③正中神经及肱动、静脉；④肱肌（图 5–13 ～图 5–18）。

【针刺意外与预防】针刺时，医者押手拇指按压该动脉，拇指甲放置于肱二头肌腱内侧缘处，然后沿拇指甲边缘进针，以避开动脉。

4. Quze (PC 3)

【Location】On the transverse crease of the elbow, and in the depression of the ulnar edge of the tendon of biceps brachii.

【Method】Avoid the axillary a., puncture perpendicularly 1-1.5 cun, or prick with a three-edged needle to cause bleeding.

【Indications】Angina, palpitations, timorousness, stomachache, vomiting, diarrhea, febrile disease, sunstroke, and spasmodic pain of the elbow and arm.

【Stratified anatomy】①Skin; ②Subcutaneous tissue (There are branches of the medial antebrachial cutaneous n..); ③Median n. and brachial a. & v.; ④Brachialis m. (Fig.5-13 ~ Fig.5-18).

【Cautions】When needling, the acupuncturist presses the artery with the thumb of his pressing hand and places the thumb nail on the inner edge of the tendon of biceps brachii and then the needle is inserted along the edge of the thumb nail to avoid the artery.

五、少海

【定位】肘横纹上，肱骨内上髁与肘横纹内侧端连线的中点。

【操作】直刺 0.5 ～ 1 寸。

【主治】头痛，癔病，心痛，腋胁痛，肘臂痛麻。

【进针层次】①皮肤；②皮下组织（内有前臂内侧皮神经的分支和贵要静脉）；③旋前圆肌；④正中神经及尺侧返动、静脉；⑤肱肌（图 5–13 ～图 5–18）。

5. Shaohai (HT 3)

【Location】On the transverse crease of the elbow, and at the midpoint of the line connecting the medial epicondyle of the humerus and the inner end of the transverse crease of the elbow.

【Method】Puncture perpendicularly 0.5-1 cun.

【Indications】Headache, hysteria, angina, pain in the axilla and hypochondrium, and pain and numbness in the elbow and arm.

【Stratified anatomy】①Skin; ②Subcutaneous tissue (There are branches of the medial antebrachial cutaneous n. and basilic v..); ③Pronator teres m.; ④Median n. and ulnar recurrent a. & v.; ⑤Brachialis m. (Fig.5-13 ~ Fig.5-18).

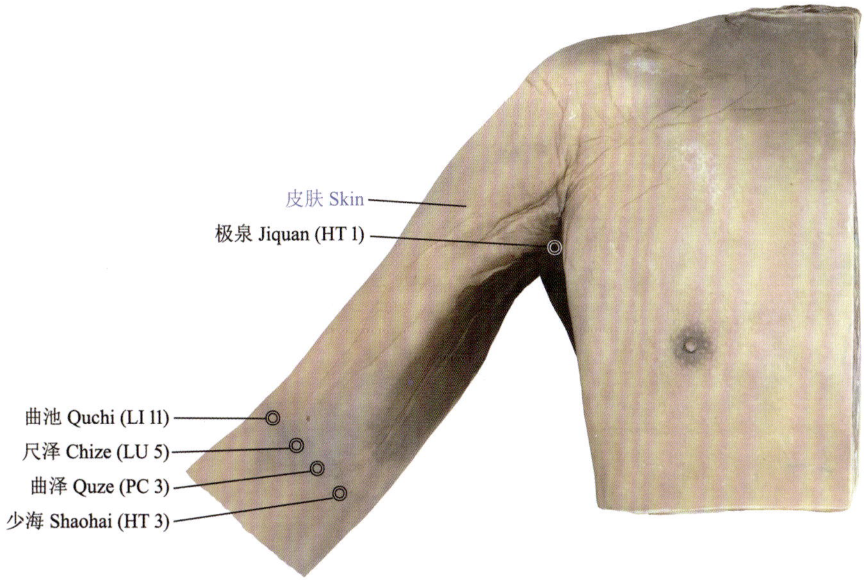
皮肤 Skin
极泉 Jiquan (HT 1)
曲池 Quchi (LI 11)
尺泽 Chize (LU 5)
曲泽 Quze (PC 3)
少海 Shaohai (HT 3)

图 5–13 肩臂前面腧穴层次解剖（1）

Fig.5-13 Layered anatomy of acupoints on the anterior aspect of the shoulder and arm (1)

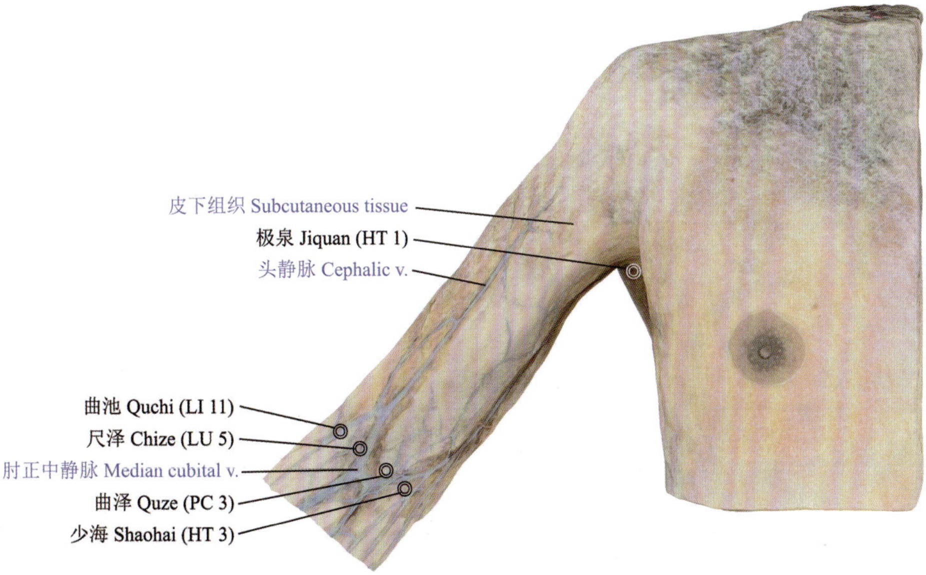
皮下组织 Subcutaneous tissue
极泉 Jiquan (HT 1)
头静脉 Cephalic v.
曲池 Quchi (LI 11)
尺泽 Chize (LU 5)
肘正中静脉 Median cubital v.
曲泽 Quze (PC 3)
少海 Shaohai (HT 3)

图 5–14 肩臂前面腧穴层次解剖（2）

Fig.5-14 Layered anatomy of acupoints on the anterior aspect of the shoulder and arm (2)

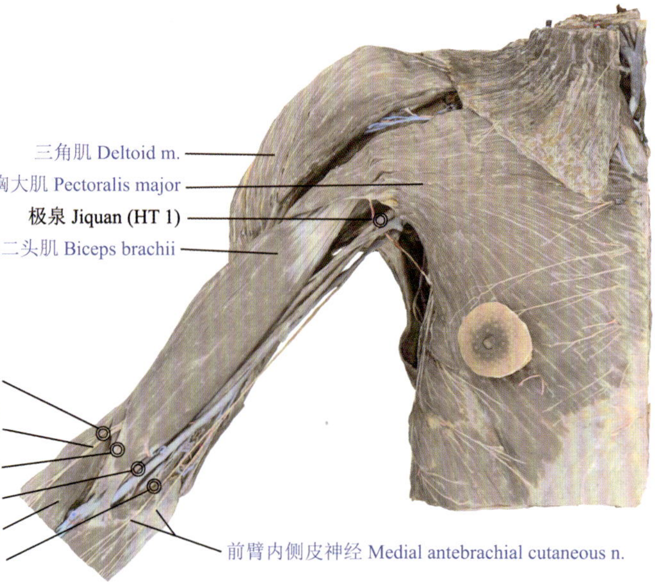
三角肌 Deltoid m.
胸大肌 Pectoralis major
极泉 Jiquan (HT 1)
肱二头肌 Biceps brachii
曲池 Quchi (LI 11)
前臂外侧皮神经
Lateral antebrachial cutaneous n.
尺泽 Chize (LU 5)
曲泽 Quze (PC 3)
肱桡肌 Brachioradialis m.
少海 Shaohai (HT 3)
前臂内侧皮神经 Medial antebrachial cutaneous n.

图 5–15　肩臂前面腧穴层次解剖（3）

Fig.5-15　Layered anatomy of acupoints on the anterior aspect of the shoulder and arm (3)

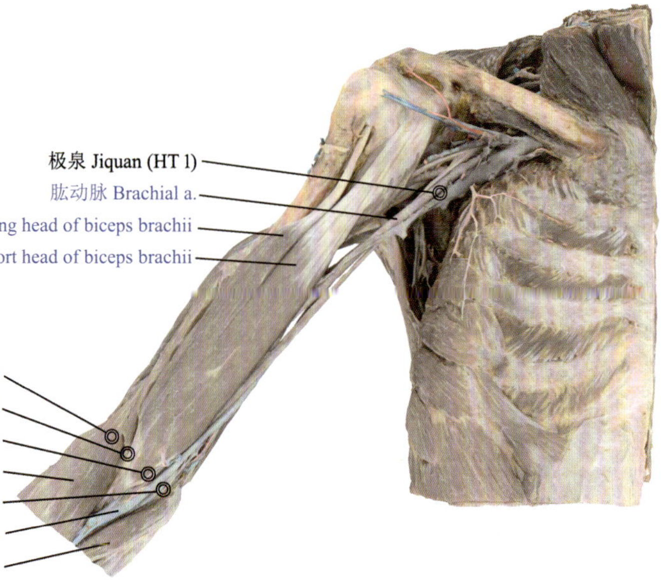
极泉 Jiquan (HT 1)
肱动脉 Brachial a.
肱二头肌长头 Long head of biceps brachii
肱二头肌短头 Short head of biceps brachii
曲池 Quchi (LI 11)
尺泽 Chize (LU 5)
曲泽 Quze (PC 3)
肱桡肌 Brachioradialis m.
少海 Shaohai (HT 3)
肱静脉 Brachial v.
旋前圆肌 Pronator teres m.

图 5–16　肩臂前面腧穴层次解剖（4）

Fig.5-16　Layered anatomy of acupoints on the anterior aspect of the shoulder and arm (4)

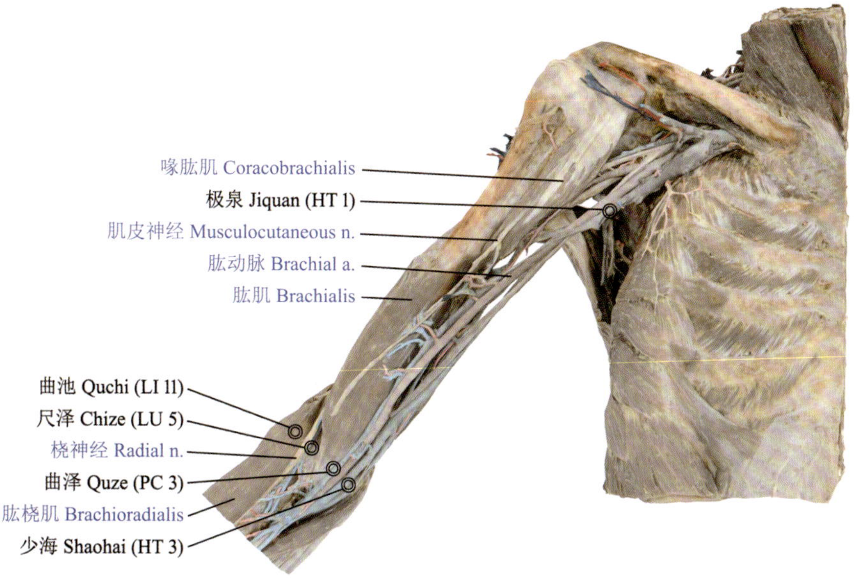
喙肱肌 Coracobrachialis
极泉 Jiquan (HT 1)
肌皮神经 Musculocutaneous n.
肱动脉 Brachial a.
肱肌 Brachialis
曲池 Quchi (LI 11)
尺泽 Chize (LU 5)
桡神经 Radial n.
曲泽 Quze (PC 3)
肱桡肌 Brachioradialis
少海 Shaohai (HT 3)

图 5–17　肩臂前面腧穴层次解剖（5）

Fig.5-17　Layered anatomy of acupoints on the anterior aspect of the shoulder and arm (5)

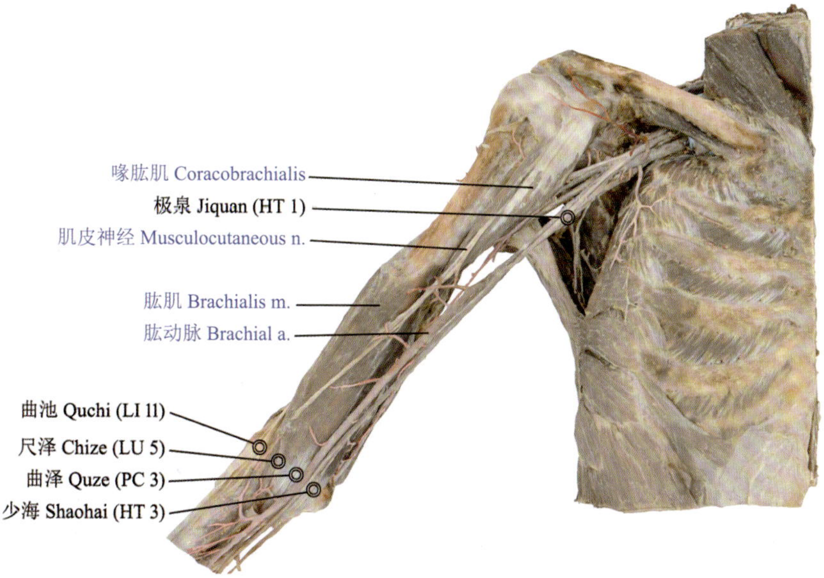
喙肱肌 Coracobrachialis
极泉 Jiquan (HT 1)
肌皮神经 Musculocutaneous n.
肱肌 Brachialis m.
肱动脉 Brachial a.
曲池 Quchi (LI 11)
尺泽 Chize (LU 5)
曲泽 Quze (PC 3)
少海 Shaohai (HT 3)

图 5–18　肩臂前面腧穴层次解剖（6）

Fig.5-18　Layered anatomy of acupoints on the anterior aspect of the shoulder and arm (6)

第四节　前臂前面腧穴

Section 4　Acupoints on the anterior aspect of the forearm

一、孔最

【定位】腕横纹上 7 寸，当尺泽与太渊穴的连线上。

【操作】直刺 0.5 ～ 0.8 寸。

【主治】咳嗽，气喘，咽喉肿痛，肘臂挛痛，热病无汗，头痛，痔疾。

【进针层次】①皮肤；②皮下组织（内有前臂外侧皮神经的分支、桡神经的浅支和头静脉的属支）；③肱桡肌；④桡侧腕屈肌；⑤桡神经的浅支及桡动、静脉；⑥指浅屈肌与旋前圆肌；⑦拇长屈肌（图 5–19 ～图 5–26）。

1. Kongzui (LU 6)

【Location】7 cun above the transverse crease of the elbow, and on the line connecting Chize (LU 5) and Taiyuan (LU 9).

【Method】Puncture perpendicularly 0.5-0.8 cun.

【Indications】Cough, panting, sore throat, spasmodic pain in the elbow and arm, febrile disease with anhidrosis, headache, and hemorrhoids.

【Stratified anatomy】①Skin; ②Subcutaneous tissue (There are branches of the lateral antebrachial cutaneous n., superficial branch of the radial n. and tributaries of the cephalic v..); ③Brachioradialis m.; ④Flexor carpi radialis m.; ⑤Superficial branch of radial n., radial a. & v.; ⑥Flexor digitorum superficialis and pronator teres m.; ⑦Flexor pollicis longus m. (Fig.5-19 ~ Fig.5-26).

二、郄门

【定位】腕横纹上 5 寸，掌长肌腱与桡侧腕屈肌腱之间。

【操作】直刺 0.5 ～ 1 寸。

【主治】心痛，心悸，心烦，胸痛，咳血，呕血，衄血，癫痫。

【进针层次】①皮肤；②皮下组织（内有前臂外侧皮神经的分支和前臂正中静脉）；③桡侧腕屈肌腱和掌长肌腱之间；④指浅屈肌；⑤正中神经；⑥指深屈肌（图 5–19 ～图 5–26）。

2. Ximen (PC 4)

【Location】5 cun above the transverse crease of the wrist, and between the tendons of the long palmar m. and the flexor carpi radialis m..

【Method】Puncture perpendicularly 0.5-1 cun.

【Indications】Angina, palpitations, dysphoria, chest pain, hemoptysis, hematemesis, bleeding from five sense organs or subcutaneous tissue, and epilepsy.

【Stratified anatomy】①Skin; ②Subcutaneous tissue (There are branches of the lateral antebrachial cutaneous n. and median antebrachial v..); ③Between the tendons of flexor carpi radialis m. and palmaris longus m.; ④Flexor digitorum superficialis m.; ⑤Median n.; ⑥Flexor digitorum profundus m. (Fig.5-19 ~ Fig.5-26).

三、间使

【定位】腕横纹上 3 寸，掌长肌腱与桡侧腕屈肌腱之间。

【操作】直刺 0.5 ～ 1 寸。

【主治】心痛，心悸，胃痛，呕吐，热病，癫狂痫，肘臂挛痛。

【进针层次】①皮肤；②皮下组织（内有前臂内、外侧皮神经的分支和前臂正中静脉）；③桡侧腕屈肌腱和掌长肌腱之间；④指浅屈肌；⑤正中神经；⑥指深屈肌；⑦旋前方肌（图 5–19 ～图 5–26）。

3. Jianshi (PC 5)

【Location】3 cun above the transverse crease of the wrist, and between the tendons of the long palmar m. and the flexor carpi radialis m..

【Method】Puncture perpendicularly 0.5-1 cun.

【Indications】Angina, palpitations, stomachache, vomiting, febrile disease, insanity, mania, epilepsy, and spasmodic pain of the elbow and arm.

【Stratified anatomy】①Skin; ②Subcutaneous tissue (There are branches of the medial and lateral antebrachial cutaneous n. and median antebrachial v..); ③Between the tendons of flexor carpi radialis m. and palmaris longus m.; ④Flexor digitorum superficialis m.; ⑤Median n.; ⑥Flexor digitorum profundus m.; ⑦Pronator quadratus m. (Fig.5-19 ~ Fig.5-26).

四、内关

【定位】腕横纹上 2 寸，掌长肌腱与桡侧腕屈肌腱之间。

【操作】直刺 0.5 ～ 1 寸。

【主治】心痛，心悸，胸闷，胃痛，呕吐，呃逆，胁痛，中风，失眠，眩晕，郁证，癫狂痫，偏头痛，肘臂挛痛。

【进针层次】①皮肤；②皮下组织（内有前臂内、外侧皮神经的分支和前臂正中静脉）；③桡侧腕屈肌腱和掌长肌腱之间；④指浅屈肌；⑤正中神经；⑥指深屈肌；⑦旋前方肌（图 5–19 ～图 5–26）。

4. Neiguan (PC 6)

【Location】2 cun above the transverse crease of the wrist, and between the tendons of the long palmar m. and the flexor carpi radialis m..

【Method】Puncture perpendicularly 0.5-1 cun.

【Indications】Angina, palpitations, stuffy chest, stomachache, vomiting, hiccup, pain in the hypochondrium, wind stroke, insomnia, vertigo, depression, insanity, mania, epilepsy, migraine, and spasmodic pain in the elbow and arm.

【Stratified anatomy】①Skin; ②Subcutaneous tissue (There are branches of the medial and lateral antebrachial cutaneous n. and median antebrachial v..); ③Between the tendons of flexor carpi radialis m. and palmaris longus m.; ④Flexor digitorum superficialis m.; ⑤Median n.; ⑥Flexor digitorum profundus m.; ⑦Pronator quadratus m. (Fig.5-19 ~ Fig.5-26).

五、列缺

【定位】在桡骨茎突上方，腕横纹上 1.5 寸；或两虎口交叉，示指尖下取穴。

【操作】向肘部斜刺 0.3 ～ 1 寸。

【主治】咳嗽，气喘，咽喉肿痛，头痛，口眼㖞斜，项强，齿痛。

【进针层次】①皮肤；②皮下组织（内有前臂外侧皮神经的分支、桡神经的浅支和头静脉）；③拇长展肌腱；④肱桡肌腱；⑤旋前方肌（图 5–19 ～图 5–26）。

5. Lieque (LU 7)

【Location】Above the radius styloid process, 1.5 cun above the carpal crease; Or under the tip of the index finger, when the left and right hukou of both hands are intercrossed and the index finger are pressed on another styloid process behind the wrist of the radius.

【Method】Puncture obliquely 0.5-1 cun toward the elbow.

【Indications】Cough, panting, sore throat, headache, deviated mouth and eye, stiffness in the neck, and toothache.

【Stratified anatomy】①Skin; ②Subcutaneous tissue (There are branches of the lateral antebrachial cutaneous n., superficial branch of radial n. and cephalic v..); ③Tendon of abductor pollicis longus; ④Tendon of brachioradialis; ⑤Pronator quadratus m. (Fig.5-19 ~ Fig.5-26).

六、通里

【定位】腕横纹上 1 寸，尺侧腕屈肌腱的桡侧缘。

【操作】直刺 0.3 ～ 0.5 寸。

【主治】心悸，怔忡，舌强不语，暴喑，腕臂痛。

【进针层次】①皮肤；②皮下组织（内有前臂内侧皮神经的分支和贵要静脉的属

支）；③尺侧腕屈肌和指浅屈肌之间；④尺神经及尺动、静脉；⑤指深屈肌；⑥旋前方肌（图 5–19 ～图 5–26）。

6. Tongli (HT 5)

【Location】1 cun above the carpal crease, and on the radial aspect of the flexor carpi ulnaris tendon.

【Method】Puncture perpendicularly 0.3-0.5 cun.

【Indications】Palpitations, fearful throbbing, aphasia with stiff tongue, sudden loss of voice, and pain in the wrist and arm.

【Stratified anatomy】①Skin; ②Subcutaneous tissue (There are branches of the medial antebrachial cutaneous n. and tributaries of basilic v..); ③Between the flexor carpi ulnaris and flexor digitorum superficialis; ④Ulnar n., a. & v.; ⑤Flexor digitorum profundus m.; ⑥Pronator quadratus m. (Fig.5-19 ~ Fig.5-26).

七、阴郄

【定位】腕横纹上 0.5 寸，尺侧腕屈肌腱的桡侧缘。

【操作】避开尺动脉，直刺 0.3 ～ 0.5 寸。

【主治】心痛，心悸，吐血，衄血，骨蒸盗汗，暴喑。

【进针层次】①皮肤；②皮下组织（内有前臂内侧皮神经的分支和贵要静脉的属支）；③尺侧腕屈肌腱；④尺神经及尺动、静脉（图 5–19 ～图 5–26）。

7. Yinxi (HT 6)

【Location】0.5 cun above the carpal crease, and on the radial aspect of the tendon of the flexor carpi ulnaris.

【Method】Avoid the ulnar a., puncture perpendicularly 0.3-0.5 cun.

【Indications】Angina, palpitations, hematemesis, bleeding from five sense organs or subcutaneous tissue, tidal fever and night sweating, and sudden loss of voice.

【Stratified anatomy】①Skin; ②Subcutaneous tissue (There are branches of the medial antebrachial cutaneous n. and tributaries of the basilic v..); ③Tendon of the flexor carpi ulnaris; ④Ulnar n., a. and v. (Fig.5-19 ~ Fig.5-26).

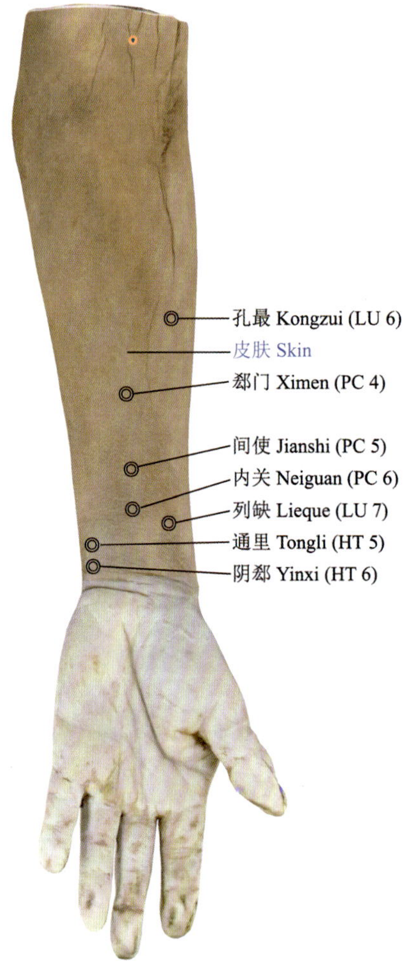
孔最 Kongzui (LU 6)
皮肤 Skin
郄门 Ximen (PC 4)
间使 Jianshi (PC 5)
内关 Neiguan (PC 6)
列缺 Lieque (LU 7)
通里 Tongli (HT 5)
阴郄 Yinxi (HT 6)

图 5–19　前臂前面腧穴层次解剖（1）
Fig.5-19　Layered anatomy of acupoints on the anterior aspect of the forearm (1)

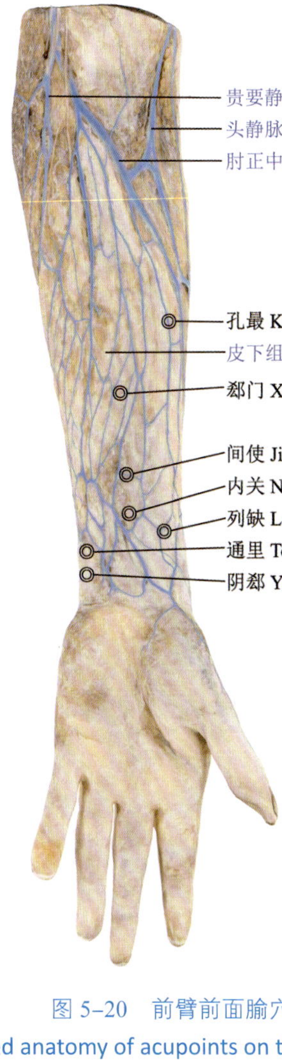
贵要静脉 Basilic v.
头静脉 Cephalic v.
肘正中静脉 Median cubital v.
孔最 Kongzui (LU 6)
皮下组织 Subcutaneous tissue
郄门 Ximen (PC 4)
间使 Jianshi (PC 5)
内关 Neiguan (PC 6)
列缺 Lieque (LU 7)
通里 Tongli (HT 5)
阴郄 Yinxi (HT 6)

图 5-20　前臂前面腧穴层次解剖（2）

Fig.5-20　Layered anatomy of acupoints on the anterior aspect of the forearm (2)

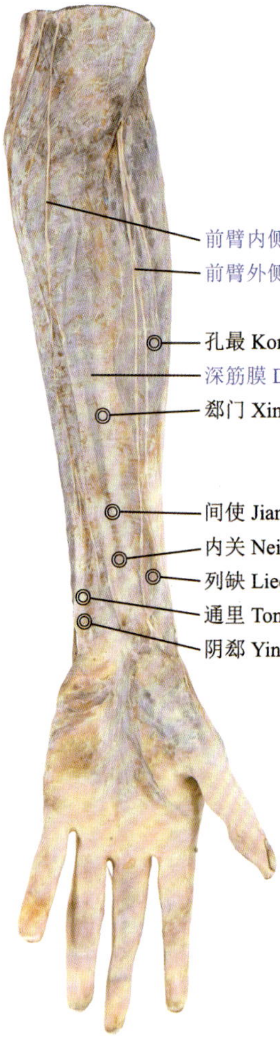
前臂内侧皮神经 Medial antebrachial cutaneous n.
前臂外侧皮神经 Lateral antebrachial cutaneous n.
孔最 Kongzui (LU 6)
深筋膜 Deep fascia
郄门 Ximen (PC 4)
间使 Jianshi (PC 5)
内关 Neiguan (PC 6)
列缺 Lieque (LU 7)
通里 Tongli (HT 5)
阴郄 Yinxi (HT 6)

图 5–21　前臂前面腧穴层次解剖（3）

Fig.5-21　Layered anatomy of acupoints on the anterior aspect of the forearm (3)

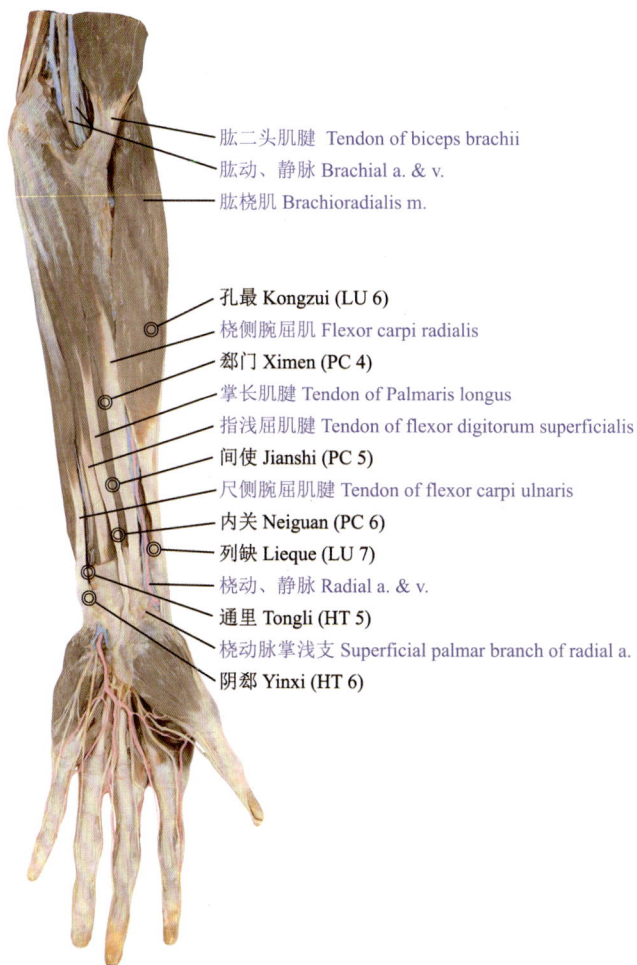

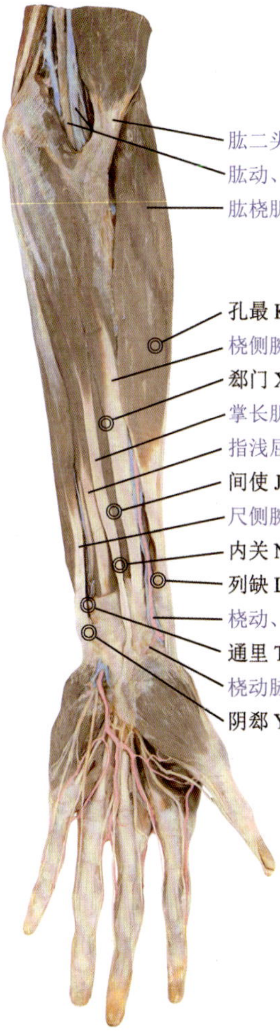
肱二头肌腱 Tendon of biceps brachii
肱动、静脉 Brachial a. & v.
肱桡肌 Brachioradialis m.
孔最 Kongzui (LU 6)
桡侧腕屈肌 Flexor carpi radialis
郄门 Ximen (PC 4)
掌长肌腱 Tendon of Palmaris longus
指浅屈肌腱 Tendon of flexor digitorum superficialis
间使 Jianshi (PC 5)
尺侧腕屈肌腱 Tendon of flexor carpi ulnaris
内关 Neiguan (PC 6)
列缺 Lieque (LU 7)
桡动、静脉 Radial a. & v.
通里 Tongli (HT 5)
桡动脉掌浅支 Superficial palmar branch of radial a.
阴郄 Yinxi (HT 6)

图 5–22　前臂前面腧穴层次解剖（4）

Fig.5-22　Layered anatomy of acupoints on the anterior aspect of the forearm (4)

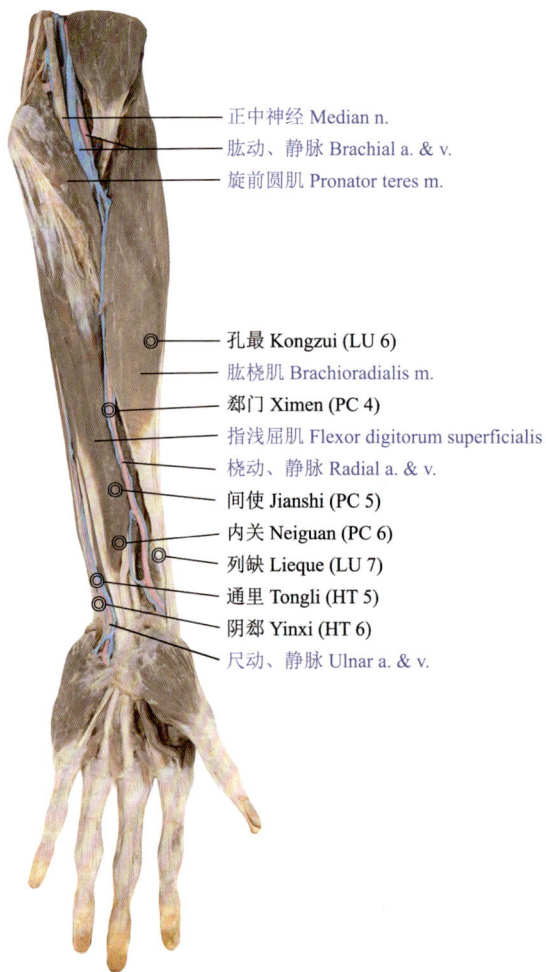

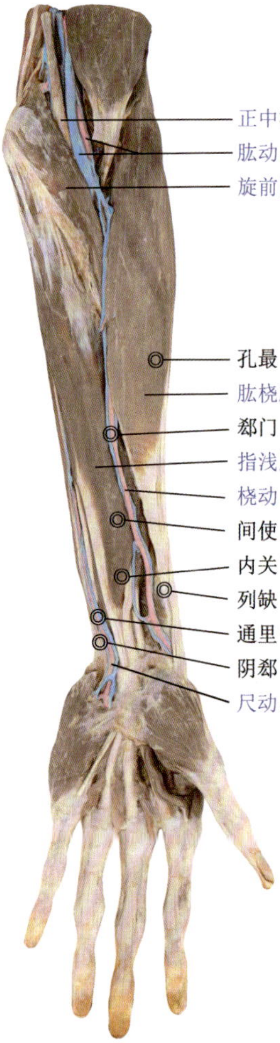
正中神经 Median n.
肱动、静脉 Brachial a. & v.
旋前圆肌 Pronator teres m.
孔最 Kongzui (LU 6)
肱桡肌 Brachioradialis m.
郄门 Ximen (PC 4)
指浅屈肌 Flexor digitorum superficialis
桡动、静脉 Radial a. & v.
间使 Jianshi (PC 5)
内关 Neiguan (PC 6)
列缺 Lieque (LU 7)
通里 Tongli (HT 5)
阴郄 Yinxi (HT 6)
尺动、静脉 Ulnar a. & v.

图 5–23　前臂前面腧穴层次解剖（5）

Fig.5-23　Layered anatomy of acupoints on the anterior aspect of the forearm (5)

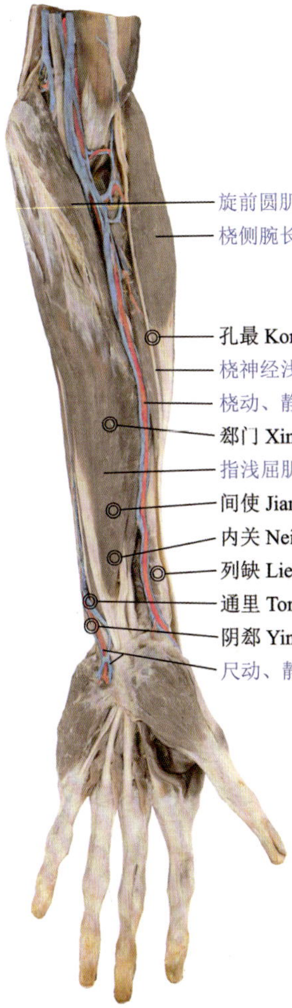
旋前圆肌 Pronator teres m.
桡侧腕长伸肌 Extensor carpiradialis longus m.
孔最 Kongzui (LU 6)
桡神经浅支 Superficial branch of radial n.
桡动、静脉 Radial a. & v.
郄门 Ximen (PC 4)
指浅屈肌 Flexor digitorum superficialis m.
间使 Jianshi (PC 5)
内关 Neiguan (PC 6)
列缺 Lieque (LU 7)
通里 Tongli (HT 5)
阴郄 Yinxi (HT 6)
尺动、静脉 Ulnar a. & v.

图 5-24　前臂前面腧穴层次解剖（6）

Fig.5-24　Layered anatomy of acupoints on the anterior aspect of the forearm (6)

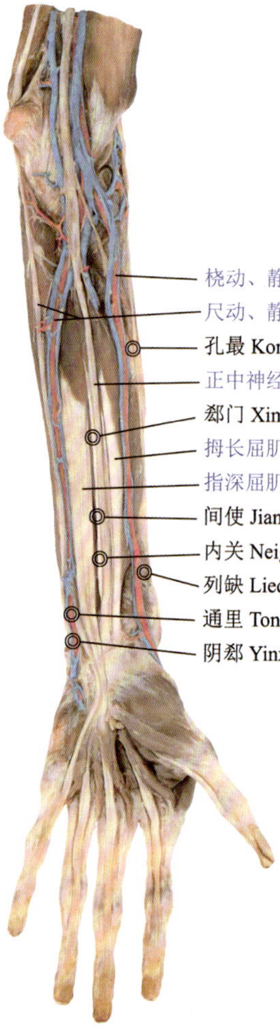
桡动、静脉 Radial a. & v.
尺动、静脉和尺神经 Ulnar a. , v. & n.
孔最 Kongzui (LU 6)
正中神经 Median n.
郄门 Ximen (PC 4)
拇长屈肌 Flexor pollicis longus m.
指深屈肌 Flexor digitorum profundus m.
间使 Jianshi (PC 5)
内关 Neiguan (PC 6)
列缺 Lieque (LU 7)
通里 Tongli (HT 5)
阴郄 Yinxi (HT 6)

图 5–25　前臂前面腧穴层次解剖（7）

Fig.5-25　Layered anatomy of acupoints on the anterior aspect of the forearm (7)

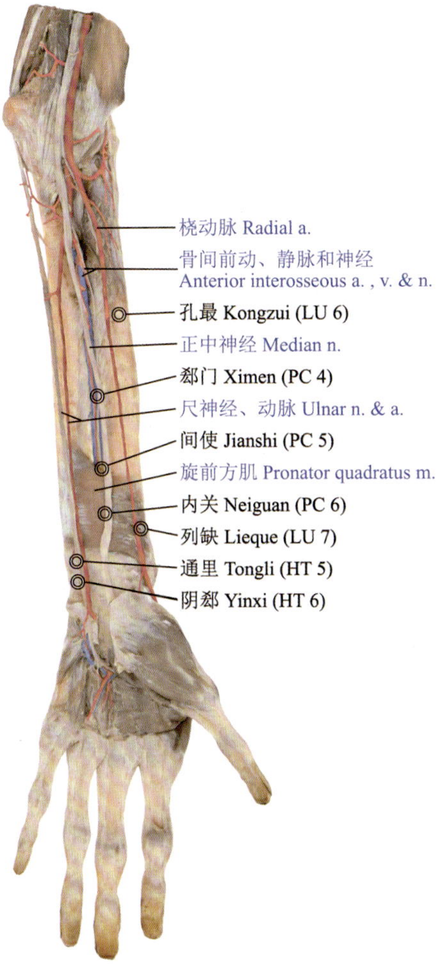
桡动脉 Radial a.
骨间前动、静脉和神经
Anterior interosseous a. , v. & n.
孔最 Kongzui (LU 6)
正中神经 Median n.
郄门 Ximen (PC 4)
尺神经、动脉 Ulnar n. & a.
间使 Jianshi (PC 5)
旋前方肌 Pronator quadratus m.
内关 Neiguan (PC 6)
列缺 Lieque (LU 7)
通里 Tongli (HT 5)
阴郄 Yinxi (HT 6)

图 5-26　前臂前面腧穴层次解剖（8）
Fig.5-26　Layered anatomy of acupoints on the anterior aspect of the forearm (8)

第五节　前臂后面腧穴

Section 5　Acupoints on the posterior aspect of the forearm

一、小海

【定位】尺骨鹰嘴与肱骨内上髁之间凹陷中。

【操作】直刺 0.3 ～ 0.5 寸。

【主治】肘臂挛痛，癫痫。

【进针层次】①皮肤；②皮下组织（内有前臂内侧皮神经和臂内侧皮神经的分支）；③尺神经及尺侧上副动、静脉（图 5–27 ～图 5–34）。

1. Xiaohai (SI 8)

【Location】In the depression of the olecranon of the ulna and the medial epicondyle of the humerus.

【Method】Puncture perpendicularly 0.3-0.5 cun.

【Indications】Spasmodic pain of the elbow and arm, and epilepsy.

【Stratified anatomy】①Skin; ②Subcutaneous tissue (There are branches of the medial antebrachial cutaneous n. and medial brachial cutaneous n..); ③Ulnar n., superior ulnar collateral a. & v. (Fig.5-27 ~ Fig.5-34).

二、手三里

【定位】肘横纹下 2 寸，阳溪与曲池的连线上。

【操作】直刺 0.8 ～ 1.2 寸。

【主治】肩臂痛麻，上肢不遂，腹痛，腹泻，齿痛，颊肿。

【进针层次】①皮肤；②皮下组织（内有前臂外侧皮神经的分支和头静脉）；③桡侧腕长伸肌；④桡侧腕短伸肌；⑤指伸肌；⑥旋后肌和桡神经的深支（图 5–27 ～图 5–34）。

2. Shousanli (LI 10)

【Location】2 cun below the cubital crease, and on the line connecting Yangxi (LI 5) and Quchi (LI 11).

【Method】Puncture perpendicularly 0.8-1.2 cun.

【Indications】Pain and numbness in the shoulder and arm, paralysis of upper limbs, abdominal pain, diarrhea, toothache, and swelling in the cheek.

【Stratified anatomy】①Skin; ②Subcutaneous tissue (There are branches of the lateral antebrachial cutaneous n. and cephalic v..); ③Extensor carpi radialis longus; ④Extensor carpi radialis brevis m.; ⑤Extensor digitorum m.; ⑥Supinator, deep branch of the radial n. (Fig.5-27 ~ Fig.5-34).

三、支正

【定位】腕背侧横纹上 5 寸，当阳谷与小海穴的连线上。

【操作】直刺 0.5 ～ 0.8 寸。

【主治】头痛，目眩，热病，癫狂，项强，肘臂疼痛。

【进针层次】①皮肤；②皮下组织（内有前臂内侧皮神经的分支和贵要静脉的属支）；③尺侧腕屈肌；④指深屈肌（图 5–27 ～图 5–34）。

3. Zhizheng (SI 7)

【Location】5 cun above the dorsal transverse crease of the wrist, and on the line connecting Yanggu (SI 5) and Xiaohai (SI 8).

【Method】Puncture perpendicularly 0.5-0.8 cun.

【Indications】Headache, blurred vision, febrile disease, insanity and mania, stiffness in the neck, and pain in the elbow and arm.

【Stratified anatomy】①Skin; ②Subcutaneous tissue (There are branches of the medial antebrachial cutaneous n. and tributaries of the basilic v..); ③Flexor carpi ulnaris m.; ④Flexor digitorum profundus m. (Fig.5-27 ~ Fig.5-34).

四、偏历

【定位】腕背侧横纹上 3 寸，当阳溪与曲池穴的连线上。

【操作】直刺 0.5 ～ 0.8 寸。

【主治】目赤，耳聋，鼻衄，咽喉肿痛，水肿，手臂酸痛。

【进针层次】①皮肤；②皮下组织（内有前臂外侧皮神经的分支、桡神经的浅支和头静脉的属支）；③桡侧腕长伸肌腱和拇短伸肌；④拇长展肌腱（图 5–27 ～图 5–34）。

4. Pianli (LI 6)

【Location】3 cun above the dorsal transverse crease of the wrist, and on the line connecting Yangxi (LI 5) and Quchi (LI 11).

【Method】Puncture perpendicularly 0.5-0.8 cun.

【Indications】Redness in the eye, deafness, epistaxis, sore throat, edema, and soreness in the hand and arm.

【Stratified anatomy】①Skin; ②Subcutaneous tissue (There are branches of the lateral antebrachial cutaneous n., superficial branch of the radial n. and tributaries of the cephalic v..); ③Tendon of extensor carpiradialis longus and extensor pollicis brevis m.; ④Tendon of abductor pollicis longus (Fig.5-27 ~ Fig.5-34).

五、支沟

【定位】腕背侧横纹上 3 寸，桡骨与尺骨之间的中点。

【操作】直刺 0.5 ～ 1 寸。

【主治】热病，便秘，胁肋疼痛，落枕，暴喑，耳鸣，耳聋，肘臂疼痛。

【进针层次】①皮肤；②皮下组织（内有前臂后皮神经的分支，头静脉和贵要静脉的属支）；③小指伸肌；④拇长伸肌；⑤骨间后动、静脉和神经（图 5–27 ～图 5–34）。

5. Zhigou (TE 6)

【Location】3 cun above the dorsal transverse crease of the wrist, and at the midpoint between the ulna and radius.

【Method】Puncture perpendicularly 0.5-1 cun.

【Indications】Febrile disease, constipation, pain in the hypochondrium, stiff neck, sudden loss of voice, tinnitus, deafness, and pain in the elbow and arm.

【Stratified anatomy】①Skin; ②Subcutaneous tissue (There are branches of the posterior antebrachial cutaneous n., tributaries of the cephalic v. and basilic v..); ③Extensor digiti minimi m.; ④Extensor pollicis longus m.; ⑤Posterior interosseous n., a. & v. (Fig.5-27 ~ Fig.5-34).

六、外关

【定位】腕背侧横纹上 2 寸，桡骨与尺骨之间的中点。

【操作】直刺 0.5 ～ 1 寸。

【主治】热病，偏头痛，目赤肿痛，耳鸣，耳聋，胸胁痛，上肢痿痹。

【进针层次】①皮肤；②皮下组织（内有前臂后皮神经的分支，头静脉和贵要静脉的属支）；③指伸肌和小指伸肌；④骨间后动、静脉和神经；⑤拇长伸肌（图 5–27 ～图 5–34）。

6. Waiguan (TE 5)

【Location】2 cun above the dorsal transverse crease of the wrist, and at the midpoint between the ulna and radius.

【Method】Puncture perpendicularly 0.5-1 cun.

【Indications】Febrile disease, migraine, pain and swelling in the eyes, tinnitus, deafness, pain in the chest and hypochondrium, and flaccidity and impediment of the upper limb.

【Stratified anatomy】①Skin; ②Subcutaneous tissue (There are branches of the posterior antebrachial cutaneous n., tributaries of the cephalic v. and basilic v..); ③Extensor digitorum m. and extensor digiti minimi m.; ④Posterior interosseous n., a. & v.; ⑤Extensor pollicis longus m.. (Fig.5-27 ~ Fig.5-34).

七、养老

【定位】腕背侧横纹上 1 寸，尺骨头桡侧凹陷中。

【操作】掌心向胸，直刺 0.5 ～ 0.8 寸。

【主治】目视不明，头痛，面痛，项强，肩背肘臂疼痛，急性腰痛。

【进针层次】①皮肤；②皮下组织（内有前臂后皮神经的分支）；③指伸肌腱与小指伸肌腱之间（图 5–27 ～图 5–34）。

7. Yanglao (SI 6)

【Location】1 cun above the dorsal transverse crease of the wrist, and in the depression of the radial border of the ulnar head.

【Method】The patient's palm is straight to the chest, puncture perpendicularly 0.5-0.8 cun.

【Indications】Blurred vision, headache, facial pain, stiffness in the neck, pain in the shoulder, back, elbow and arm, and acute lumbago.

【Stratified anatomy】①Skin; ②Subcutaneous tissue (There are branches of the posterior antebrachial cutaneous n..); ③Between the tendons of extensor digitorum m. and extensor digiti minimi m. (Fig.5-27 ~ Fig.5-34).

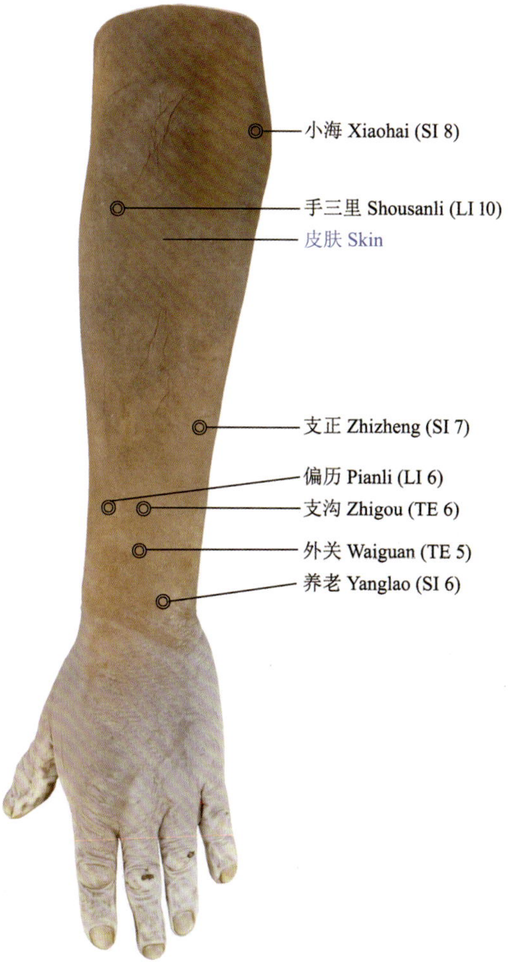
小海 Xiaohai (SI 8)
手三里 Shousanli (LI 10)
皮肤 Skin
支正 Zhizheng (SI 7)
偏历 Pianli (LI 6)
支沟 Zhigou (TE 6)
外关 Waiguan (TE 5)
养老 Yanglao (SI 6)

图 5–27　前臂后面腧穴层次解剖（1）

Fig.5-27　Layered anatomy of acupoints on the posterior aspect of the forearm (1)

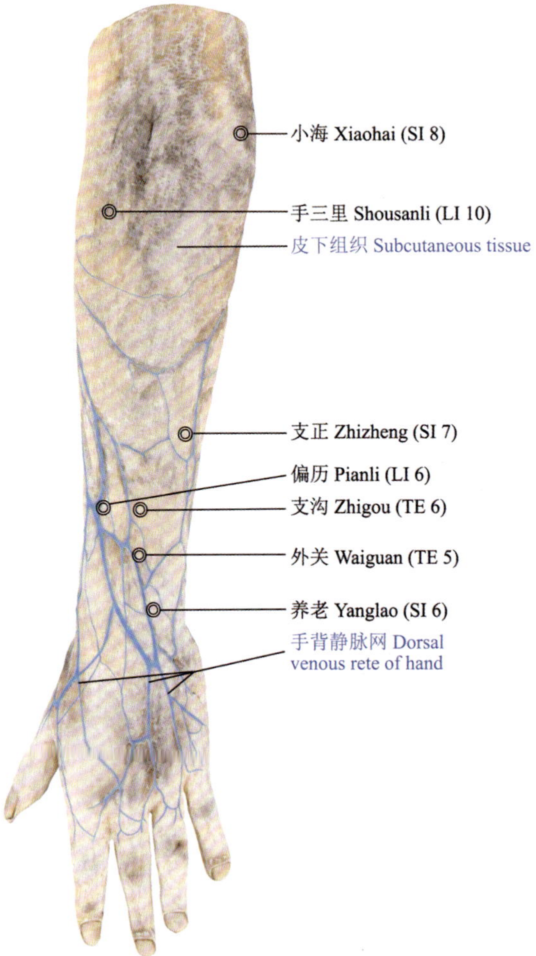
小海 Xiaohai (SI 8)
手三里 Shousanli (LI 10)
皮下组织 Subcutaneous tissue
支正 Zhizheng (SI 7)
偏历 Pianli (LI 6)
支沟 Zhigou (TE 6)
外关 Waiguan (TE 5)
养老 Yanglao (SI 6)
手背静脉网 Dorsal venous rete of hand

图 5-28　前臂后面腧穴层次解剖（2）

Fig.5-28　Layered anatomy of acupoints on the posterior aspect of the forearm (2)

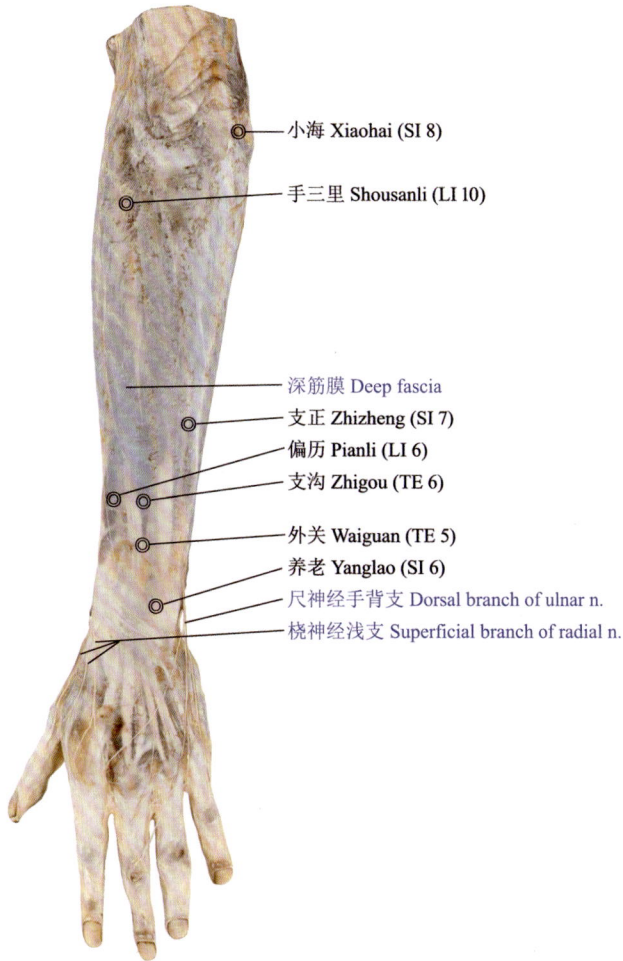

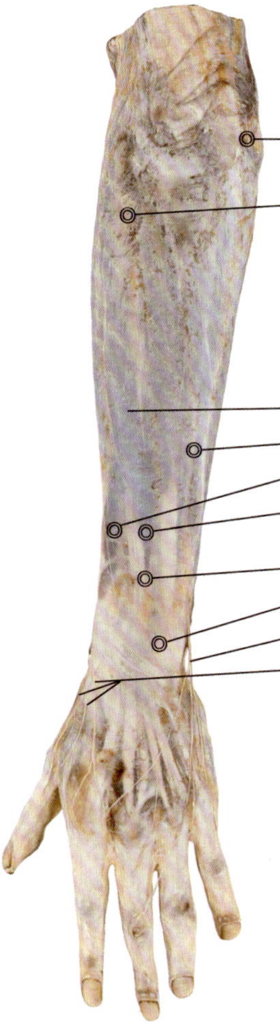
小海 Xiaohai (SI 8)
手三里 Shousanli (LI 10)
深筋膜 Deep fascia
支正 Zhizheng (SI 7)
偏历 Pianli (LI 6)
支沟 Zhigou (TE 6)
外关 Waiguan (TE 5)
养老 Yanglao (SI 6)
尺神经手背支 Dorsal branch of ulnar n.
桡神经浅支 Superficial branch of radial n.

图 5–29　前臂后面腧穴层次解剖（3）
Fig.5-29　Layered anatomy of acupoints on the posterior aspect of the forearm (3)

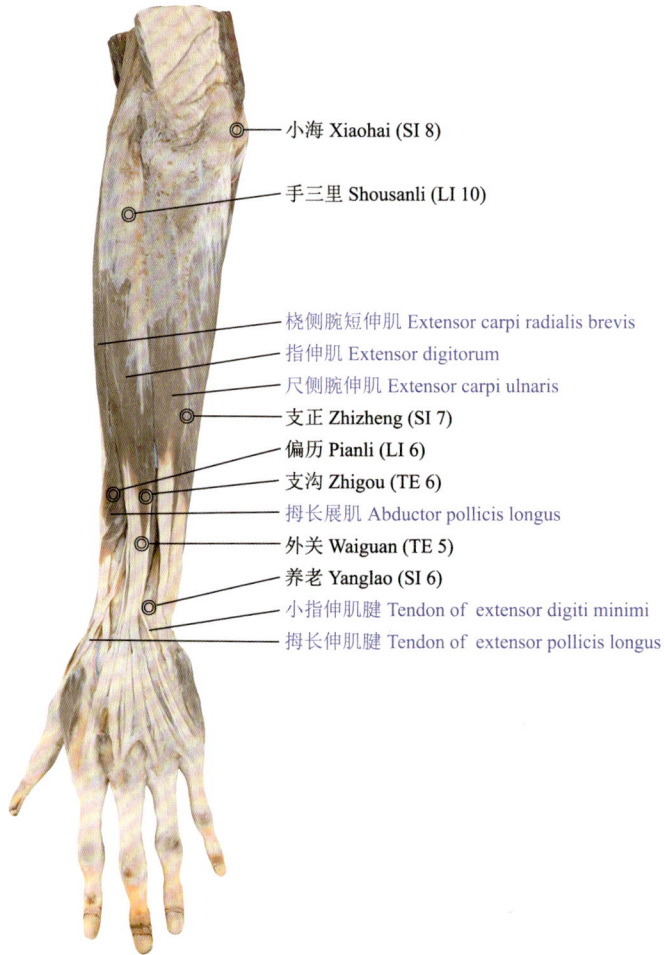

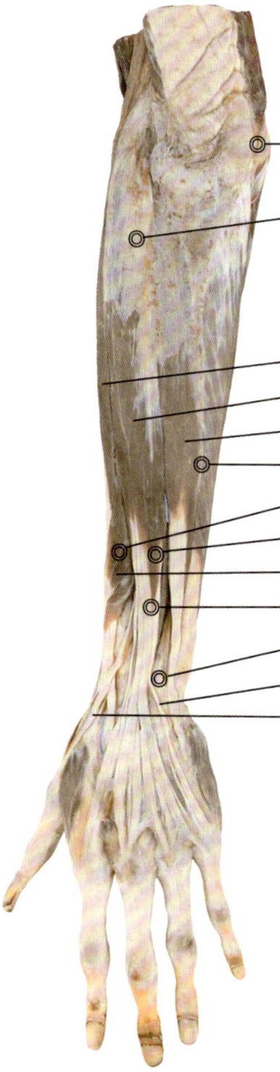
小海 Xiaohai (SI 8)
手三里 Shousanli (LI 10)
桡侧腕短伸肌 Extensor carpi radialis brevis
指伸肌 Extensor digitorum
尺侧腕伸肌 Extensor carpi ulnaris
支正 Zhizheng (SI 7)
偏历 Pianli (LI 6)
支沟 Zhigou (TE 6)
拇长展肌 Abductor pollicis longus
外关 Waiguan (TE 5)
养老 Yanglao (SI 6)
小指伸肌腱 Tendon of extensor digiti minimi
拇长伸肌腱 Tendon of extensor pollicis longus

图 5–30　前臂后面腧穴层次解剖（4）

Fig.5-30　Layered anatomy of acupoints on the posterior aspect of the forearm (4)

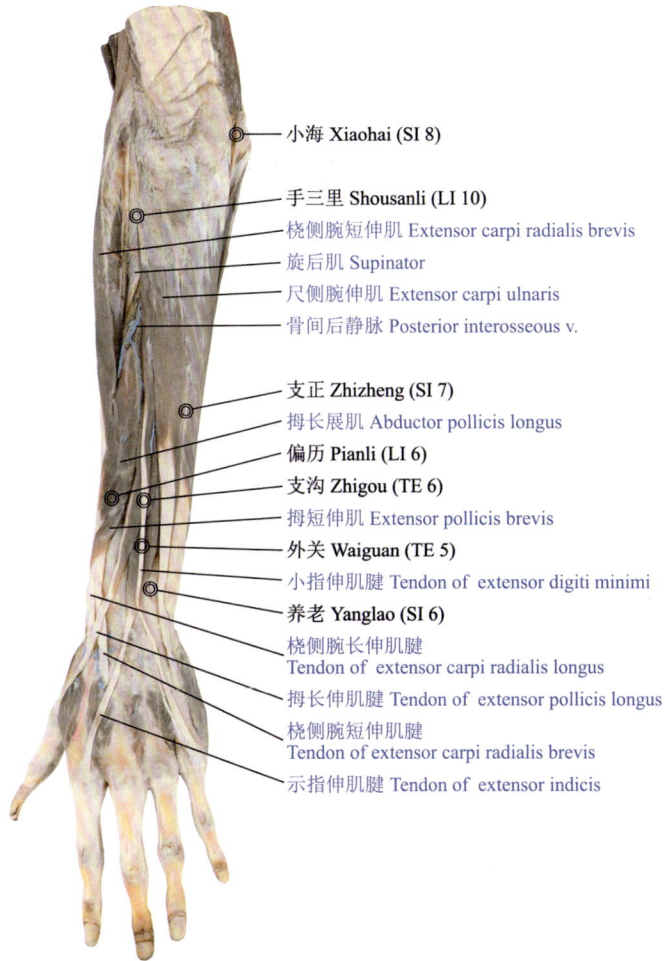

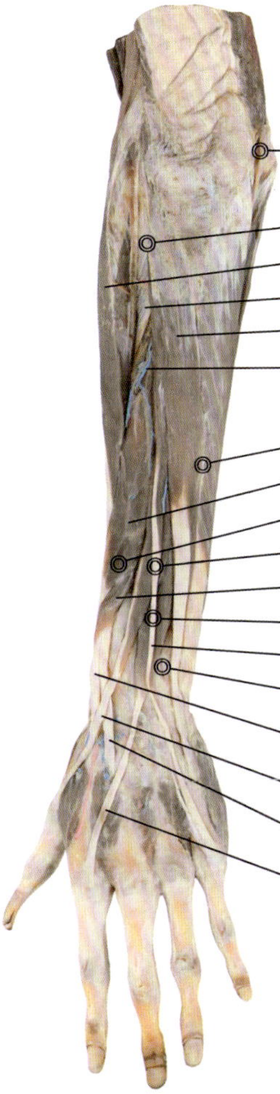
小海 Xiaohai (SI 8)
手三里 Shousanli (LI 10)
桡侧腕短伸肌 Extensor carpi radialis brevis
旋后肌 Supinator
尺侧腕伸肌 Extensor carpi ulnaris
骨间后静脉 Posterior interosseous v.
支正 Zhizheng (SI 7)
拇长展肌 Abductor pollicis longus
偏历 Pianli (LI 6)
支沟 Zhigou (TE 6)
拇短伸肌 Extensor pollicis brevis
外关 Waiguan (TE 5)
小指伸肌腱 Tendon of extensor digiti minimi
养老 Yanglao (SI 6)
桡侧腕长伸肌腱
Tendon of extensor carpi radialis longus
拇长伸肌腱 Tendon of extensor pollicis longus
桡侧腕短伸肌腱
Tendon of extensor carpi radialis brevis
示指伸肌腱 Tendon of extensor indicis

图 5-31 前臂后面腧穴层次解剖（5）

Fig.5-31 Layered anatomy of acupoints on the posterior aspect of the forearm (5)

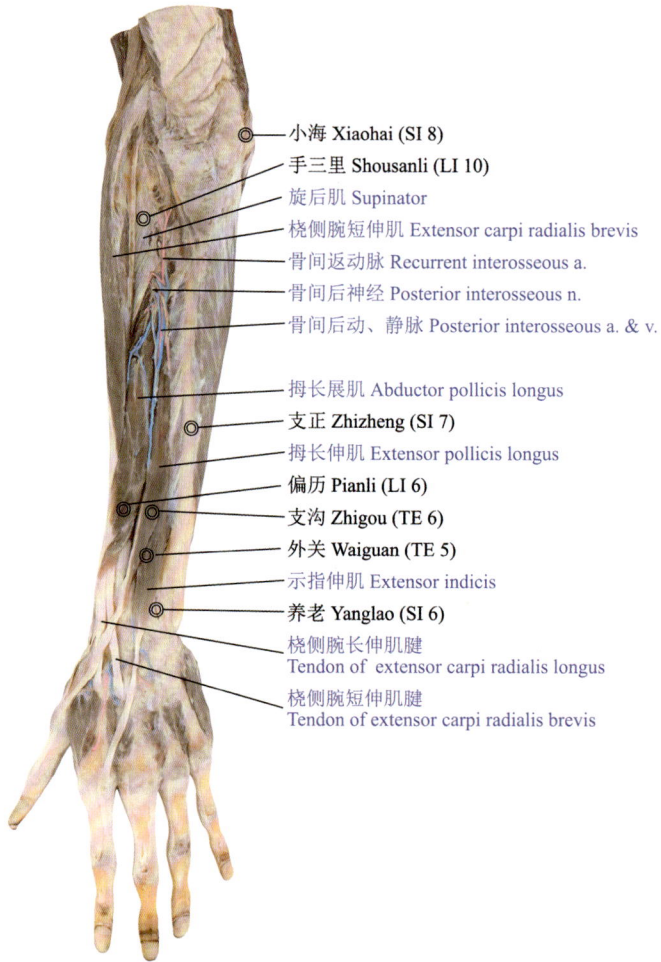

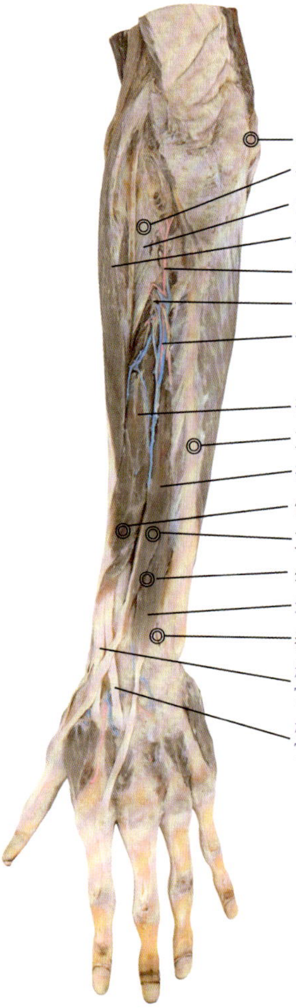
小海 Xiaohai (SI 8)
手三里 Shousanli (LI 10)
旋后肌 Supinator
桡侧腕短伸肌 Extensor carpi radialis brevis
骨间返动脉 Recurrent interosseous a.
骨间后神经 Posterior interosseous n.
骨间后动、静脉 Posterior interosseous a. & v.
拇长展肌 Abductor pollicis longus
支正 Zhizheng (SI 7)
拇长伸肌 Extensor pollicis longus
偏历 Pianli (LI 6)
支沟 Zhigou (TE 6)
外关 Waiguan (TE 5)
示指伸肌 Extensor indicis
养老 Yanglao (SI 6)
桡侧腕长伸肌腱
Tendon of extensor carpi radialis longus
桡侧腕短伸肌腱
Tendon of extensor carpi radialis brevis

图 5-32　前臂后面腧穴层次解剖（6）

Fig.5-32　Layered anatomy of acupoints on the posterior aspect of the forearm (6)

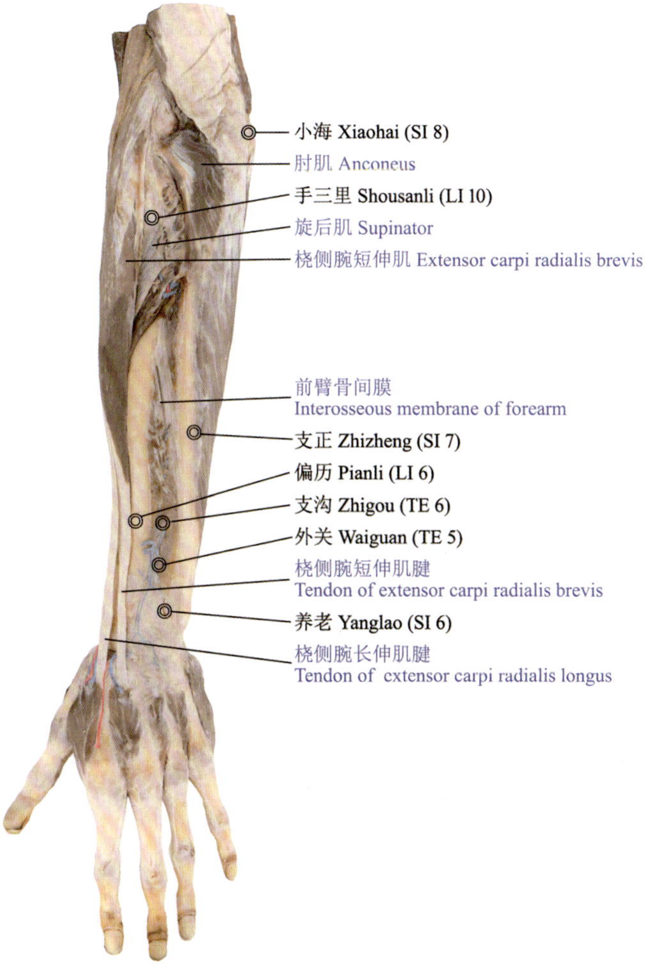
小海 Xiaohai (SI 8)
肘肌 Anconeus
手三里 Shousanli (LI 10)
旋后肌 Supinator
桡侧腕短伸肌 Extensor carpi radialis brevis
前臂骨间膜
Interosseous membrane of forearm
支正 Zhizheng (SI 7)
偏历 Pianli (LI 6)
支沟 Zhigou (TE 6)
外关 Waiguan (TE 5)
桡侧腕短伸肌腱
Tendon of extensor carpi radialis brevis
养老 Yanglao (SI 6)
桡侧腕长伸肌腱
Tendon of extensor carpi radialis longus

图 5–33　前臂后面腧穴层次解剖（7）

Fig.5-33　Layered anatomy of acupoints on the posterior aspect of the forearm (7)

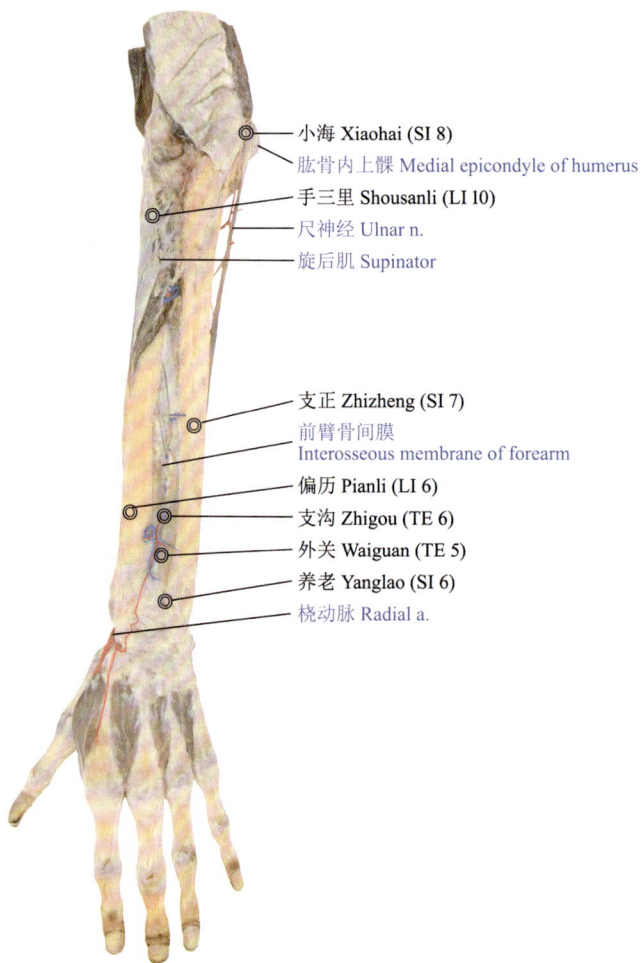

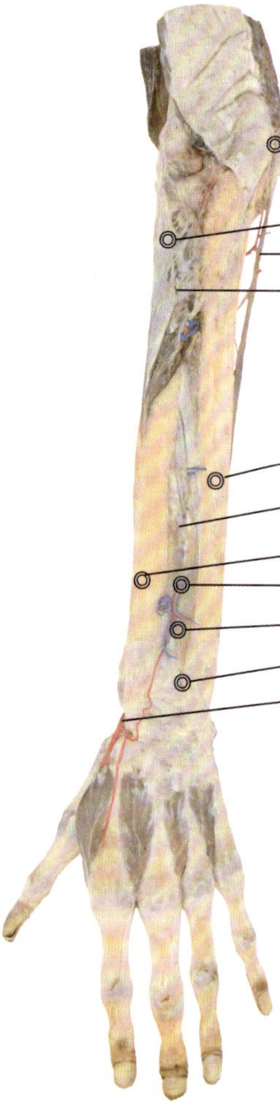
小海 Xiaohai (SI 8)
肱骨内上髁 Medial epicondyle of humerus
手三里 Shousanli (LI 10)
尺神经 Ulnar n.
旋后肌 Supinator
支正 Zhizheng (SI 7)
前臂骨间膜
Interosseous membrane of forearm
偏历 Pianli (LI 6)
支沟 Zhigou (TE 6)
外关 Waiguan (TE 5)
养老 Yanglao (SI 6)
桡动脉 Radial a.

图 5–34　前臂后面腧穴层次解剖（8）

Fig.5-34　Layered anatomy of acupoints on the posterior aspect of the forearm (8)

第六节　腕手掌腧穴

Section 6　Acupoints on the wrist and palm

一、太渊

【定位】桡骨茎突与手舟骨之间，拇长展肌腱尺侧凹陷中；或腕横纹桡侧端，桡动脉搏动处。

【操作】避开桡动脉，直刺 0.2 ～ 0.3 寸。

【主治】咳嗽，气喘，咳血，胸背痛，无脉症。

【进针层次】①皮肤；②皮下组织（内有前臂外侧皮神经的分支，桡神经的浅支，头静脉及桡动脉的掌浅支）；③桡侧腕屈肌腱和拇长展肌腱之间；④桡动、静脉（图 5–35 ～图 5–44）。

【针刺意外与预防】针刺时，医者押手拇指按压桡动脉，拇指甲放置于拇长展肌腱尺侧缘处，然后刺手沿拇指甲边缘进针，以避开该动脉。

1. Taiyuan (LU 9)

【Location】Between the styloid process of the radius and the scaphoidbone, and in the ulnar depression of the abductor pollicis longus tendon; Or at the radial end of the wrist crease, and at the pulsating site of the radial a..

【Method】Avoid the radial a., puncture perpendicularly 0.2-0.3 cun.

【Indications】Cough, panting, hemoptysis, pain in the chest and back, and pulseless disease.

【Stratified anatomy】①Skin; ②Subcutaneous tissue (There are branches of the lateral antebrachial cutaneous n., superficial branch of radial n., cephalic v. and superficial palmar branch of radial a..); ③Between the tendons of flexor carpi radialis and abductor pollicis longus; ④Radial a. & v. (Fig.5-35 ~ Fig.5-44).

【Cautions】When needling, the acupuncturist presses radial artery with the thumb of his pressing hand, and places the thumb nail on the ulnar edge of the abductor pollicis longus tendon, and then inserts the needle along the edge of the thumb nail to avoid the artery.

二、大陵

【定位】腕横纹中，掌长肌腱与桡侧腕屈肌腱之间。

【操作】直刺 0.3 ～ 0.5 寸。

【主治】心痛，心悸，胃痛，呕吐，胸胁胀痛，喜笑悲恐，癫狂痫，手臂挛痛。

【进针层次】①皮肤；②皮下组织（内有正中神经掌支的分支）；③桡侧腕屈肌腱和掌长

肌腱之间；④正中神经；⑤拇长屈肌腱与指浅、深屈肌腱之间（图 5–35 ～图 5–44）。

2. Daling (PC 7)

【Location】On the wrist transverse crease, and between the tendon of flexor carpi radialis and palmaris longus.

【Method】Puncture perpendicularly 0.3-0.5 cun.

【Indications】Angina, palpitations, stomachache, vomiting, distension and pain in the chest and hypochondrium, insanity, mania, epilepsy, and spasmodic pain of the hand and arm.

【Stratified anatomy】①Skin; ②Subcutaneous tissue (There are branches of the palmar branch of the median n..); ③Between the tendon of flexor carpi radialis and palmaris longus; ④Median n.; ⑤Between flexor pollicis longus and flexor digitorum superficialis & profundus tendons (Fig.5-35 ~ Fig.5-44).

三、神门

【定位】腕横纹尺侧端，尺侧腕屈肌腱的桡侧缘。

【操作】避开尺动脉，直刺 0.3 ～ 0.5 寸。

【主治】心痛，惊悸，怔忡，心烦，健忘，失眠，痴呆，癫狂，眩晕，胸胁痛。

【进针层次】①皮肤；②皮下组织（内有前臂内侧皮神经的分支和尺神经掌支）；③尺侧腕屈肌腱；④尺神经及尺动、静脉（图 5–35 ～图 5–44）。

【针刺意外与预防】针刺时，医者押手拇指按压尺动脉，拇指甲放置于尺侧腕屈肌腱的桡侧缘处，然后刺手沿拇指甲边缘进针，以避开该动脉。

3. Shenmen (HT 7)

【Location】On the ulnar border of the wrist transverse crease, and on the radial edge of the flexor carpi ulnaris tendon.

【Method】Avoid the ulnar a., puncture perpendicularly 0.3-0.5 cun.

【Indications】Angina, palpitations, fearful throbbing, dysphoria, forgetfulness, insomnia, dementia, insanity and mania, vertigo, and pain in the chest and hypochondrium.

【Stratified anatomy】①Skin; ②Subcutaneous tissue (There are branches of the medial antebrachial cutaneous n. and palmar branch of ulnar n..); ③Flexor carpi ulnaris tendon; ④Ulnar n., a. & v. (Fig.5-35 ~ Fig.5-44).

【Cautions】When needling, the acupuncturist presses the ulnar a. with the thumb of his pressing hand, and places the thumb nail on the radial edge of the flexor carpi ulnaris tendon, and then inserts the needle along the edge of the thumb nail to avoid the artery.

四、劳宫

【定位】第 2、第 3 掌骨之间偏第 3 掌骨，握拳屈指中指尖下。

【操作】直刺 0.3 ～ 0.5 寸。

【主治】中风昏迷，中暑，癫狂痫，心痛，心烦，呕吐，口疮，口臭，鹅掌风。

【进针层次】①皮肤；②皮下组织（内有正中神经掌支的分支）；③掌腱膜；④示指浅、深屈肌腱与中指浅、深屈肌腱之间；⑤第 2 蚓状肌、第 1 指掌侧总动脉和第 2 指掌侧总神经；⑥第 1 骨间掌侧肌和第 2 骨间背侧肌（图 5–35 ～图 5–44）。

4. Laogong (PC 8)

【Location】Between the 2nd and 3rd metacarpal bones, and close to the 3rd metacarpal bone, and under the tip of the middle finger when making a fist.

【Method】Puncture perpendicularly 0.3-0.5 cun.

【Indications】Apoplectic coma, sunstroke, insanity, mania, epilepsy, angina, dysphoria, vomiting, sore of tongue and mouth, halitosis, and tinea manuum.

【Stratified anatomy】①Skin; ②Subcutaneous tissue (There are branches for the palmar branch of the median n..); ③Palmar aponeurosis; ④Between the tendons of flexor digitorum superficialis & profundus of the index finger and middle finger; ⑤The 2nd lumbricales m., the 1st common palmar digital a. and the 2nd common palmar digital n.; ⑥The 1st palmar interossei and the 2nd dorsal interossei m. (Fig.5-35 ~ Fig.5-44).

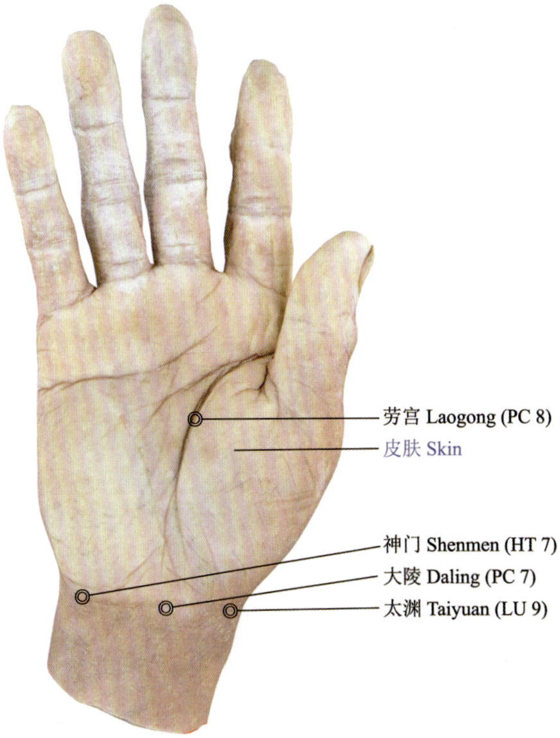

图 5–35　腕手掌腧穴层次解剖（1）

Fig.5-35　Layered anatomy of acupoints on the wrist and palm (1)

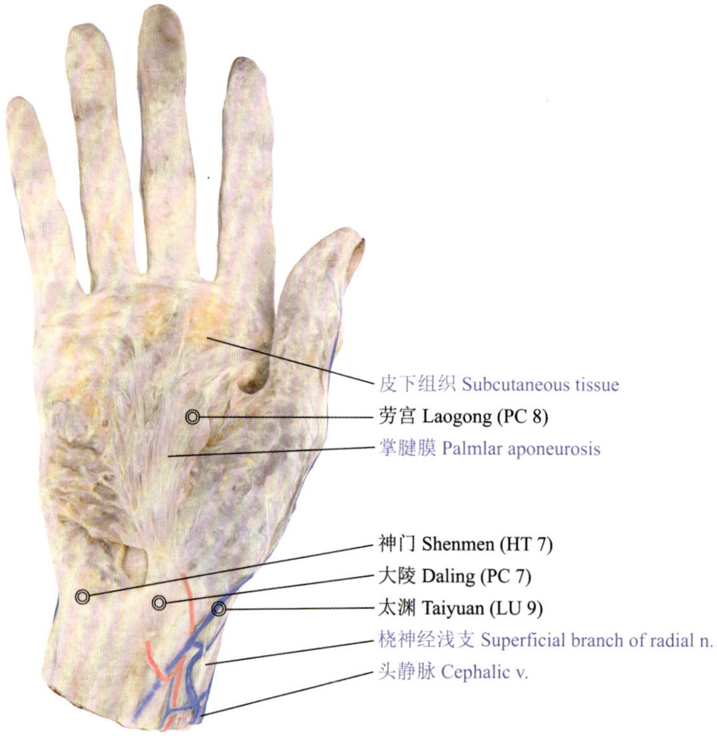
皮下组织 Subcutaneous tissue
劳宫 Laogong (PC 8)
掌腱膜 Palmlar aponeurosis
神门 Shenmen (HT 7)
大陵 Daling (PC 7)
太渊 Taiyuan (LU 9)
桡神经浅支 Superficial branch of radial n.
头静脉 Cephalic v.

图 5–36 腕手掌腧穴层次解剖（2）

Fig.5-36 Layered anatomy of acupoints on the wrist and palm (2)

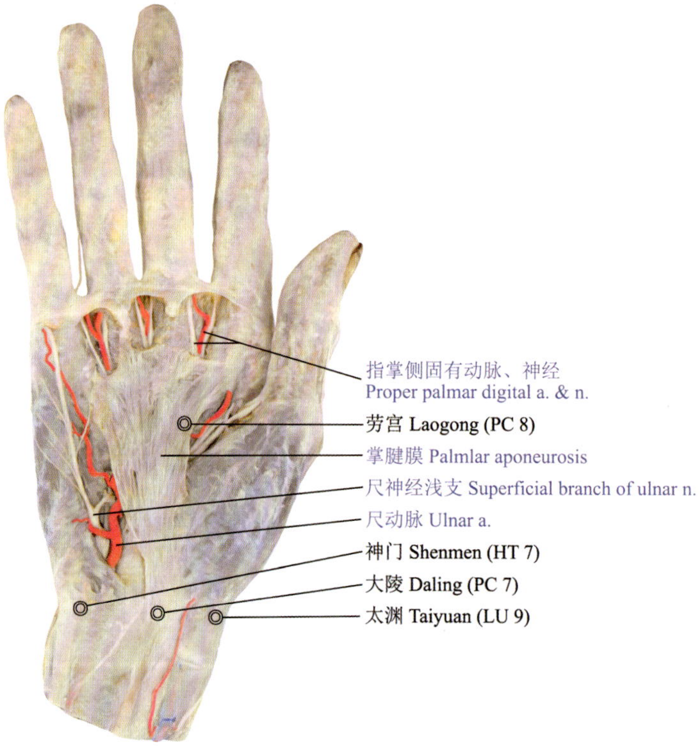
指掌侧固有动脉、神经
Proper palmar digital a. & n.
劳宫 Laogong (PC 8)
掌腱膜 Palmlar aponeurosis
尺神经浅支 Superficial branch of ulnar n.
尺动脉 Ulnar a.
神门 Shenmen (HT 7)
大陵 Daling (PC 7)
太渊 Taiyuan (LU 9)

图 5–37 腕手掌腧穴层次解剖（3）

Fig.5-37 Layered anatomy of acupoints on the wrist and palm (3)

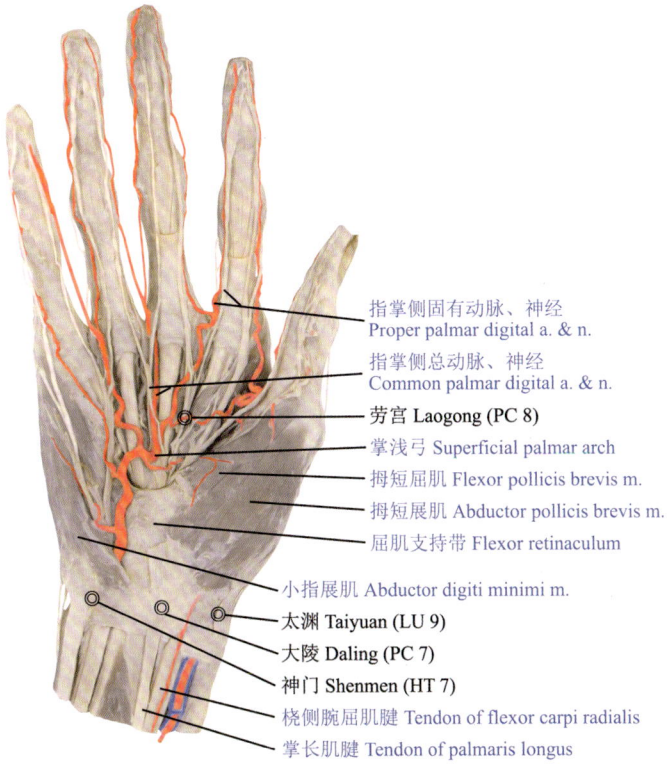

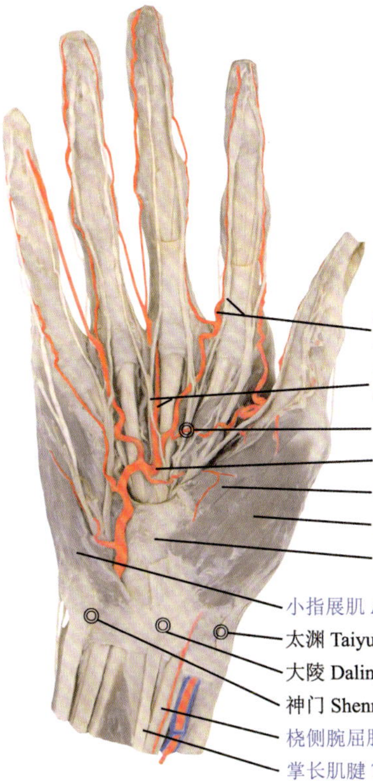
指掌侧固有动脉、神经
Proper palmar digital a. & n.
指掌侧总动脉、神经
Common palmar digital a. & n.
劳宫 Laogong (PC 8)
掌浅弓 Superficial palmar arch
拇短屈肌 Flexor pollicis brevis m.
拇短展肌 Abductor pollicis brevis m.
屈肌支持带 Flexor retinaculum
小指展肌 Abductor digiti minimi m.
太渊 Taiyuan (LU 9)
大陵 Daling (PC 7)
神门 Shenmen (HT 7)
桡侧腕屈肌腱 Tendon of flexor carpi radialis
掌长肌腱 Tendon of palmaris longus

图 5-38　腕手掌腧穴层次解剖（4）

Fig.5-38　Layered anatomy of acupoints on the wrist and palm (4)

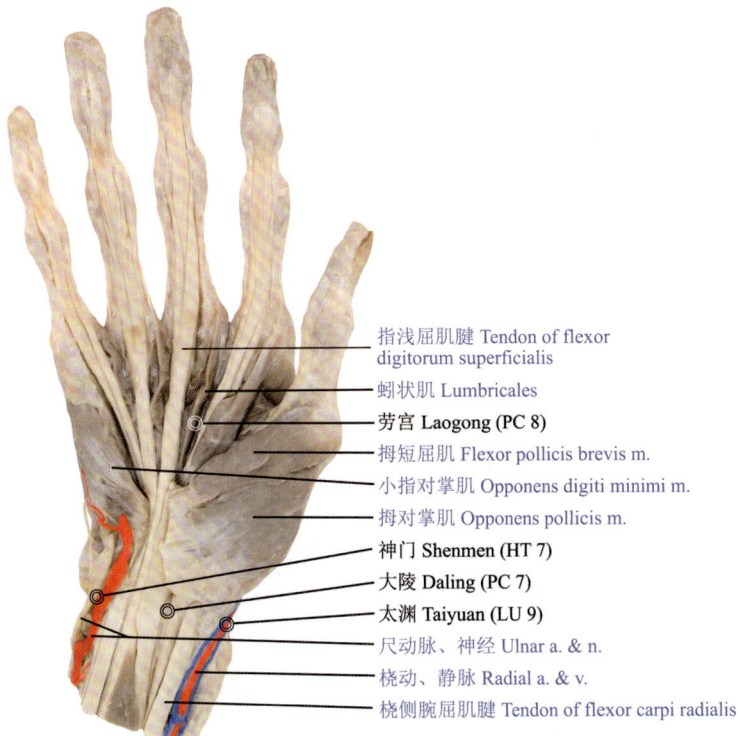

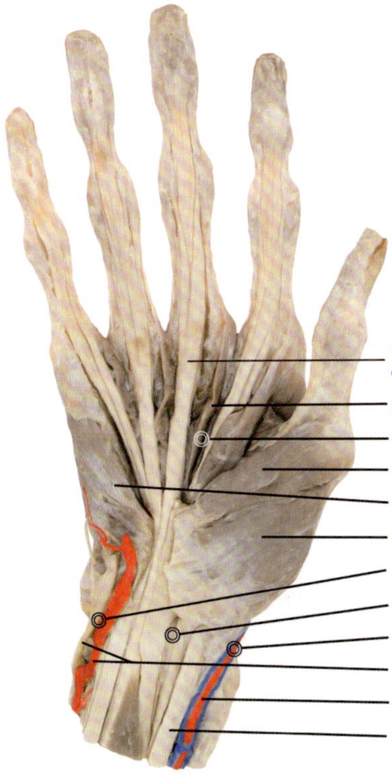
指浅屈肌腱 Tendon of flexor digitorum superficialis
蚓状肌 Lumbricales
劳宫 Laogong (PC 8)
拇短屈肌 Flexor pollicis brevis m.
小指对掌肌 Opponens digiti minimi m.
拇对掌肌 Opponens pollicis m.
神门 Shenmen (HT 7)
大陵 Daling (PC 7)
太渊 Taiyuan (LU 9)
尺动脉、神经 Ulnar a. & n.
桡动、静脉 Radial a. & v.
桡侧腕屈肌腱 Tendon of flexor carpi radialis

图 5-39　腕手掌腧穴层次解剖（5）

Fig.5-39　Layered anatomy of acupoints on the wrist and palm (5)

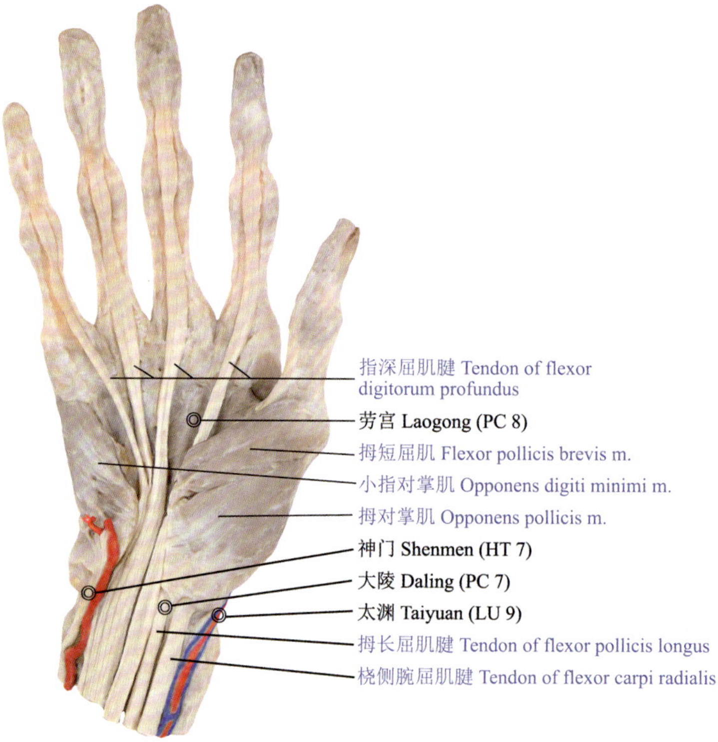

图 5–40　腕手掌腧穴层次解剖（6）

Fig.5-40　Layered anatomy of acupoints on the wrist and palm (6)

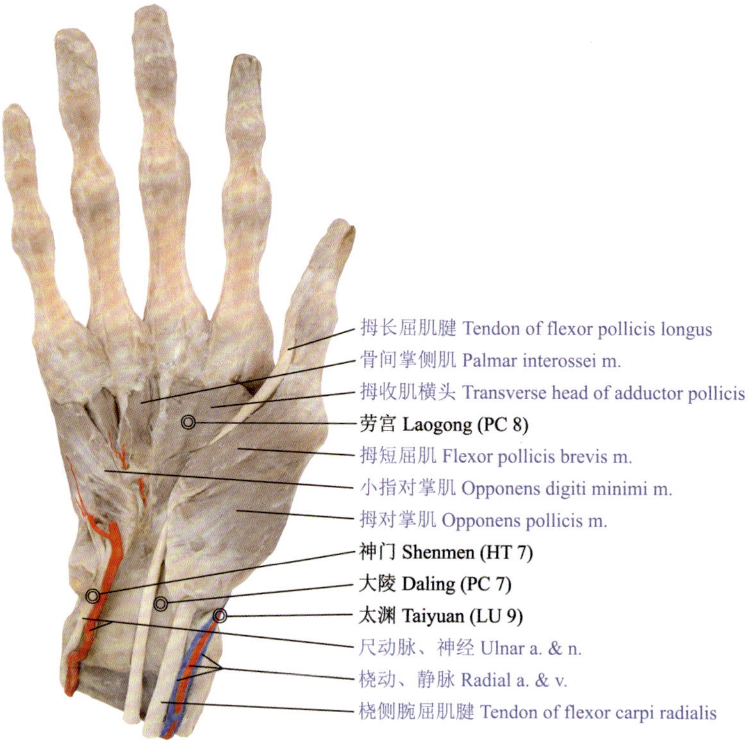

图 5–41　腕手掌腧穴层次解剖（7）

Fig.5-41　Layered anatomy of acupoints on the wrist and palm (7)

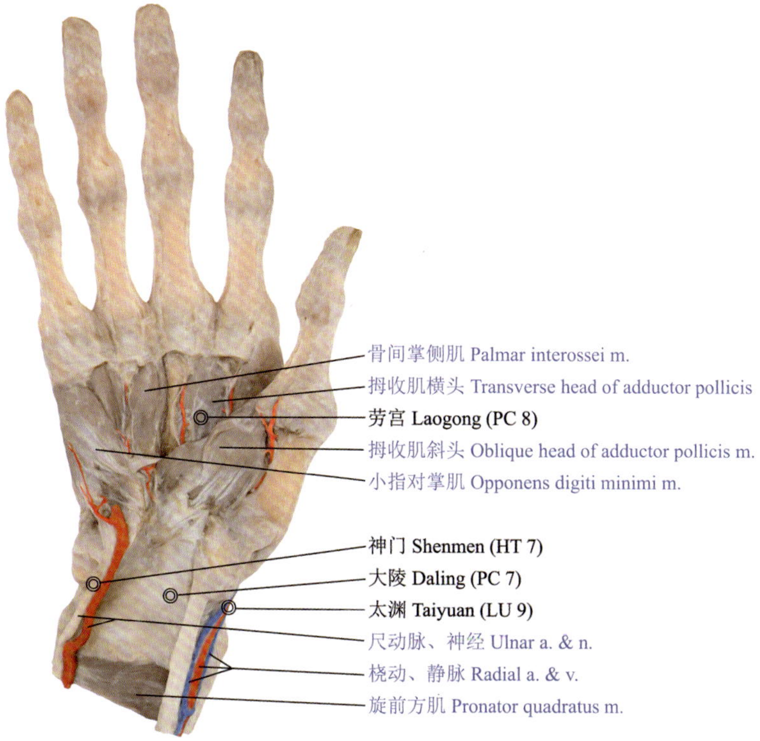
骨间掌侧肌 Palmar interossei m.
拇收肌横头 Transverse head of adductor pollicis
劳宫 Laogong (PC 8)
拇收肌斜头 Oblique head of adductor pollicis m.
小指对掌肌 Opponens digiti minimi m.
神门 Shenmen (HT 7)
大陵 Daling (PC 7)
太渊 Taiyuan (LU 9)
尺动脉、神经 Ulnar a. & n.
桡动、静脉 Radial a. & v.
旋前方肌 Pronator quadratus m.

图 5–42　腕手掌腧穴层次解剖（8）

Fig.5-42　Layered anatomy of acupoints on the wrist and palm (8)

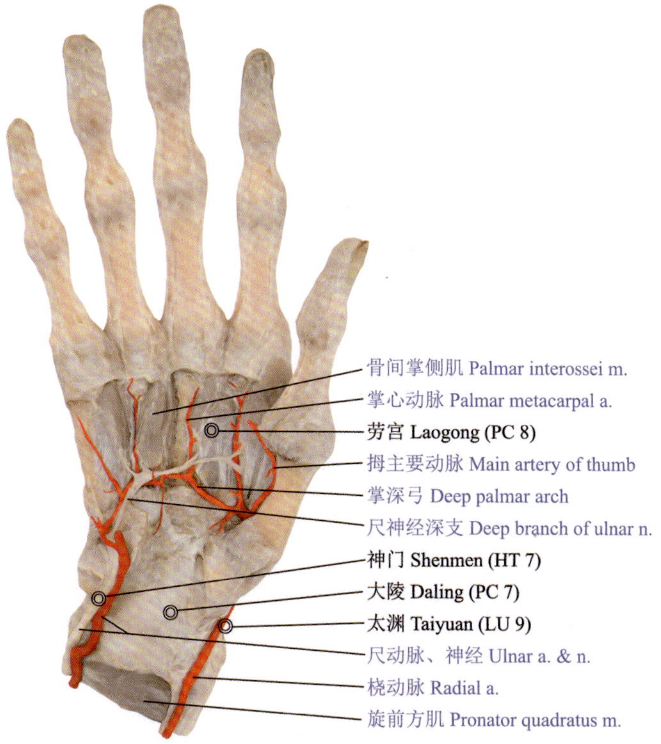
骨间掌侧肌 Palmar interossei m.
掌心动脉 Palmar metacarpal a.
劳宫 Laogong (PC 8)
拇主要动脉 Main artery of thumb
掌深弓 Deep palmar arch
尺神经深支 Deep branch of ulnar n.
神门 Shenmen (HT 7)
大陵 Daling (PC 7)
太渊 Taiyuan (LU 9)
尺动脉、神经 Ulnar a. & n.
桡动脉 Radial a.
旋前方肌 Pronator quadratus m.

图 5–43　腕手掌腧穴层次解剖（9）

Fig.5-43　Layered anatomy of acupoints on the wrist and palm (9)

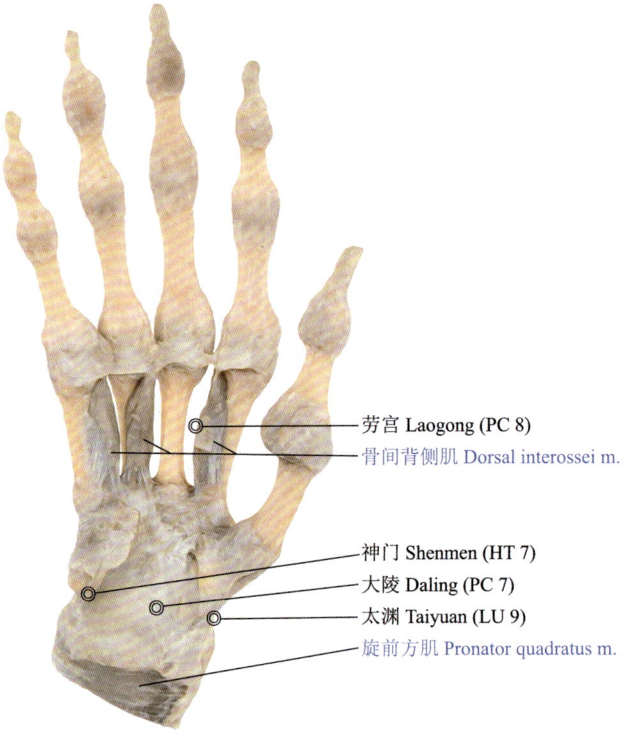

图 5-44　腕手掌腧穴层次解剖（10）
Fig.5-44　Layered anatomy of acupoints on the wrist and palm (10)

第七节　腕手背腧穴
Section 7　Acupoints on the back of the wrist and hand

一、阳溪

【定位】腕背侧横纹的桡侧端，拇指翘起，当拇短伸肌腱与拇长伸肌腱之间的凹陷中。

【操作】直刺 0.5 ～ 0.8 寸。

【主治】头痛，目赤肿痛，齿痛，咽喉肿痛，手腕痛。

【进针层次】①皮肤；②皮下组织（内有桡神经浅支的分支和头静脉）；③拇短伸肌腱和拇长伸肌腱之间；④桡侧腕长伸肌腱；⑤桡动、静脉（图 5-45 ～图 5-52）。

1. Yangxi (LI 5)

【Location】When the thumb is raised upward, the acupoint is located at the radial end of the dorsal transverse crease of the wrist, and in the depression between the extensor pollicis brevis tendon and the extensor pollicis longus tendon.

【Method】Puncture perpendicularly 0.5-0.8 cun.

【Indications】Headache, pain and swelling in the eyes, toothache, sore throat, and pain in the wrist.

【Stratified anatomy】①Skin; ②Subcutaneous tissue (There are branches of the superficial branches of the radial n., and cephalic v..); ③Between the extensor pollicis brevis tendon and the extensor pollicis longus tendon; ④Extensor carpi radialis longus tendon; ⑤Radial a. & v. (Fig.5-45 ~ Fig.5-52).

二、阳池

【定位】腕背侧横纹上，指伸肌腱的尺侧缘凹陷中。

【操作】直刺 0.3 ～ 0.5 寸。

【主治】目赤肿痛，咽喉肿痛，耳聋，消渴，腕痛，肘臂痛。

【进针层次】①皮肤；②皮下组织（内有尺神经的手背支和前臂后皮神经的分支，贵要静脉）；③指伸肌腱和小指伸肌腱之间（图 5–45 ～图 5–52）。

2. Yangchi (TE 4)

【Location】On the dorsal transverse crease of the wrist, and in the depression on the ulnar aspect of the extensor digitorum tendons.

【Method】Puncture perpendicularly 0.3-0.5 cun.

【Indications】Pain and swelling in the eyes, sore throat, deafness, wasting thirst disorder, pain in the wrist, and pain in the elbow and arm.

【Stratified anatomy】①Skin; ②Subcutaneous tissue (There are branches of the dorsal branch of the ulnar n. and posterior cutaneous n., and basilic v..); ③Between the extensor digitorum tendons and extensor digiti minimi tendon (Fig.5-45 ~ Fig.5-52).

三、腕骨

【定位】第 5 掌骨底与三角骨之间的赤白肉际凹陷中。

【操作】直刺 0.3 ～ 0.5 寸。

【主治】头项强痛，耳鸣，黄疸，消渴，热病，指挛腕痛。

【进针层次】①皮肤；②皮下组织（内有前臂内侧皮神经，尺神经掌支和尺神经手背支的分支）；③小指展肌；④豆掌韧带（图 5–45 ～图 5–52）。

3. Wangu (SI 4)

【Location】In the depression of the red and white skin between the bottom of the 5th metacarpal bone and triquetral bone.

【Method】Puncture perpendicularly 0.3-0.5 cun.

【Indications】Stiffness and pain in the head and neck, tinnitus, jaundice, wasting thirst disorder, febrile disease, and spasmodic pain in the wrist and fingers.

【Stratified anatomy】①Skin; ②Subcutaneous tissue (There are branches of the medial cutaneous n. of the forearm, palmar branch of ulnar n., and the dorsal branch of ulnar n..);

③Abductor digiti minimi m.; ④Pisometacarpal lig. (Fig.5-45 ~ Fig.5-52).

四、合谷

【定位】第 2 掌骨桡侧的中点。

【操作】直刺 0.5 ～ 1 寸。

【主治】头痛，齿痛，目赤肿痛，咽喉肿痛，鼻衄，耳聋，口噤，口㖞，发热，无汗，多汗，经闭，滞产，腹痛，便秘，上肢疼痛、不遂。

【进针层次】①皮肤；②皮下组织（内有桡神经浅支的分支和头静脉起始部）；③第 1 骨间背侧肌；④拇收肌（图 5–45 ～图 5–52）。

4. Hegu (LI 4)

【Location】At the midpoint of the radial aspect of the 2nd metacarpal bone.

【Method】Puncture perpendicularly 0.5-1 cun.

【Indications】Headache, toothache, pain and swelling in the eyes, sore throat, epistaxis, deafness, lockjaw, deviated mouth, fever, no sweating, profuse sweating, amenorrhea, delayed labour, abdominal pain, constipation, and pain and paralysis in the upper limb.

【Stratified anatomy】①Skin; ②Subcutaneous tissue (There are branches of the superficial branches of the radial n., and the beginning part of cephalic v..); ③The 1st dorsal interossei m.; ④Adductor pollcis m. (Fig.5-45 ~ Fig.5-52).

五、中渚

【定位】第 4、第 5 掌骨之间，第 4 掌指关节后凹陷中。

【操作】直刺 0.3 ～ 0.5 寸。

【主治】头痛，目赤，耳鸣，耳聋，咽喉肿痛，热病，消渴，手指屈伸不利，肘臂肩背疼痛。

【进针层次】①皮肤；②皮下组织（内有尺神经手背支的分支和手背静脉网的尺侧部）；③第 4 骨间背侧肌（图 5–45 ～图 5–52）。

5. Zhongzhu (TE 3)

【Location】Between the 4th and 5th metacarpal bones, and in the depression posterior to the 4th metacarpophalangeal joint.

【Method】Puncture perpendicularly 0.3-0.5 cun.

【Indications】Headache, redness in the eye, tinnitus, deafness, sore throat, febrile disease, wasting thirst disorder, limited finger flexion and extension, and pain in the elbow, arm, shoulder, and back.

【Stratified anatomy】①Skin; ②Subcutaneous tissue (There are branches of the dorsal branch of ulnar n. and ulnar part of the dorsal venous rete of hand.); ③The 4th dorsal interossei m. (Fig.5-45 ~ Fig.5-52).

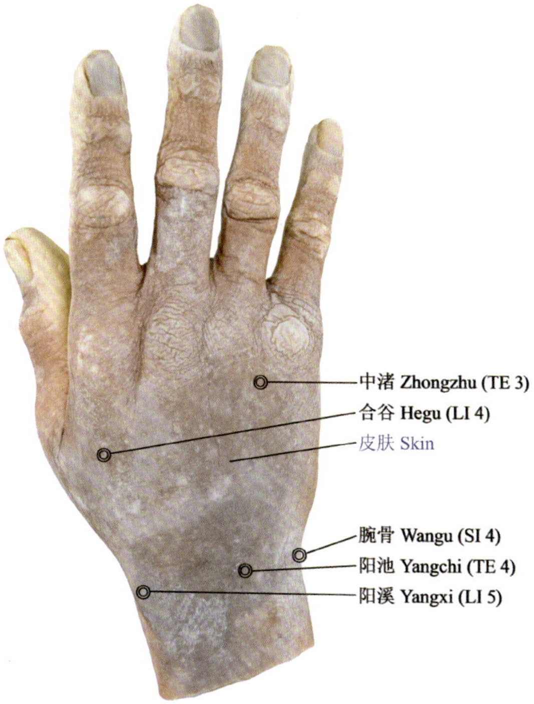

图 5-45　腕手背腧穴层次解剖（1）

Fig.5-45　Layered anatomy of acupoints on the back of the wrist and hand (1)

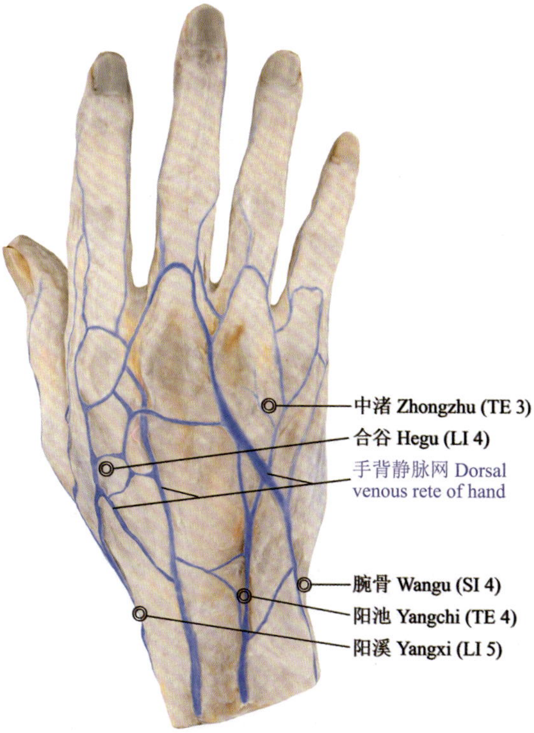

图 5-46　腕手背腧穴层次解剖（2）

Fig.5-46　Layered anatomy of acupoints on the back of the wrist and hand (2)

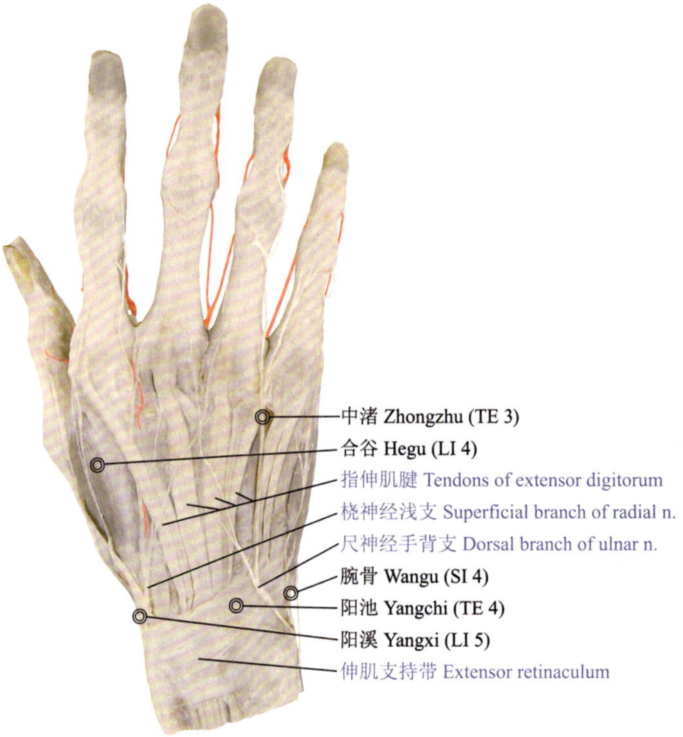
中渚 Zhongzhu (TE 3)
合谷 Hegu (LI 4)
指伸肌腱 Tendons of extensor digitorum
桡神经浅支 Superficial branch of radial n.
尺神经手背支 Dorsal branch of ulnar n.
腕骨 Wangu (SI 4)
阳池 Yangchi (TE 4)
阳溪 Yangxi (LI 5)
伸肌支持带 Extensor retinaculum

图 5–47　腕手背腧穴层次解剖（3）

Fig.5-47　Layered anatomy of acupoints on the back of the wrist and hand (3)

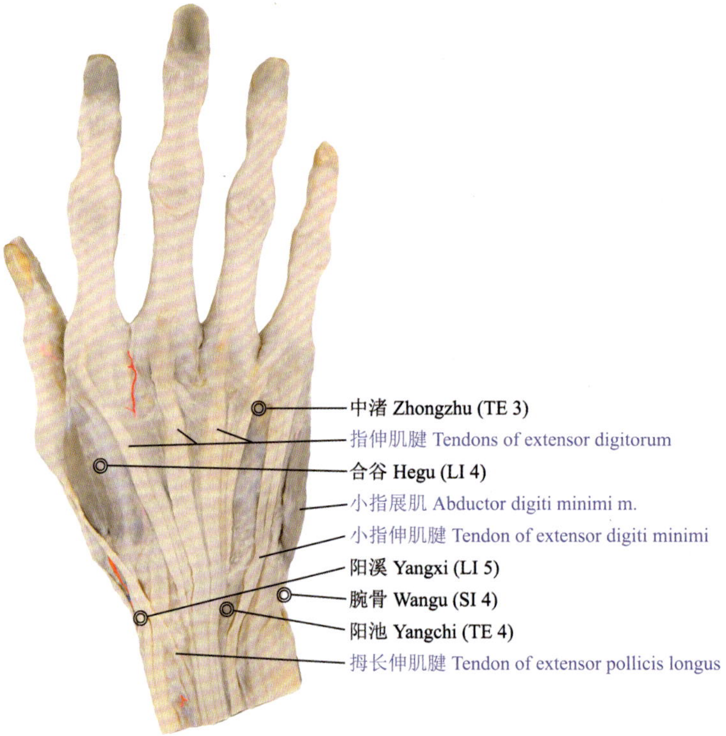
中渚 Zhongzhu (TE 3)
指伸肌腱 Tendons of extensor digitorum
合谷 Hegu (LI 4)
小指展肌 Abductor digiti minimi m.
小指伸肌腱 Tendon of extensor digiti minimi
阳溪 Yangxi (LI 5)
腕骨 Wangu (SI 4)
阳池 Yangchi (TE 4)
拇长伸肌腱 Tendon of extensor pollicis longus

图 5–48　腕手背腧穴层次解剖（4）

Fig.5-48　Layered anatomy of acupoints on the back of the wrist and hand (4)

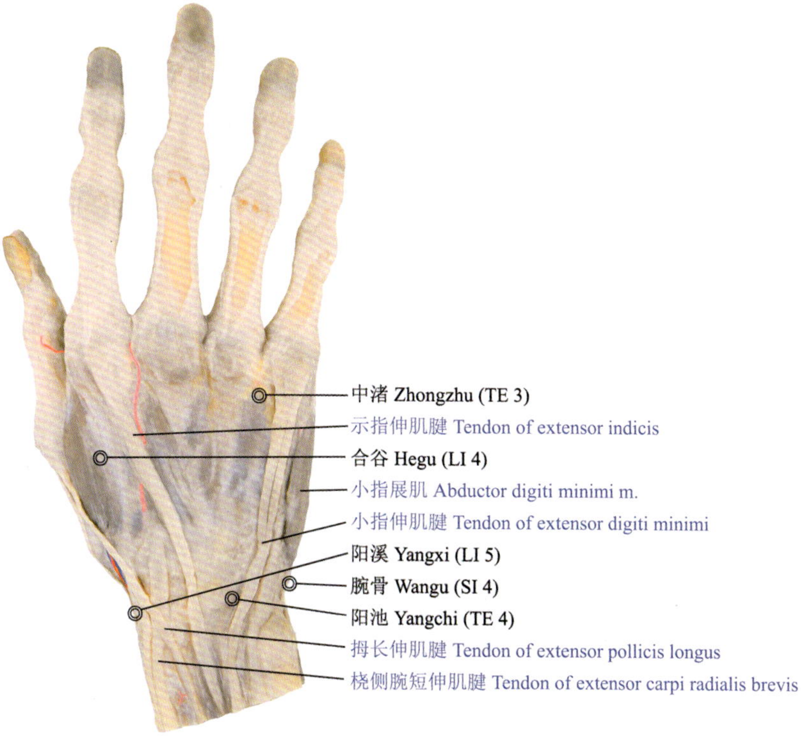
中渚 Zhongzhu (TE 3)
示指伸肌腱 Tendon of extensor indicis
合谷 Hegu (LI 4)
小指展肌 Abductor digiti minimi m.
小指伸肌腱 Tendon of extensor digiti minimi
阳溪 Yangxi (LI 5)
腕骨 Wangu (SI 4)
阳池 Yangchi (TE 4)
拇长伸肌腱 Tendon of extensor pollicis longus
桡侧腕短伸肌腱 Tendon of extensor carpi radialis brevis

图 5-49　腕手背腧穴层次解剖（5）

Fig.5-49　Layered anatomy of acupoints on the back of the wrist and hand (5)

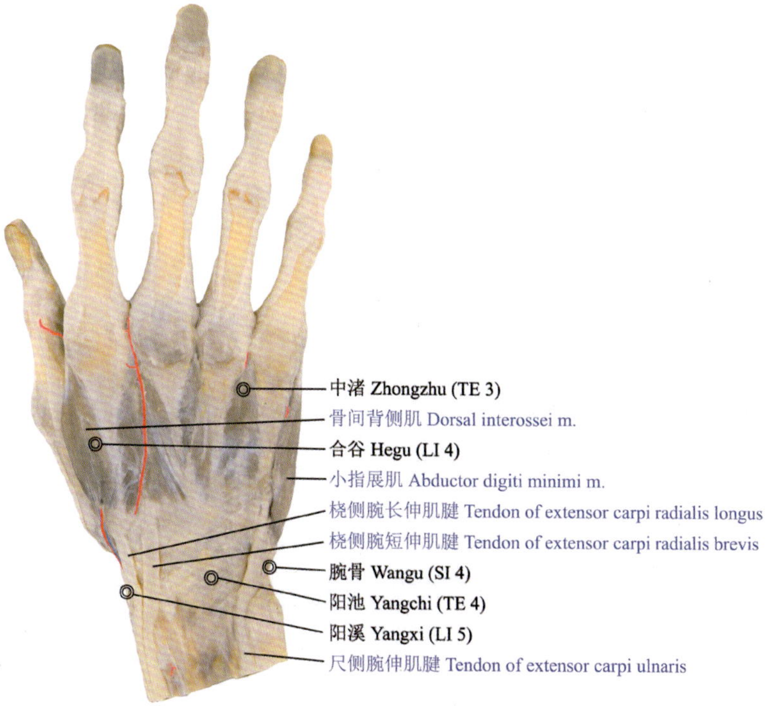
中渚 Zhongzhu (TE 3)
骨间背侧肌 Dorsal interossei m.
合谷 Hegu (LI 4)
小指展肌 Abductor digiti minimi m.
桡侧腕长伸肌腱 Tendon of extensor carpi radialis longus
桡侧腕短伸肌腱 Tendon of extensor carpi radialis brevis
腕骨 Wangu (SI 4)
阳池 Yangchi (TE 4)
阳溪 Yangxi (LI 5)
尺侧腕伸肌腱 Tendon of extensor carpi ulnaris

图 5-50　腕手背腧穴层次解剖（6）

Fig.5-50　Layered anatomy of acupoints on the back of the wrist and hand (6)

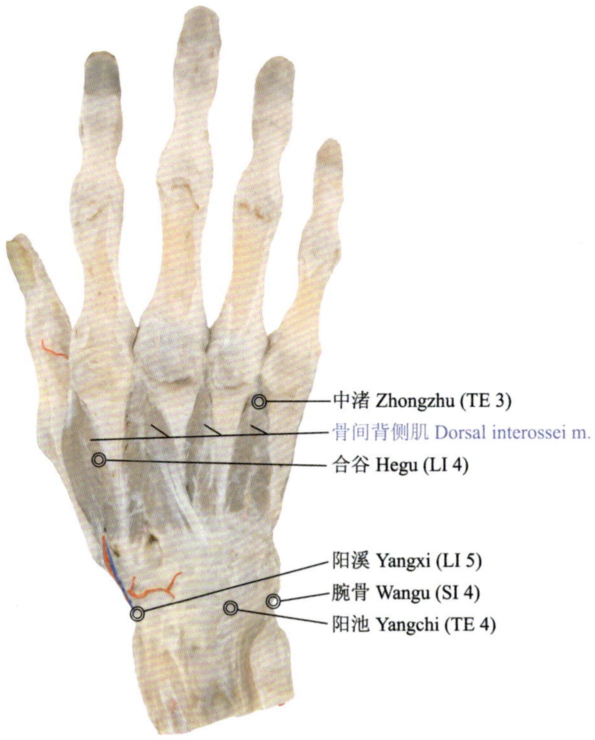
中渚 Zhongzhu (TE 3)
骨间背侧肌 Dorsal interossei m.
合谷 Hegu (LI 4)
阳溪 Yangxi (LI 5)
腕骨 Wangu (SI 4)
阳池 Yangchi (TE 4)

图 5-51　腕手背腧穴层次解剖（7）

Fig.5-51　Layered anatomy of acupoints on the back of the wrist and hand (7)

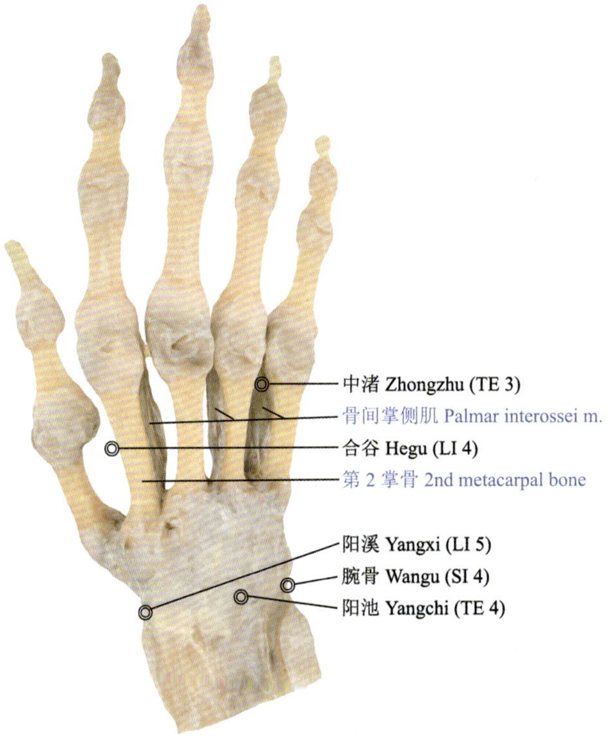
中渚 Zhongzhu (TE 3)
骨间掌侧肌 Palmar interossei m.
合谷 Hegu (LI 4)
第 2 掌骨 2nd metacarpal bone
阳溪 Yangxi (LI 5)
腕骨 Wangu (SI 4)
阳池 Yangchi (TE 4)

图 5-52　腕手背腧穴层次解剖（8）

Fig.5-52　Layered anatomy of acupoints on the back of the wrist and hand (8)

第六章　下肢腧穴层次解剖

Chapter 6　Layered Anatomy of Acupoints on the Lower Limb

第一节　大腿前面腧穴

Section 1　Acupoints on the anterior aspect of the thigh

一、阴廉

【定位】气冲穴直下2寸，耻骨结节下方。

【操作】直刺0.8～1寸。

【主治】小腹疼痛，股内侧痛，月经不调，带下。

【进针层次】①皮肤；②皮下组织（内有股神经前皮支的分支）；③长收肌；④短收肌；⑤大收肌上部（图6–1～图6–7）。

1. Yinlian (LR 11)

【Location】2 cun directly below Qichong (ST 30), and below the pubic tubercle.

【Method】Puncture perpendicularly 0.8-1 cun.

【Indications】Lower abdominal pain, medial thigh pain, irregular menstruation, and leucorrhoea.

【Stratified anatomy】①Skin; ②Subcutaneous tissue (There are branches of the anterior cutaneous branch of the femoral n..); ③Musculus adductor longus; ④The upper part of the musculus adductor magnus (Fig.6-1 ~ Fig.6-7).

二、伏兔

【定位】髌底上6寸，髂前上棘与髌底外侧端的连线上。

【操作】直刺1～2寸。

【主治】腰膝冷痛，下肢痿痹，疝气。

【进针层次】①皮肤；②皮下组织（内有股神经前皮支和股外侧皮神经的分支）；③股直肌；④旋股外侧动、静脉降支和股神经肌支；⑤股中间肌（图6–1～图6–7）。

2. Futu (ST 32)

【Location】6 cun above the base of the patella, and on the line connecting the anterosuperior iliac spine and the lateral border of the base of the patella.

【Method】Puncture perpendicularly 1-2 cun.

【Indications】Cold pain in the waist and knee, flaccidity and impediment of the lower limb, and hernia.

【Stratified anatomy】①Skin; ②Subcutaneous tissue (There are branches of the anterior cutaneous branch of femoral n. and lateral femoral cutaneous n..); ③Rectus femoris m.;

④Descending branch of the lateral femoral circumflex a. & v., muscular branch of femoral n.; ⑤Vastus intermedius m. (Fig.6-1 ~ Fig.6-7).

三、梁丘

【定位】髌底外侧端上 2 寸，股外侧肌和股直肌腱之间。

【操作】直刺 1 ～ 1.5 寸。

【主治】急性胃痛，乳痈，膝痛，下肢不遂。

【进针层次】①皮肤；②皮下组织（内有股神经前皮支和股外侧皮神经的分支）；③股直肌腱和股外侧肌之间；④旋股外侧动、静脉降支和股神经肌支；⑤股中间肌腱（图 6–1 ～图 6–7）。

3. Liangqiu (ST 34)

【Location】2 cun above the lateral border of the base of the patella, and between the musculus vastus lateralis and rectus femoris tendon.

【Method】Puncture perpendicularly 1-1.5 cun.

【Indications】Acute stomachache, acute mastitis, pain in the knee, and motor impediment in the lower limb.

【Stratified anatomy】①Skin; ②Subcutaneous tissue (There are branches of the anterior cutaneous branch of femoral n. and lateral femoral cutaneous n..); ③Between the rectus femoris tendon and musculus vastus lateralis; ④Descending branch of the lateral femoral circumflex a. & v., muscular branch of the femoral n.; ⑤Vastus intermedius tendon (Fig.6-1 ~ Fig.6-7).

四、血海

【定位】髌底内侧端上 2 寸，当股内侧肌隆起处。

【操作】直刺 1 ～ 1.2 寸。

【主治】月经不调，痛经，闭经，崩漏，瘾疹，湿疹，丹毒，膝痛，贫血。

【进针层次】①皮肤；②皮下组织（内有股神经前皮支的分支）；③股内侧肌（图 6–1 ～图 6–7）。

4. Xuehai (SP 10)

【Location】2 cun above the medial border of the base of the patella, and at the bulging area of the vastus medial m..

【Method】Puncture perpendicularly 1-1.2 cun.

【Indications】Irregular menstruation, dysmenorrhea, amenorrhea, metrorrhagia and metrostaxis, urticaria, eczema, erysipelas, pain in the knee, and anemia.

【Stratified anatomy】①Skin; ②Subcutaneous tissue (There are branches of the anterior cutaneous branch of femoral n..); ③Vastus medial m. (Fig.6-1 ~ Fig.6-7).

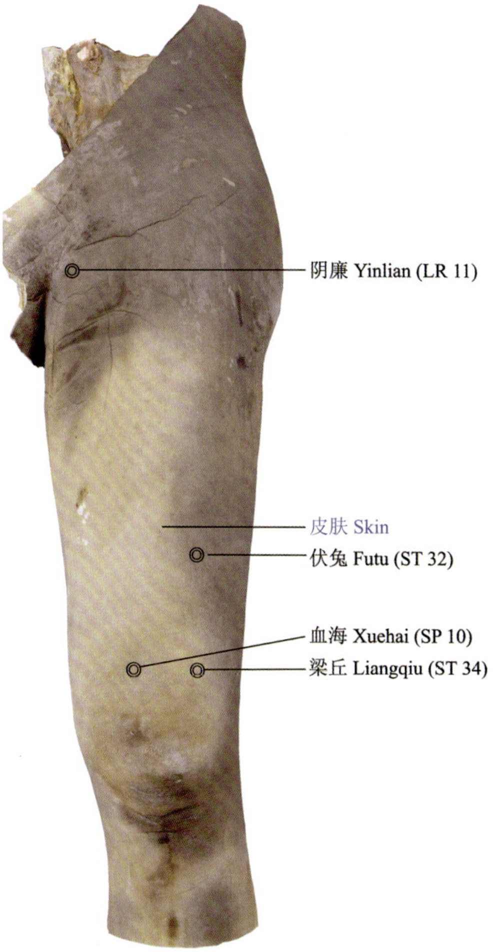

图 6-1　大腿前面腧穴层次解剖（1）
Fig.6-1　Layered anatomy of acupoints on the anterior aspect of the thigh (1)

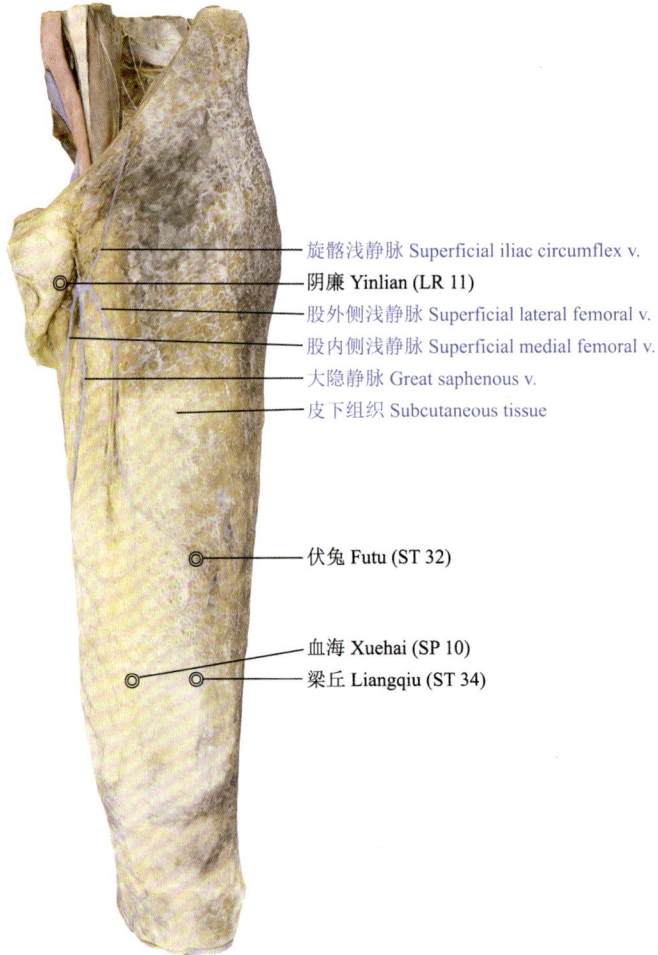

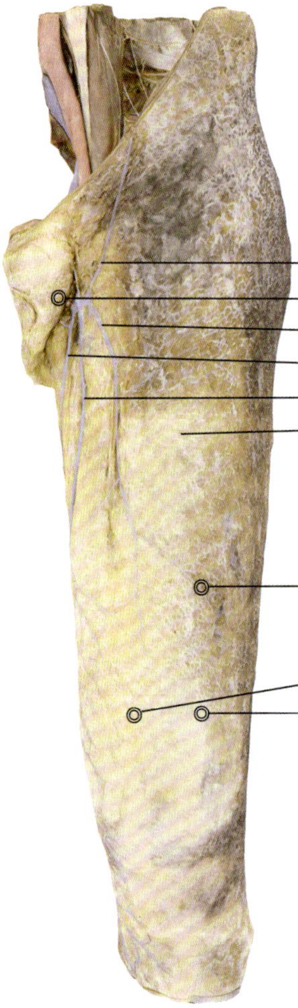
旋髂浅静脉 Superficial iliac circumflex v.
阴廉 Yinlian (LR 11)
股外侧浅静脉 Superficial lateral femoral v.
股内侧浅静脉 Superficial medial femoral v.
大隐静脉 Great saphenous v.
皮下组织 Subcutaneous tissue
伏兔 Futu (ST 32)
血海 Xuehai (SP 10)
梁丘 Liangqiu (ST 34)

图 6–2　大腿前面腧穴层次解剖（2）

Fig.6-2　Layered anatomy of acupoints on the anterior aspect of the thigh (2)

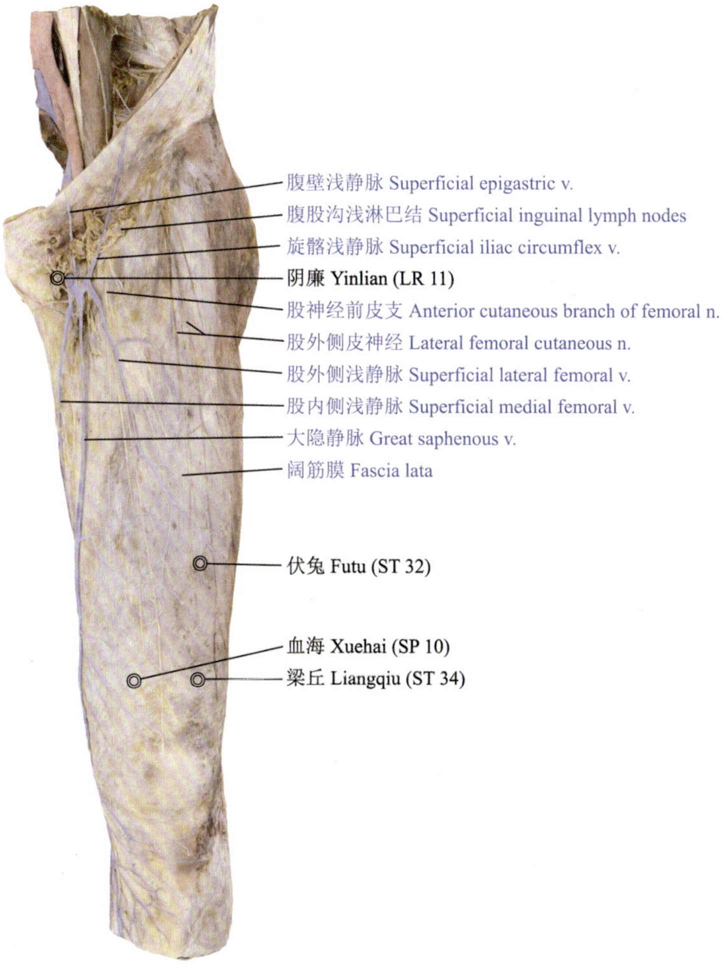
腹壁浅静脉 Superficial epigastric v.
腹股沟浅淋巴结 Superficial inguinal lymph nodes
旋髂浅静脉 Superficial iliac circumflex v.
阴廉 Yinlian (LR 11)
股神经前皮支 Anterior cutaneous branch of femoral n.
股外侧皮神经 Lateral femoral cutaneous n.
股外侧浅静脉 Superficial lateral femoral v.
股内侧浅静脉 Superficial medial femoral v.
大隐静脉 Great saphenous v.
阔筋膜 Fascia lata
伏兔 Futu (ST 32)
血海 Xuehai (SP 10)
梁丘 Liangqiu (ST 34)

图 6–3　大腿前面腧穴层次解剖（3）

Fig.6-3　Layered anatomy of acupoints on the anterior aspect of the thigh (3)

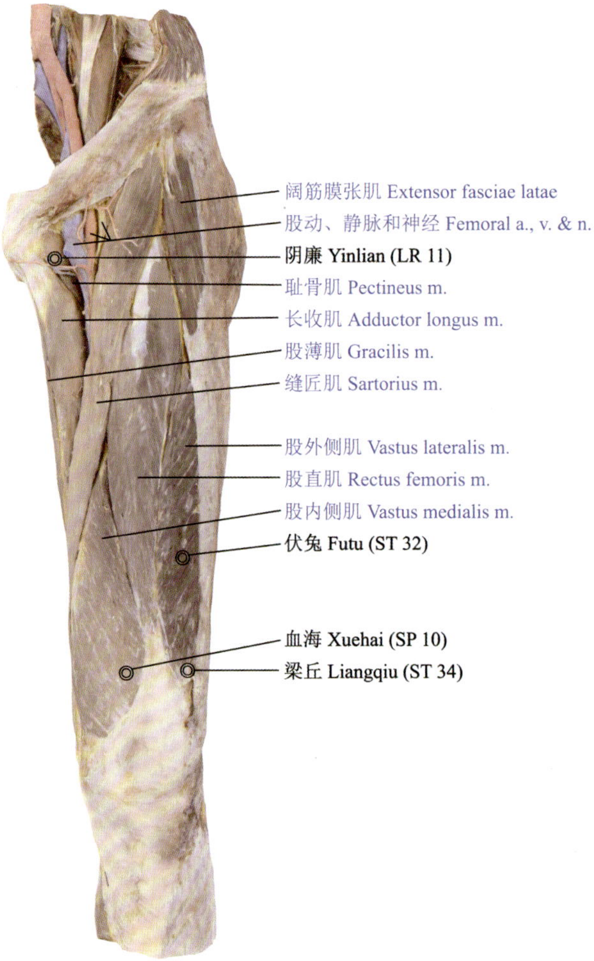
阔筋膜张肌 Extensor fasciae latae
股动、静脉和神经 Femoral a., v. & n.
阴廉 Yinlian (LR 11)
耻骨肌 Pectineus m.
长收肌 Adductor longus m.
股薄肌 Gracilis m.
缝匠肌 Sartorius m.
股外侧肌 Vastus lateralis m.
股直肌 Rectus femoris m.
股内侧肌 Vastus medialis m.
伏兔 Futu (ST 32)
血海 Xuehai (SP 10)
梁丘 Liangqiu (ST 34)

图 6–4　大腿前面腧穴层次解剖（4）

Fig.6-4　Layered anatomy of acupoints on the anterior aspect of the thigh (4)

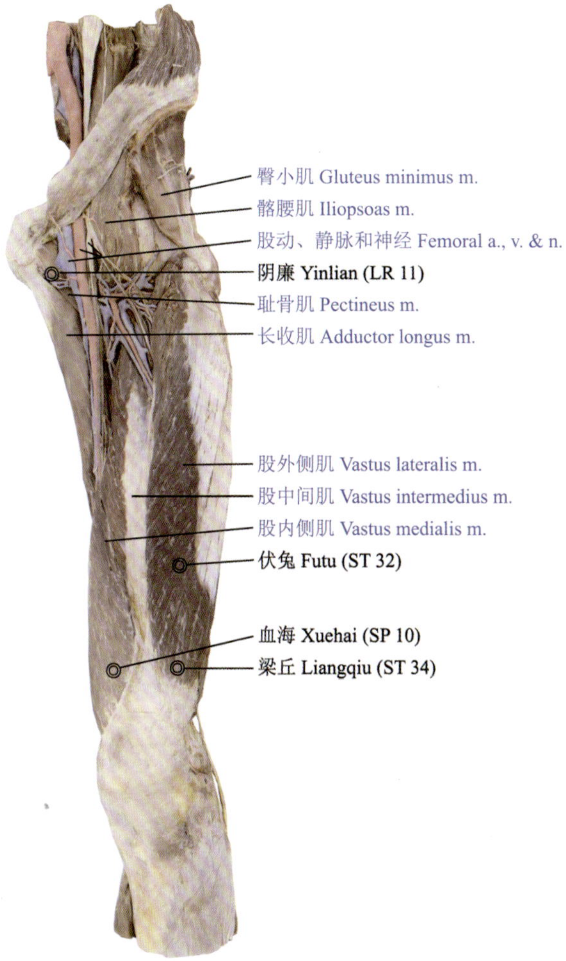
臀小肌 Gluteus minimus m.
髂腰肌 Iliopsoas m.
股动、静脉和神经 Femoral a., v. & n.
阴廉 Yinlian (LR 11)
耻骨肌 Pectineus m.
长收肌 Adductor longus m.
股外侧肌 Vastus lateralis m.
股中间肌 Vastus intermedius m.
股内侧肌 Vastus medialis m.
伏兔 Futu (ST 32)
血海 Xuehai (SP 10)
梁丘 Liangqiu (ST 34)

图 6–5　大腿前面腧穴层次解剖（5）
Fig.6-5　Layered anatomy of acupoints on the anterior aspect of the thigh (5)

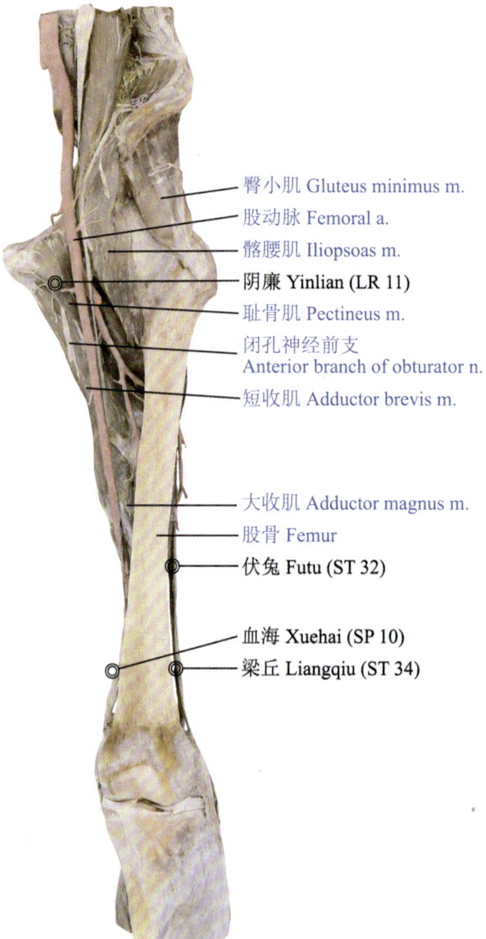
臀小肌 Gluteus minimus m.
股动脉 Femoral a.
髂腰肌 Iliopsoas m.
阴廉 Yinlian (LR 11)
耻骨肌 Pectineus m.
闭孔神经前支
Anterior branch of obturator n.
短收肌 Adductor brevis m.
大收肌 Adductor magnus m.
股骨 Femur
伏兔 Futu (ST 32)
血海 Xuehai (SP 10)
梁丘 Liangqiu (ST 34)

图 6–6　大腿前面腧穴层次解剖（6）

Fig.6-6　Layered anatomy of acupoints on the anterior aspect of the thigh (6)

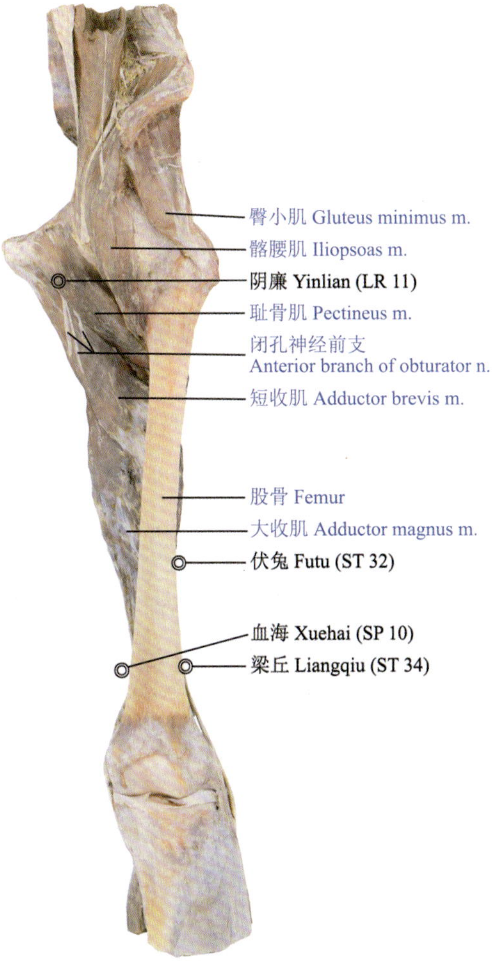

图 6-7 大腿前面腧穴层次解剖（7）

Fig.6-7 Layered anatomy of acupoints on the anterior aspect of the thigh (7)

第二节　臀部及大腿后面腧穴

Section 2　Acupoints on the posterior aspect of the buttock and thigh

一、秩边

【定位】平第 4 骶后孔，骶正中嵴旁开 3 寸。

【操作】直刺 1.5 ～ 3 寸。

【主治】腰骶痛，下肢痿痹，便秘，痔疾，阴部肿痛，小便不利。

【进针层次】①皮肤；②皮下组织（内有臀上皮神经的分支）；③臀大肌；④梨状肌和坐骨神经；⑤臀小肌（图 6–8 ～图 6–13）。

1. Zhibian (BL 54)

【Location】At the level of the 4th posterior sacral foramen, and 3 cun lateral to the sacral median ridge.

【Method】Puncture perpendicularly 1.5-3 cun.

【Indications】Pain in the loins and sacral region, flaccidity and impediment of lower limb, constipation, hemorrhoids, swelling and pain in the external genitali, and dysuria.

【Stratified anatomy】①Skin; ②Subcutaneous tissue (There are branches of the superior clunial n..); ③Gluteus maximus m.; ④Piriformis and sciatic n.; ⑤Gluteus minimus m. (Fig.6-8 ~ Fig.6-13).

二、环跳

【定位】股骨大转子最高点与骶管裂孔连线的外侧 1/3 与内侧 2/3 交点处。

【操作】直刺 2 ～ 3 寸。

【主治】腰腿痛，下肢痿痹，半身不遂。

【进针层次】①皮肤；②皮下组织（内有臀上皮神经的分支）；③臀大肌；④坐骨神经；⑤上孖肌、闭孔内肌和下孖肌（图 6–8 ～图 6–13）。

2. Huantiao (GB 30)

【Location】At the intersection point of the lateral 1/3 and medial 2/3 of the line connecting the prominence of the great trochanter and the sacral hiatus.

【Method】Puncture perpendicularly 2-3 cun.

【Indications】Pain in the lower back and leg, flaccidity and impediment of lower limb, and hemiplegia.

【Stratified anatomy】①Skin; ②Subcutaneous tissue (There are branches of the superior clunial n..); ③Gluteus maximus m.; ④Sciatic n.; ⑤Gemellus superior m., obturator intermus m. and gemellus inferior m. (Fig.6-8 ~ Fig.6-13).

三、承扶

【定位】臀股沟的中点。

【操作】直刺 1.5 ～ 2.5 寸。

【主治】腰腿痛，下肢痿痹，痔疾。

【进针层次】①皮肤；②皮下组织（内有臀下皮神经的分支）；③臀大肌；④股后皮神经；⑤股二头肌长头和半腱肌；⑥坐骨神经（图 6–8 ～图 6–13）。

3. Chengfu (BL 36)

【Location】At the midpoint of the transverse gluteal fold.

【Method】Puncture perpendicularly 1.5-2.5 cun.

【Indications】Pain in the lower back and leg, flaccidity and impediment of lower limb, and hemorrhoids.

【Stratified anatomy】①Skin; ②Subcutaneous tissue (There are branches of the inferior clunial n..); ③Gluteus maximus m.; ④Posterior clunial n.; ⑤Long head of biceps femoris m. and semitendinosus m.; ⑥Sciatic n. (Fig.6-8 ~ Fig.6-13).

四、殷门

【定位】承扶与委中连线上，承扶下 6 寸。

【操作】直刺 1.5 ～ 2.5 寸。

【主治】腰腿痛，下肢痿痹。

【进针层次】①皮肤；②皮下组织（内有股后皮神经）；③股二头肌长头和半腱肌；④坐骨神经（图 6–8 ～图 6–13）。

4. Yinmen (BL 37)

【Location】At the line connecting Chengfu (BL 36) acupoint and Weizhong (BL 40) acupoint, and 6 cun below Chengfu (BL 36) acupoint.

【Method】Puncture perpendicularly 1.5-2.5 cun.

【Indications】Pain in the lower back and leg, and flaccidity and impediment of lower limb.

【Stratified anatomy】①Skin; ②Subcutaneous tissue (There are branches of the posterior femoral cutaneous n..); ③Long head of the biceps femoris m. and semitendinosus m.; ④Sciatic n. (Fig.6-8 ~ Fig.6-13).

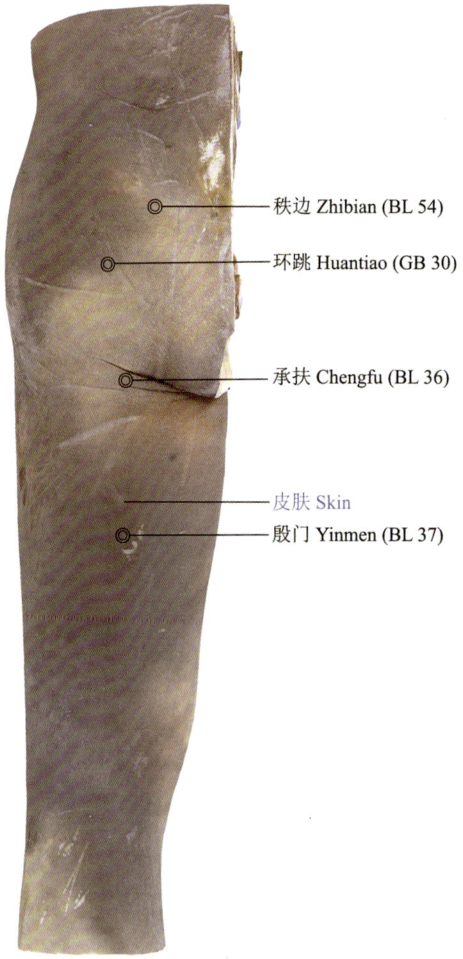

图 6-8　臀部及大腿后面腧穴层次解剖（1）
Fig.6-8　Layered anatomy of acupoints on the posterior aspect of the buttock and thigh (1)

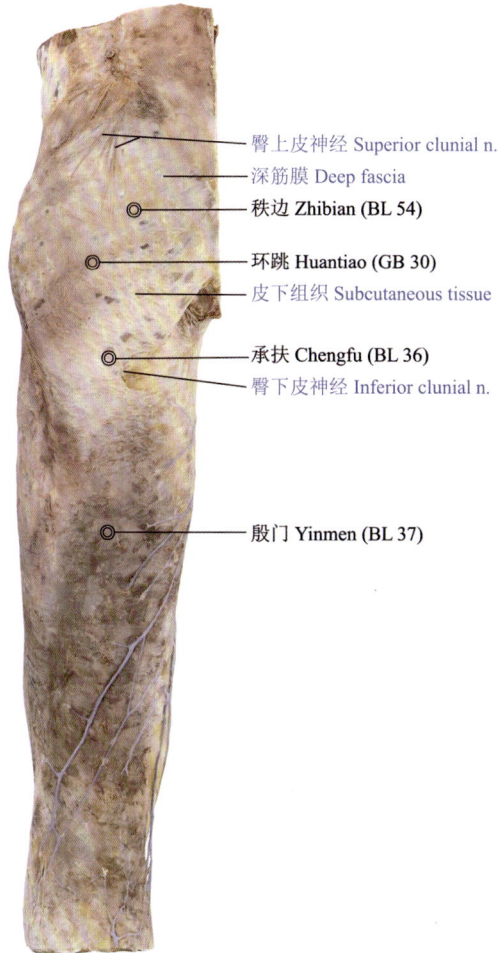

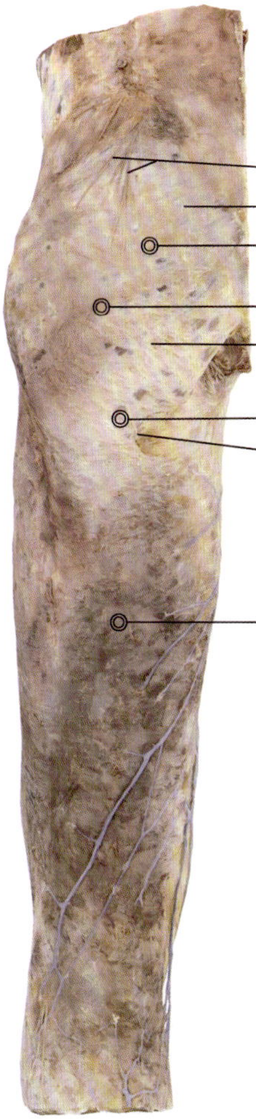
臀上皮神经 Superior clunial n.
深筋膜 Deep fascia
秩边 Zhibian (BL 54)
环跳 Huantiao (GB 30)
皮下组织 Subcutaneous tissue
承扶 Chengfu (BL 36)
臀下皮神经 Inferior clunial n.
殷门 Yinmen (BL 37)

图 6–9　臀部及大腿后面腧穴层次解剖（2）
Fig.6-9　Layered anatomy of acupoints on the posterior aspect of the buttock and thigh (2)

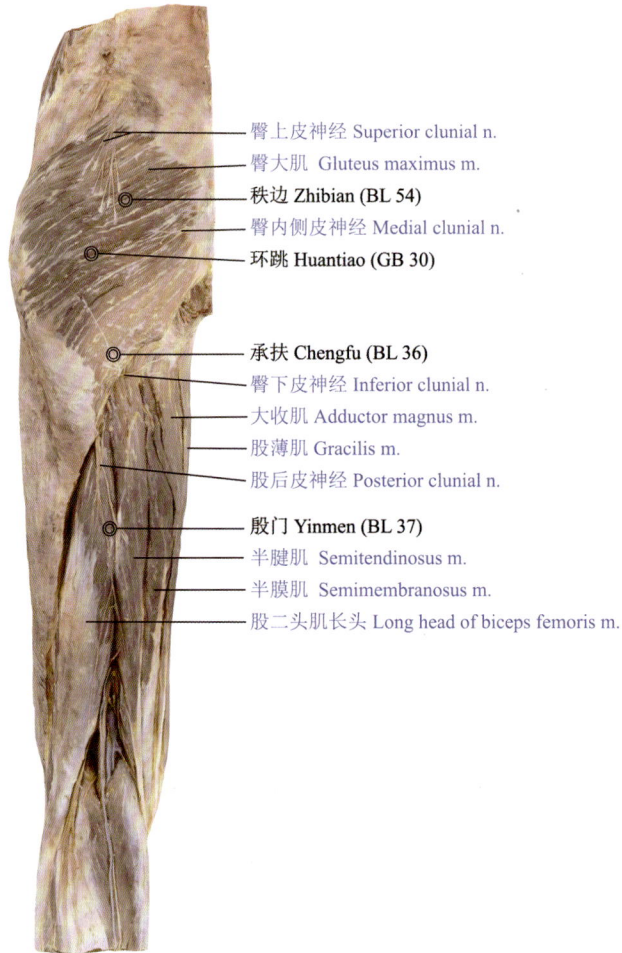

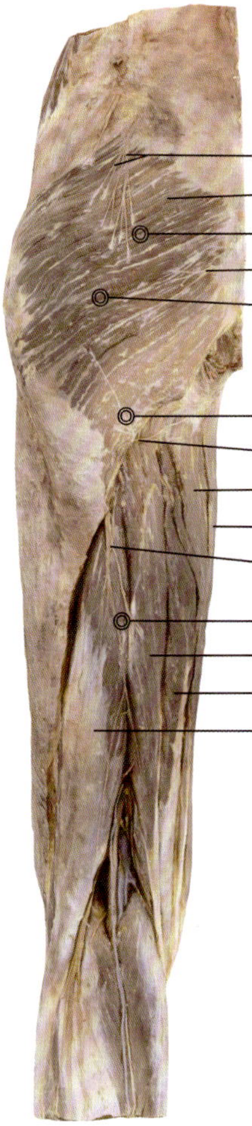
臀上皮神经 Superior clunial n.
臀大肌 Gluteus maximus m.
秩边 Zhibian (BL 54)
臀内侧皮神经 Medial clunial n.
环跳 Huantiao (GB 30)
承扶 Chengfu (BL 36)
臀下皮神经 Inferior clunial n.
大收肌 Adductor magnus m.
股薄肌 Gracilis m.
股后皮神经 Posterior clunial n.
殷门 Yinmen (BL 37)
半腱肌 Semitendinosus m.
半膜肌 Semimembranosus m.
股二头肌长头 Long head of biceps femoris m.

图 6–10　臀部及大腿后面腧穴层次解剖（3）

Fig.6-10　Layered anatomy of acupoints on the posterior aspect of the buttock and thigh (3)

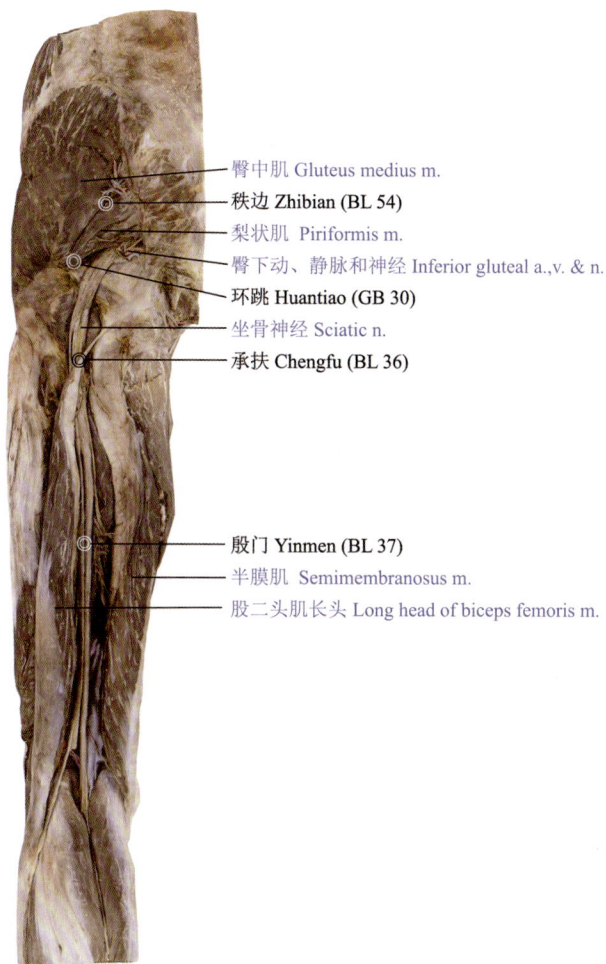

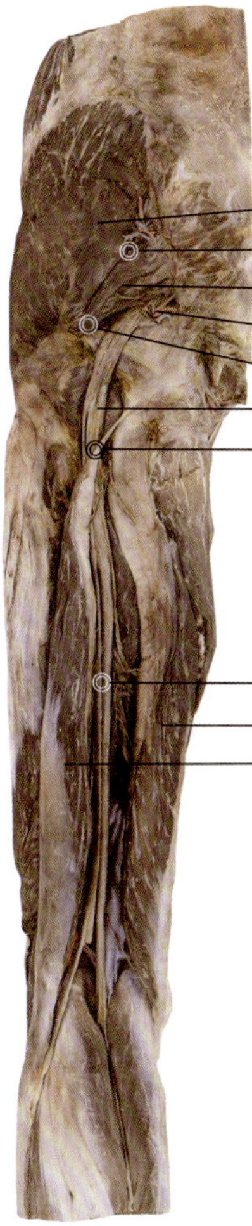
臀中肌 Gluteus medius m.
秩边 Zhibian (BL 54)
梨状肌 Piriformis m.
臀下动、静脉和神经 Inferior gluteal a.,v. & n.
环跳 Huantiao (GB 30)
坐骨神经 Sciatic n.
承扶 Chengfu (BL 36)
殷门 Yinmen (BL 37)
半膜肌 Semimembranosus m.
股二头肌长头 Long head of biceps femoris m.

图 6–11　臀部及大腿后面腧穴层次解剖（4）

Fig.6-11　Layered anatomy of acupoints on the posterior aspect of the buttock and thigh (4)

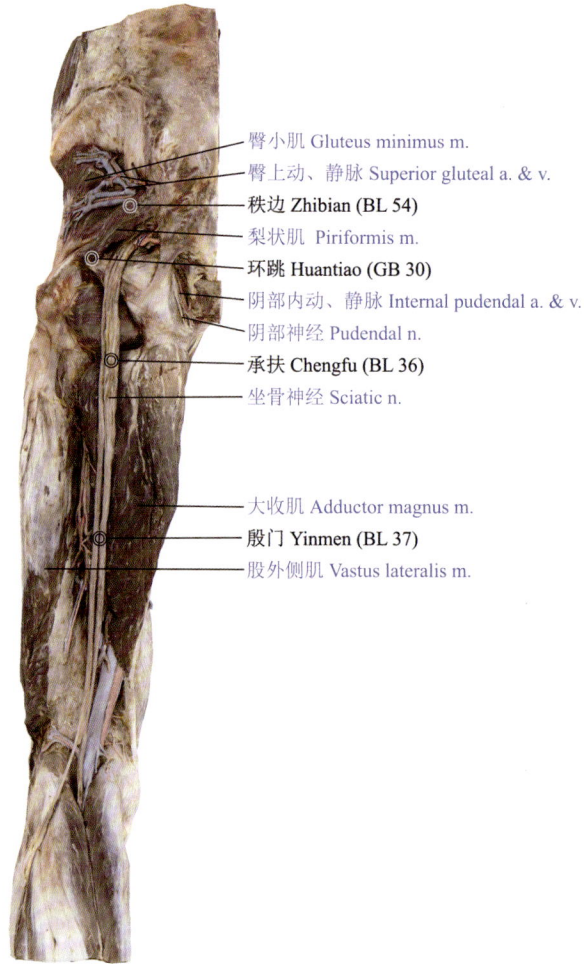

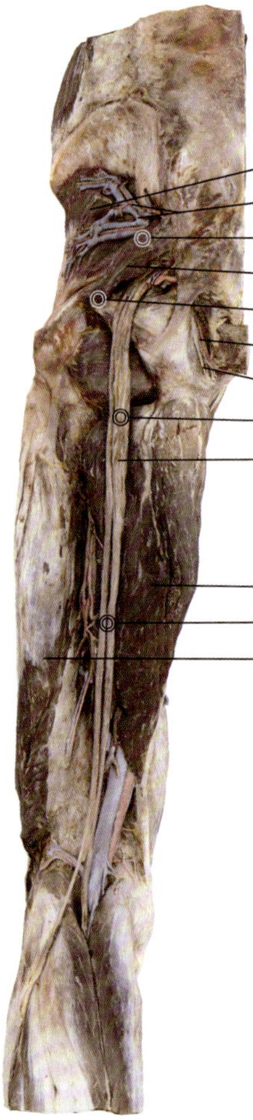
臀小肌 Gluteus minimus m.
臀上动、静脉 Superior gluteal a. & v.
秩边 Zhibian (BL 54)
梨状肌 Piriformis m.
环跳 Huantiao (GB 30)
阴部内动、静脉 Internal pudendal a. & v.
阴部神经 Pudendal n.
承扶 Chengfu (BL 36)
坐骨神经 Sciatic n.
大收肌 Adductor magnus m.
殷门 Yinmen (BL 37)
股外侧肌 Vastus lateralis m.

图 6–12　臀部及大腿后面腧穴层次解剖（5）

Fig.6-12　Layered anatomy of acupoints on the posterior aspect of the buttock and thigh (5)

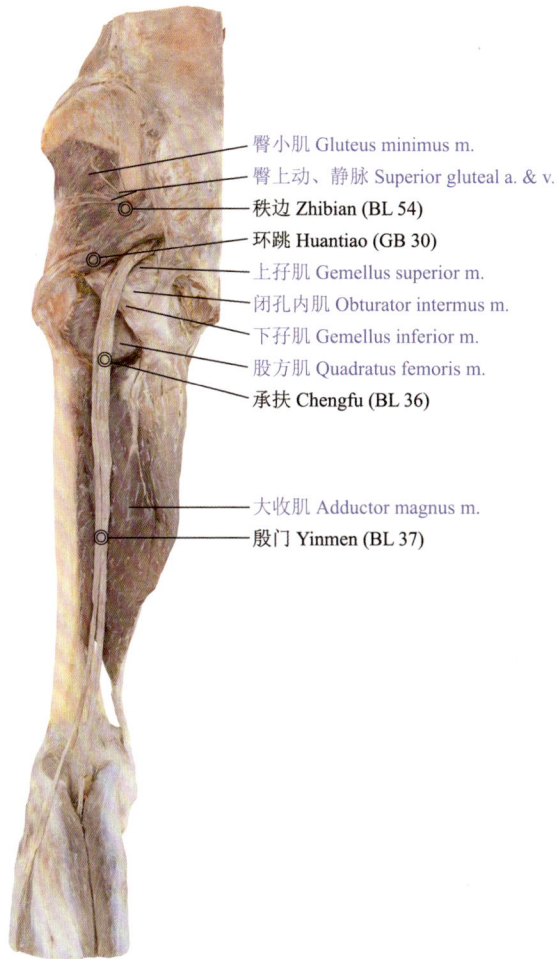

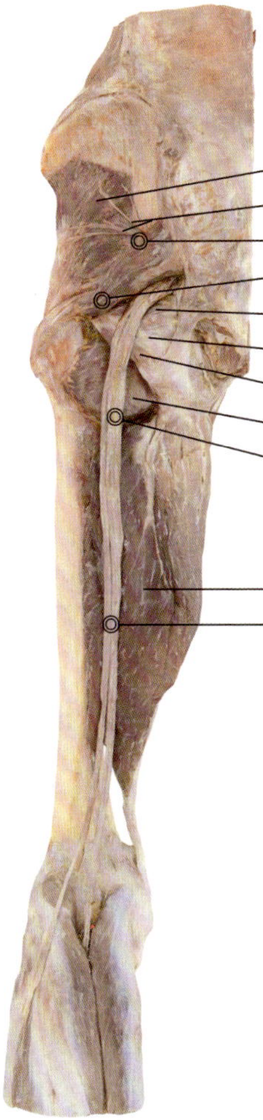
臀小肌 Gluteus minimus m.
臀上动、静脉 Superior gluteal a. & v.
秩边 Zhibian (BL 54)
环跳 Huantiao (GB 30)
上孖肌 Gemellus superior m.
闭孔内肌 Obturator intermus m.
下孖肌 Gemellus inferior m.
股方肌 Quadratus femoris m.
承扶 Chengfu (BL 36)
大收肌 Adductor magnus m.
殷门 Yinmen (BL 37)

图 6–13　臀部及大腿后面腧穴层次解剖（6）

Fig.6-13　Layered anatomy of acupoints on the posterior aspect of the buttock and thigh (6)

第三节　大腿外侧面腧穴

Section 3　Acupoints on the lateral aspect of the thigh

一、居髎

【定位】髂前上棘与股骨大转子最高点连线的中点处。

【操作】直刺 1 ～ 1.5 寸。

【主治】腰胯疼痛，下肢痿痹，疝气，少腹痛。

【进针层次】①皮肤；②皮下组织（内有髂腹下神经的外侧皮支）；③阔筋膜；④臀中肌；⑤臀小肌（图 6–14 ～图 6–20）。

1. Juliao (GB 29)

【Location】At the midpoint of the line connecting the anterosuperior iliac spine and the prominence of the great trochanter.

【Method】Puncture perpendicularly 1-1.5 cun.

【Indications】Pain in the loins and hip, flaccidity and impediment of lower limb, hernia, and pain in the lower abdomen.

【Stratified anatomy】①Skin; ②Subcutaneous tissue (There are lateral cutaneous branch of the iliohypogastric n..); ③Fascia lata; ④Gluteus medius m.; ⑤Gluteus minimus m. (Fig.6-14 ~ Fig.6-20).

二、风市

【定位】直立垂手，掌心贴于大腿外侧时，中指尖下，髂胫束后缘。

【操作】直刺 1 ～ 1.5 寸。

【主治】下肢痿痹，半身不遂，遍身瘙痒。

【进针层次】①皮肤；②皮下组织（内有股外侧皮神经的分支）；③髂胫束；④股外侧肌；⑤股中间肌（图 6–14 ～图 6–20）。

2. Fengshi (GB 31)

【Location】Standing upright with the palm pressed against the outer thigh, the acupoint is located below the middle fingertip, and at the posterior edge of the iliotibial tract.

【Method】Puncture perpendicularly 1-1.5 cun.

【Indications】Flaccidity and impediment of lower limb, hemiplegia, and general pruritus.

【Stratified anatomy】①Skin; ②Subcutaneous tissue (There are branches of the lateral femoral cutaneous n..); ③Iliotibial tract; ④Vastus lateralis m.; ⑤Vastus intermedius m. (Fig.6-14 ~ Fig.6-20).

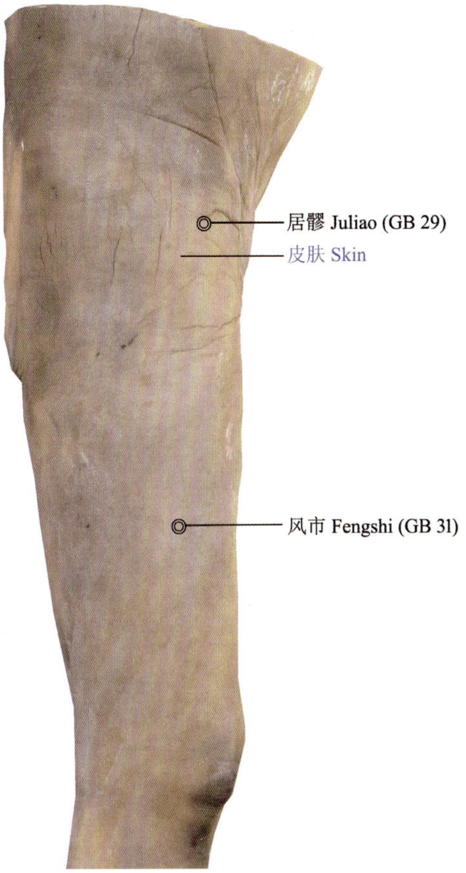

图 6–14　大腿外侧面腧穴层次解剖（1）
Fig.6-14　Layered anatomy of acupoints on the lateral aspect of the thigh (1)

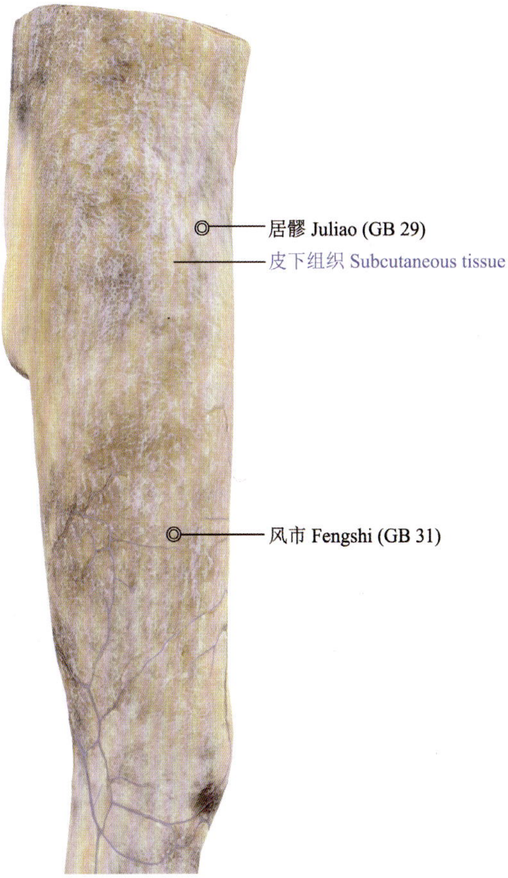

图 6–15　大腿外侧面腧穴层次解剖（2）
Fig.6-15　Layered anatomy of acupoints on the lateral aspect of the thigh (2)

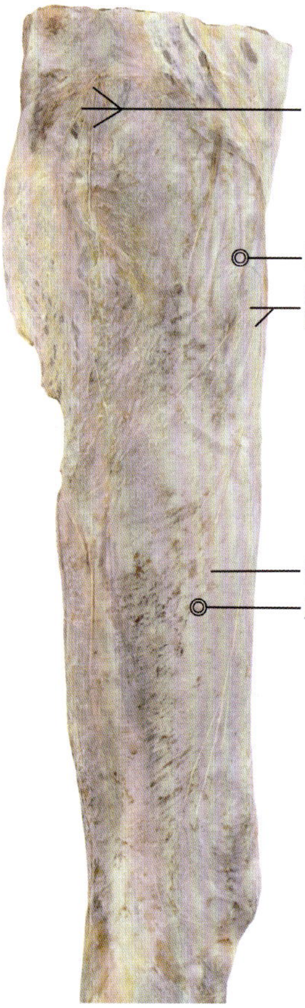
臀上皮神经 Superior clunial n.
居髎 Juliao (GB 29)
股外侧皮神经
Lateral femoral cutaneous n.
阔筋膜 Fascia lata
风市 Fengshi (GB 31)

图 6–16　大腿外侧面腧穴层次解剖（3）
Fig.6-16　Layered anatomy of acupoints on the lateral aspect of the thigh (3)

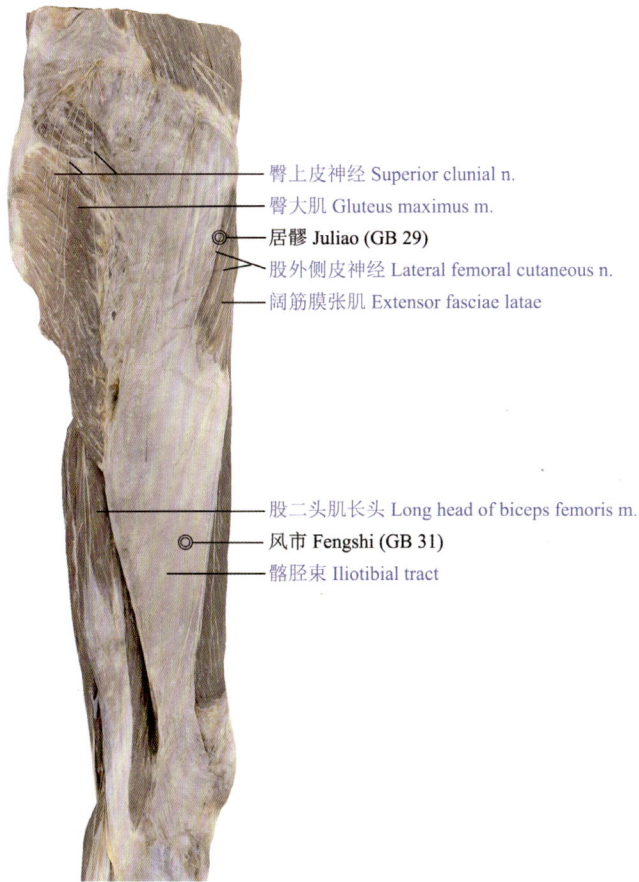

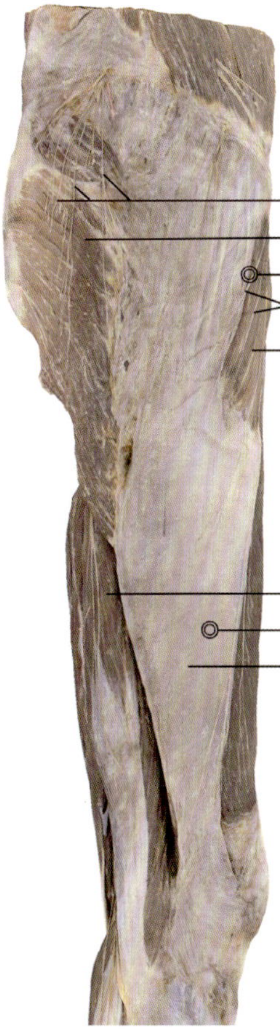
臀上皮神经 Superior clunial n.
臀大肌 Gluteus maximus m.
居髎 Juliao (GB 29)
股外侧皮神经 Lateral femoral cutaneous n.
阔筋膜张肌 Extensor fasciae latae
股二头肌长头 Long head of biceps femoris m.
风市 Fengshi (GB 31)
髂胫束 Iliotibial tract

图 6-17 大腿外侧面腧穴层次解剖（4）

Fig.6-17 Layered anatomy of acupoints on the lateral aspect of the thigh (4)

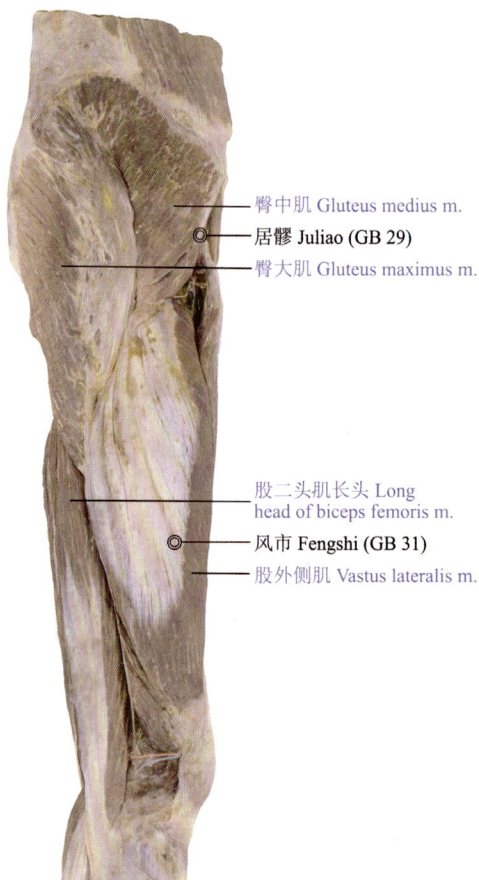

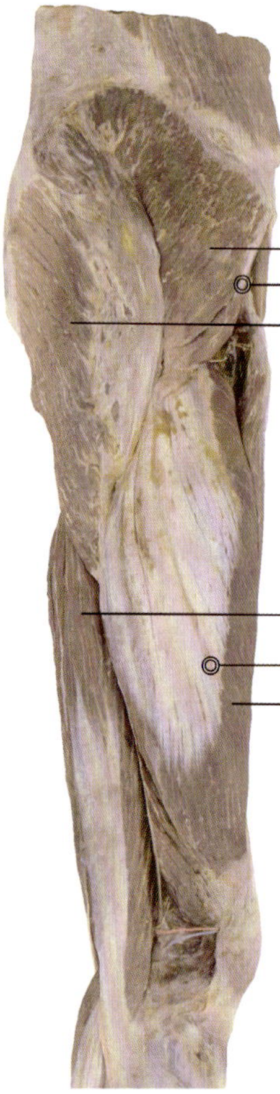
臀中肌 Gluteus medius m.
居髎 Juliao (GB 29)
臀大肌 Gluteus maximus m.
股二头肌长头 Long head of biceps femoris m.
风市 Fengshi (GB 31)
股外侧肌 Vastus lateralis m.

图 6–18　大腿外侧面腧穴层次解剖（5）
Fig.6-18　Layered anatomy of acupoints on the lateral aspect of the thigh (5)

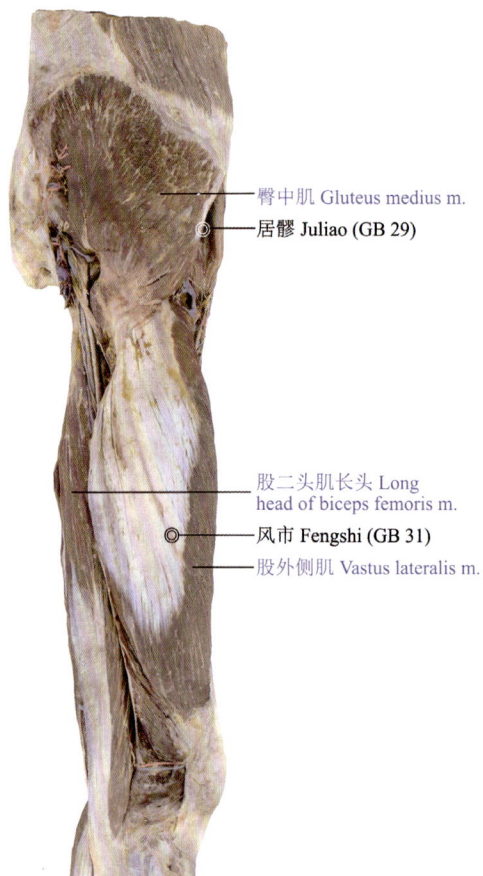

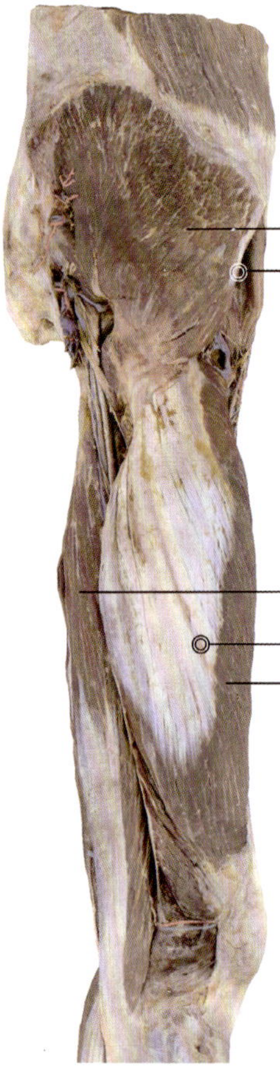
臀中肌 Gluteus medius m.
居髎 Juliao (GB 29)
股二头肌长头 Long head of biceps femoris m.
风市 Fengshi (GB 31)
股外侧肌 Vastus lateralis m.

图 6–19　大腿外侧面腧穴层次解剖（6）
Fig.6-19　Layered anatomy of acupoints on the lateral aspect of the thigh (6)

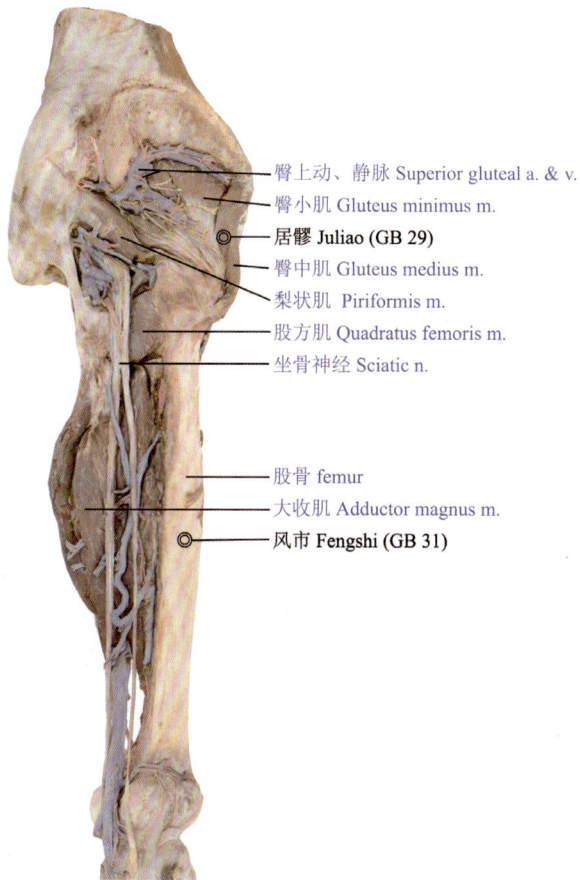

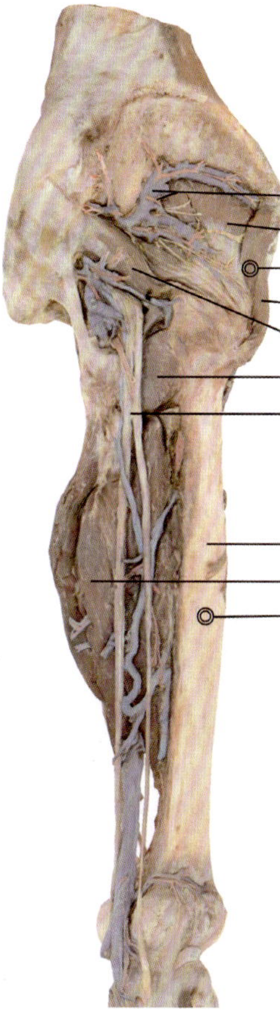
臀上动、静脉 Superior gluteal a. & v.
臀小肌 Gluteus minimus m.
居髎 Juliao (GB 29)
臀中肌 Gluteus medius m.
梨状肌 Piriformis m.
股方肌 Quadratus femoris m.
坐骨神经 Sciatic n.
股骨 femur
大收肌 Adductor magnus m.
风市 Fengshi (GB 31)

图 6–20　大腿外侧面腧穴层次解剖（7）
Fig.6-20　Layered anatomy of acupoints on the lateral aspect of the thigh (7)

第四节　小腿前面腧穴

Section 4　Acupoints on the anterior aspect of the lower leg

一、犊鼻

【定位】髌韧带外侧凹陷中。

【操作】屈膝 90°，向后内斜刺 1 ～ 1.5 寸。

【主治】膝痛，下肢痿痹。

【进针层次】①皮肤；②皮下组织（内有腓肠外侧皮神经和股神经前皮支的分支）；③髌韧带与髌外侧支持带之间；④膝关节囊；⑤翼状襞（图 6–21 ～图 6–28）。

1. Dubi (ST 35)

【Location】In the depression lateral to the patellar ligament.

【Method】Puncture obliquely backward 1-1.5 cun with the patient's knee flexed 90°.

【Indications】Pain in the knee, flaccidity and impediment of lower limb.

【Stratified anatomy】①Skin; ②Subcutaneous tissue (There are branches of the lateral sural cutaneous n. and the anterior cutaneous branch of femoral n..); ③Between the patellar lig. and the lateral patellar retinaculum; ④Capsula articularis genus; ⑤Alar folds (Fig.6-21 ~ Fig.6-28).

二、足三里

【定位】犊鼻下 3 寸，犊鼻与解溪穴的连线上。

【操作】直刺 1 ～ 2 寸。

【主治】胃痛，呕吐，腹胀，腹痛，肠鸣，完谷不化，泄泻，便秘，痢疾，乳痈，虚劳羸瘦，咳嗽，气喘，心悸，气短，头晕，失眠，癫狂，膝痛，下肢痿痹，水肿。

【进针层次】①皮肤；②皮下组织（内有腓肠外侧皮神经的分支）；③胫骨前肌；④腓深神经及胫前动、静脉；⑤小腿骨间膜；⑥胫骨后肌（图 6–21 ～图 6–28）。

2. Zusanli (ST 36)

【Location】3 cun below Dubi (ST 35) acupoint, and on the line connecting Dubi (ST 35) acupoint and Jiexi (ST 41) acupoint.

【Method】Puncture perpendicularly 1-2 cun.

【Indications】Stomachache, vomiting, abdominal distension, abdominal pain, borborygmus, diarrhea with undigested food, diarrhea, constipation, dysentery, acute mastitis, deficiency-consumption, cough, panting, palpitations, short breath, dizziness, insomnia, insanity and mania, knee pain, flaccidity and impediment of lower limb, and edema.

【Stratified anatomy】①Skin; ②Subcutaneous tissue (There are branches of the lateral sural cutaneous n..); ③Tibialis anterior m.; ④Deep peroneal n., anterior tibial a. & v.; ⑤Crural interosseous membrane; ⑥Tibialis posterior m. (Fig.6-21 ~ Fig.6-28).

三、上巨虚

【定位】犊鼻下 6 寸，犊鼻与解溪穴的连线上。

【操作】直刺 1 ～ 1.5 寸。

【主治】腹痛，肠痈，泄泻，便秘，下肢痿痹。

【进针层次】①皮肤；②皮下组织（内有腓肠外侧皮神经的分支）；③胫骨前肌；④腓深神经及胫前动、静脉；⑤小腿骨间膜；⑥胫骨后肌（图 6–21 ～图 6–28）。

3. Shangjuxu (ST 37)

【Location】6 cun below Dubi (ST 35) acupoint, and on the line connecting Dubi (ST 35) acupoint and Jiexi (ST 41) acupoint.

【Method】Puncture perpendicularly 1-1.5 cun.

【Indications】Abdominal pain, intestinal carbuncle, diarrhea, constipation, and flaccidity and impediment of lower limb.

【Stratified anatomy】①Skin; ②Subcutaneous tissue (There are branches of the lateral sural cutaneous n..); ③Tibialis anterior m.; ④Deep peroneal n., anterior tibial a. & v.; ⑤Crural interosseous membrane; ⑥Tibialis posterior m. (Fig.6-21 ~ Fig.6-28).

四、下巨虚

【定位】犊鼻下 9 寸，犊鼻与解溪穴的连线上。

【操作】直刺 1 ～ 1.5 寸。

【主治】腹痛，腰脊痛引睾丸，泄泻，便秘，乳痈，下肢痿痹。

【进针层次】①皮肤；②皮下组织（内有腓肠外侧皮神经的分支）；③胫骨前肌；④腓深神经及胫前动、静脉；⑤小腿骨间膜；⑥胫骨后肌（图 6–21 ～图 6–28）。

4. Xiajuxu (ST 39)

【Location】9 cun below Dubi (ST 35) acupoint, and on the line connecting Dubi (ST 35) acupoint and Jiexi (ST 41) acupoint.

【Method】Puncture perpendicularly 1-1.5 cun.

【Indications】Abdominal pain, pain in the low back and spine involving the testicles, diarrhea, constipation, acute mastitis, and flaccidity and impediment of lower limb.

【Stratified anatomy】①Skin; ②Subcutaneous tissue (There are branches of the lateral sural cutaneous n..); ③Tibialis anterior m.; ④Deep peroneal n., anterior tibial a. & v.; ⑤Crural interosseous membrane; ⑥Tibialis posterior m. (Fig.6-21 ~ Fig.6-28).

五、条口

【定位】犊鼻下 8 寸，犊鼻与解溪穴的连线上。

【操作】直刺 1 ～ 2 寸。

【主治】下肢痿痹，跗肿，转筋，肩臂痛。

【进针层次】①皮肤；②皮下组织（内有腓肠外侧皮神经的分支）；③胫骨前肌；④腓深神经及胫前动、静脉；⑤小腿骨间膜；⑥胫骨后肌（图 6–21 ～图 6–28）。

5. Tiaokou (ST 38)

【Location】8 cun below Dubi (ST 35) acupoint, and on the line connecting Dubi (ST 35) acupoint and Jiexi (ST 41) acupoint.

【Method】Puncture perpendicularly 1-2 cun.

【Indications】Flaccidity and impediment of lower limb, swelling of foot, spasm, and pain in the shoulder and arm.

【Stratified anatomy】①Skin; ②Subcutaneous tissue (There are branches of the lateral sural cutaneous n..); ③Tibialis anterior m.; ④Deep peroneal n., anterior tibial a. & v.; ⑤Crural interosseous membrane; ⑥Tibialis posterior m. (Fig.6-21 ~ Fig.6-28).

六、丰隆

【定位】外踝尖上 8 寸，犊鼻与外踝尖连线的中点；或条口穴外侧一横指。

【操作】直刺 1 ～ 1.5 寸。

【主治】痰多，咳嗽，哮喘，头痛，眩晕，癫狂痫，下肢痿痹。

【进针层次】①皮肤；②皮下组织（内有腓肠外侧皮神经的分支）；③趾长伸肌；④踇长伸肌；⑤小腿骨间膜；⑥胫骨后肌（图 6–21 ～图 6–28）。

6. Fenglong (ST 40)

【Location】8 cun above the outer ankle tip, and at the midpoint of the line connecting the Dubi (ST 35) and the outer ankle tip; Or one finger-breadth lateral to Tiaokou (ST 38).

【Method】Puncture perpendicularly 1-1.5 cun.

【Indications】Profuse phlegm, cough, asthma, headache, vertigo, insanity, mania, epilepsy, and flaccidity and impediment of lower limb.

【Stratified anatomy】①Skin; ②Subcutaneous tissue (There are branches of the lateral sural cutaneous n..); ③Extensor digitorum longus m.; ④Extensor hallucis longus m.; ⑤Crural interosseous membrane; ⑥Tibialis posterior m. (Fig.6-21 ~ Fig.6-28).

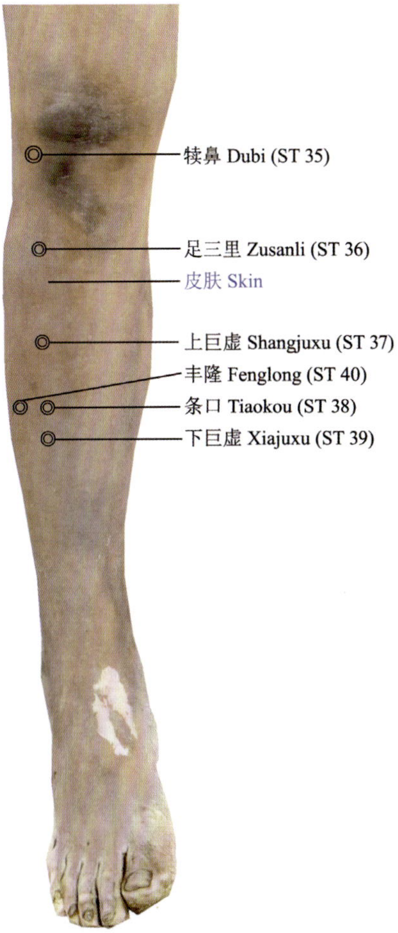

图 6–21　小腿前面腧穴层次解剖（1）
Fig.6-21　Layered anatomy of acupoints on the anterior aspect of the lower leg (1)

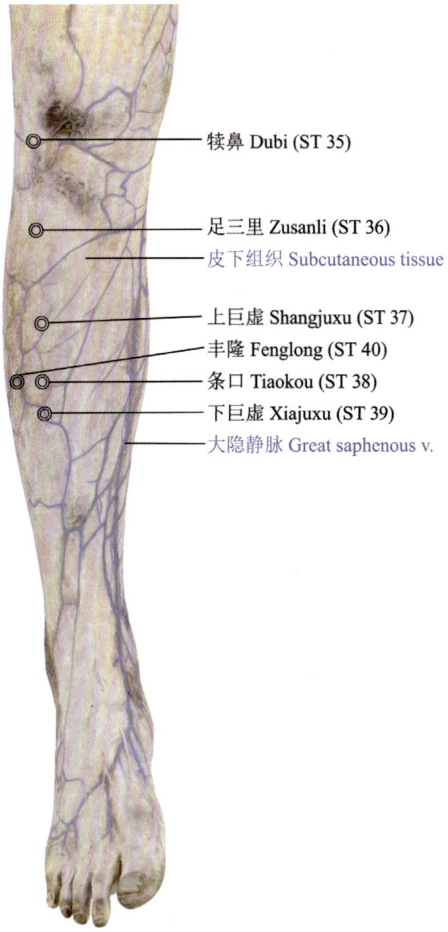

图 6–22　小腿前面腧穴层次解剖（2）
Fig.6-22　Layered anatomy of acupoints on the anterior aspect of the lower leg (2)

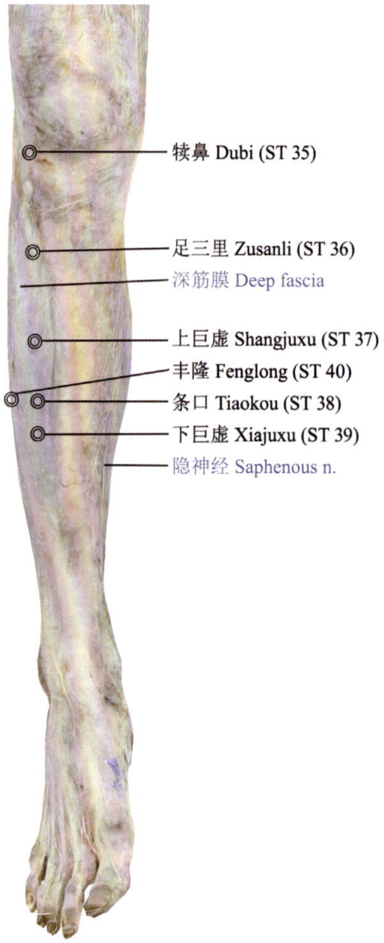
犊鼻 Dubi (ST 35)
足三里 Zusanli (ST 36)
深筋膜 Deep fascia
上巨虚 Shangjuxu (ST 37)
丰隆 Fenglong (ST 40)
条口 Tiaokou (ST 38)
下巨虚 Xiajuxu (ST 39)
隐神经 Saphenous n.

图 6–23　小腿前面腧穴层次解剖（3）
Fig.6-23　Layered anatomy of acupoints on the anterior aspect of the lower leg (3)

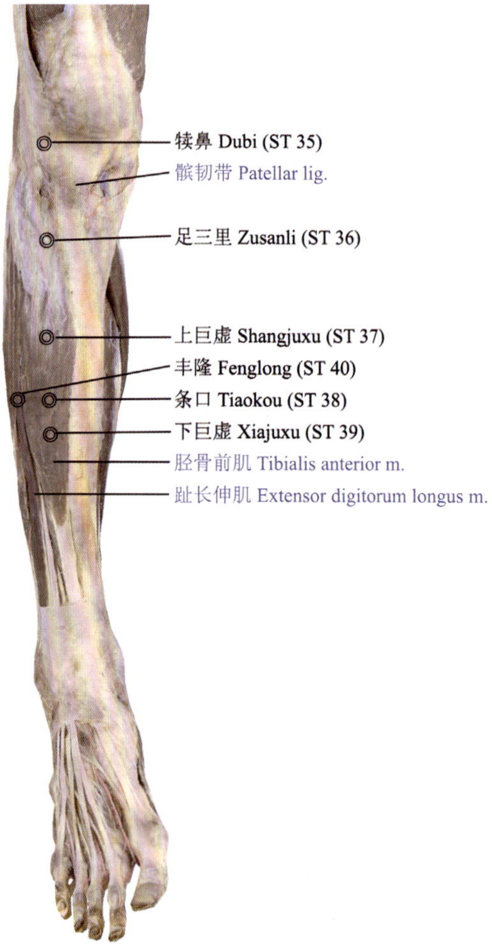
犊鼻 Dubi (ST 35)
髌韧带 Patellar lig.
足三里 Zusanli (ST 36)
上巨虚 Shangjuxu (ST 37)
丰隆 Fenglong (ST 40)
条口 Tiaokou (ST 38)
下巨虚 Xiajuxu (ST 39)
胫骨前肌 Tibialis anterior m.
趾长伸肌 Extensor digitorum longus m.

图 6–24　小腿前面腧穴层次解剖（4）
Fig.6-24　Layered anatomy of acupoints on the anterior aspect of the lower leg (4)

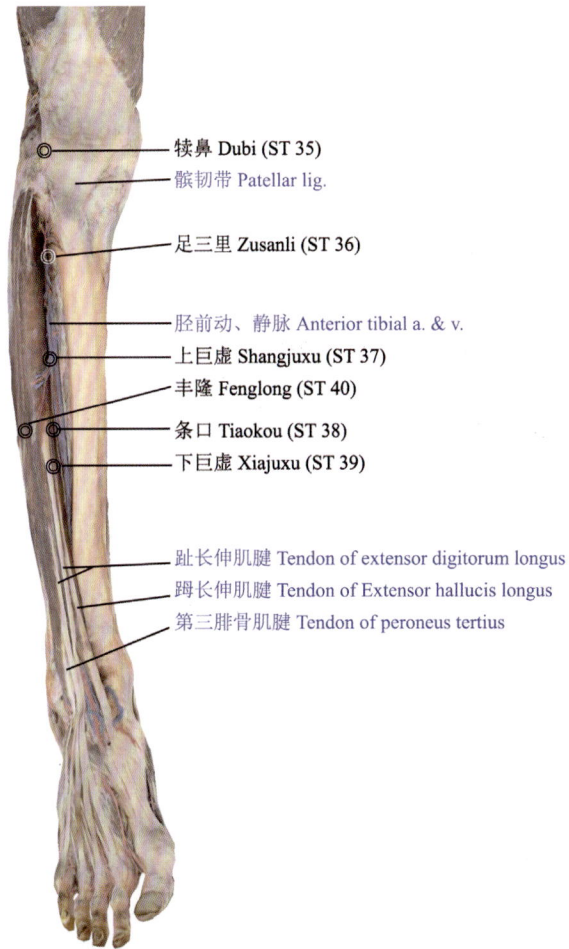

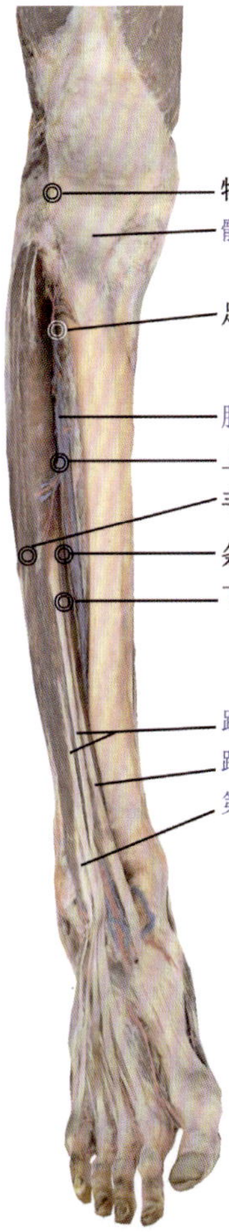
犊鼻 Dubi (ST 35)
髌韧带 Patellar lig.
足三里 Zusanli (ST 36)
胫前动、静脉 Anterior tibial a. & v.
上巨虚 Shangjuxu (ST 37)
丰隆 Fenglong (ST 40)
条口 Tiaokou (ST 38)
下巨虚 Xiajuxu (ST 39)
趾长伸肌腱 Tendon of extensor digitorum longus
蹞长伸肌腱 Tendon of Extensor hallucis longus
第三腓骨肌腱 Tendon of peroneus tertius

图 6–25　小腿前面腧穴层次解剖（5）

Fig.6-25　Layered anatomy of acupoints on the anterior aspect of the lower leg (5)

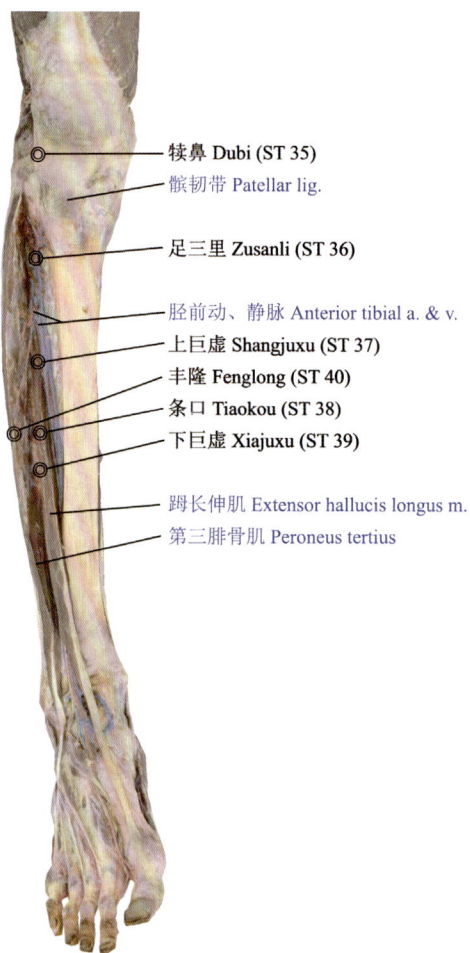

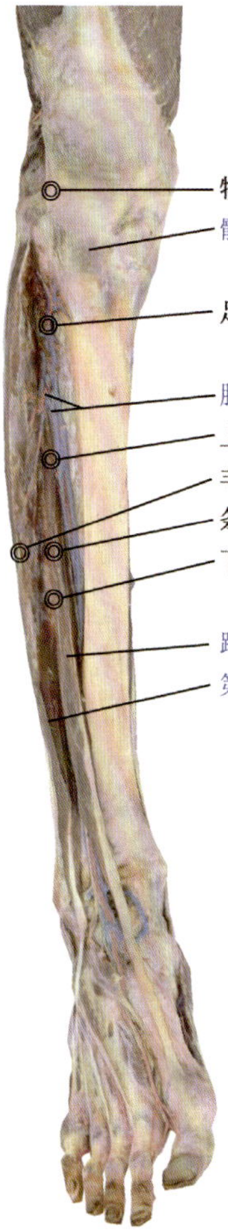

图 6–26　小腿前面腧穴层次解剖（6）

Fig.6-26　Layered anatomy of acupoints on the anterior aspect of the lower leg (6)

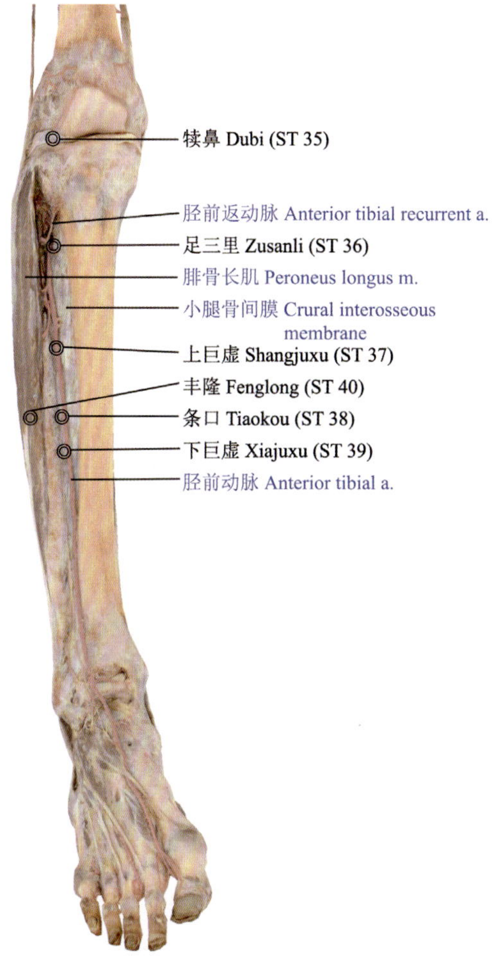
犊鼻 Dubi (ST 35)
胫前返动脉 Anterior tibial recurrent a.
足三里 Zusanli (ST 36)
腓骨长肌 Peroneus longus m.
小腿骨间膜 Crural interosseous membrane
上巨虚 Shangjuxu (ST 37)
丰隆 Fenglong (ST 40)
条口 Tiaokou (ST 38)
下巨虚 Xiajuxu (ST 39)
胫前动脉 Anterior tibial a.

图 6–27 小腿前面腧穴层次解剖（7）
Fig.6-27 Layered anatomy of acupoints on the anterior aspect of the lower leg (7)

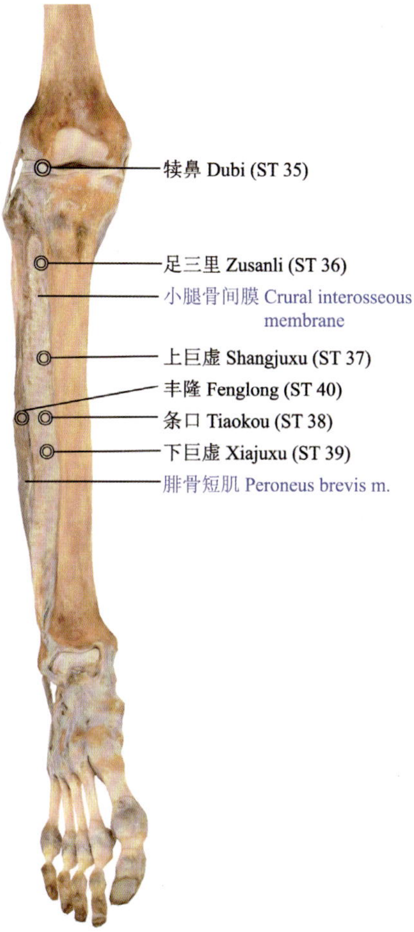
犊鼻 Dubi (ST 35)
足三里 Zusanli (ST 36)
小腿骨间膜 Crural interosseous membrane
上巨虚 Shangjuxu (ST 37)
丰隆 Fenglong (ST 40)
条口 Tiaokou (ST 38)
下巨虚 Xiajuxu (ST 39)
腓骨短肌 Peroneus brevis m.

图 6–28 小腿前面腧穴层次解剖（8）
Fig.6-28 Layered anatomy of acupoints on the anterior aspect of the lower leg (8)

第五节　小腿后面腧穴

Section 5　Acupoints on the posterior aspect of the lower leg

一、委中

【定位】腘横纹中点，当股二头肌腱与半腱肌腱中间。

【操作】直刺 0.5 ～ 1 寸，或点刺出血。

【主治】腰痛，下肢痿痹，半身不遂，腘筋挛急，腹痛，吐泻，小便不利，遗尿，瘾疹。

【进针层次】①皮肤；②皮下组织（内有小隐静脉、腓肠内侧皮神经和股后皮神经的分支）；③腓肠肌内、外侧头之间；④胫神经及腘动、静脉（图 6–29 ～图 6–36）。

【针刺意外与预防】该穴深面有腘动、静脉，若刺中动脉，针尖有搏动感；若大幅度提插捻转，则可能引起大的血肿。由于血管神经在腘窝内由浅入深和由外侧向内侧排列的顺序是胫神经、腘静脉和腘动脉，因此进针时不宜偏内侧，以免刺中血管。

1. Weizhong (BL 40)

【Location】At the midpoint of the transverse crease of the popliteal fossa, and between the tendons of the biceps femoris and the semitendinosus.

【Method】Puncture perpendicularly 0.5-1 cun, or prick with a three-edged needle to cause bleeding.

【Indications】Lumbago, flaccidity and impediment of lower limb, hemiplegia, spasm in the popliteal tendon, abdominal pain, vomiting, diarrhea, dysuria, enuresis, and urticaria.

【Stratified anatomy】①Skin; ②Subcutaneous tissue (There are small saphenous v., medial sural cutaneous n., and branches of the posterior femoral cutaneous n..); ③Between medial head and lateral head of gastrocnemius; ④Tibial n. and popliteal a. & v. (Fig.6-29 ~ Fig.6-36).

【Cautions】There are popliteal a. & v. in the deep surface of the acupoint. If the artery is stabbed, a pulsating feeling can appear in the the tip of the needle. If it is manipulated with intense lifting-thrusting and twirling, it may cause a large hematoma. Because the blood vessels and nerves arranged from shallow to deep and from the outside to the inside are the tibial nerve, popliteal v. and popliteal a. in the popliteal fossa, it is not appropriate to insert the needle at the inner side of the popliteal fossa to avoid stabbing blood vessels.

二、委阳

【定位】腘横纹外侧端，当股二头肌腱的内侧缘。

【操作】直刺 0.5 ～ 1 寸。

【主治】腹满，水肿，小便不利，腰脊强痛，下肢痿痹。

【进针层次】①皮肤；②皮下组织（内有股后皮神经的分支和腓肠外侧皮神经）；③股二头肌；④腓总神经；⑤腓肠肌外侧头；⑥腘肌起始腱（图 6–29 ～图 6–36）。

2. Weiyang (BL 39)

【Location】At the lateral end of the transverse popliteal crease, and at the medial edge of the biceps femoris tendon.

【Method】Puncture perpendicularly 0.5-1 cun.

【Indications】Abdominal distension, edema, dysuria, stiffness and pain in the loins and spine, and flaccidity and impediment of lower limb.

【Stratified anatomy】①Skin; ②Subcutaneous tissue (There are branches of the posterior femoral cutaneous n., and lateral sural cutaneous n..); ③Biceps femoris m.; ④Common peroneal n.; ⑤Lateral head of gastrocnemius; ⑥Popliteus muscle's origin tendon (Fig.6-29 ~ Fig.6-36).

三、承山

【定位】腓肠肌肌腹与肌腱交角处。

【操作】直刺 1 ～ 1.5 寸。

【主治】痔疾，便秘，腰腿拘急、疼痛。

【进针层次】①皮肤；②皮下组织（内有腓肠内侧皮神经的分支和小隐静脉）；③腓肠肌；④比目鱼肌；⑤胫神经及胫后动、静脉（图 6–29 ～图 6–36）。

3. Chengshan (BL 57)

【Location】In the intersection area betwwen the belly and tendon of the gastrocnemius.

【Method】Puncture perpendicularly 1-1.5 cun.

【Indications】Hemorrhoids, constipation, and spasmodic pain in the loins and legs.

【Stratified anatomy】①Skin; ②Subcutaneous tissue (There are branches of the medial sural cutaneous n., and small saphenous v..); ③Gastrocnemius; ④Soleus; ⑤Tibial n. and posterior tibial a. & v. (Fig.6-29 ~ Fig.6-36).

四、飞扬

【定位】昆仑穴直上 7 寸，承山穴外下方 1 寸处。

【操作】直刺 1 ～ 1.5 寸。

【主治】头痛，目眩，鼻塞，鼻衄，腰腿疼痛，下肢无力，痔疾。

【进针层次】①皮肤；②皮下组织（内有腓肠外侧皮神经的分支）；③腓肠肌；④比目鱼肌；⑤踇长屈肌（图 6–29 ～图 6–36）。

4. Feiyang (BL 58)

【Location】7 cun directly above Kunlun (BL 60) acupoint, and 1 cun lateroinferior to

Chengshan (BL 57) acupoint.

【Method】Puncture perpendicularly 1-1.5 cun.

【Indications】Headache, dizziness, nasal obstruction, epistaxis, pain in the loins and legs, weakness in the lower limb, and hemorrhoids.

【Stratified anatomy】①Skin; ②Subcutaneous tissue (There are branches of the lateral sural cutaneous n..); ③Gastrocnemius; ④Soleus; ⑤Flexor hallucis longus m. (Fig.6-29 ~ Fig.6-36).

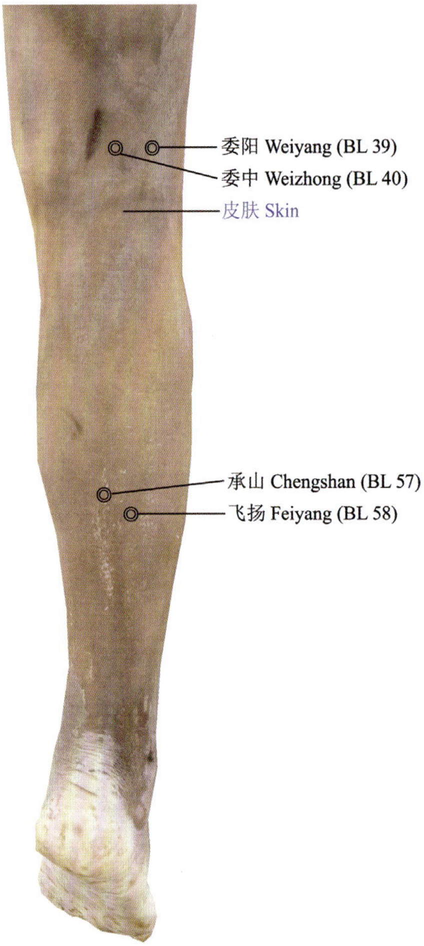

图 6–29　小腿后面腧穴层次解剖（1）
Fig.6-29　Layered anatomy of acupoints on the posterior aspect of the lower leg (1)

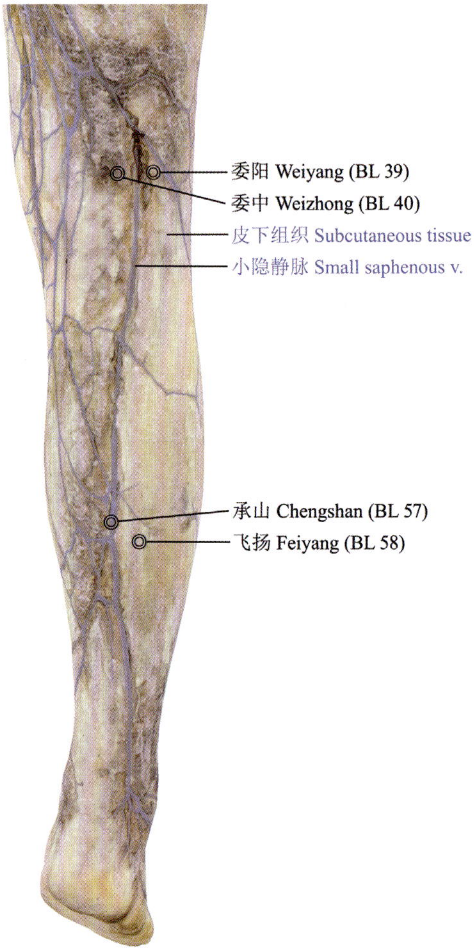

图 6–30　小腿后面腧穴层次解剖（2）
Fig.6-30　Layered anatomy of acupoints on the posterior aspect of the lower leg (2)

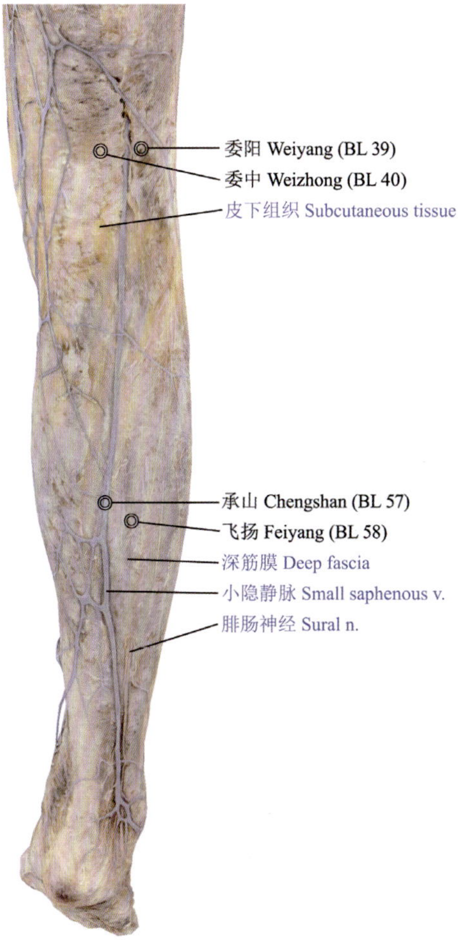
委阳 Weiyang (BL 39)
委中 Weizhong (BL 40)
皮下组织 Subcutaneous tissue
承山 Chengshan (BL 57)
飞扬 Feiyang (BL 58)
深筋膜 Deep fascia
小隐静脉 Small saphenous v.
腓肠神经 Sural n.

图 6–31　小腿后面腧穴层次解剖（3）
Fig.6-31　Layered anatomy of acupoints on the posterior aspect of the lower leg (3)

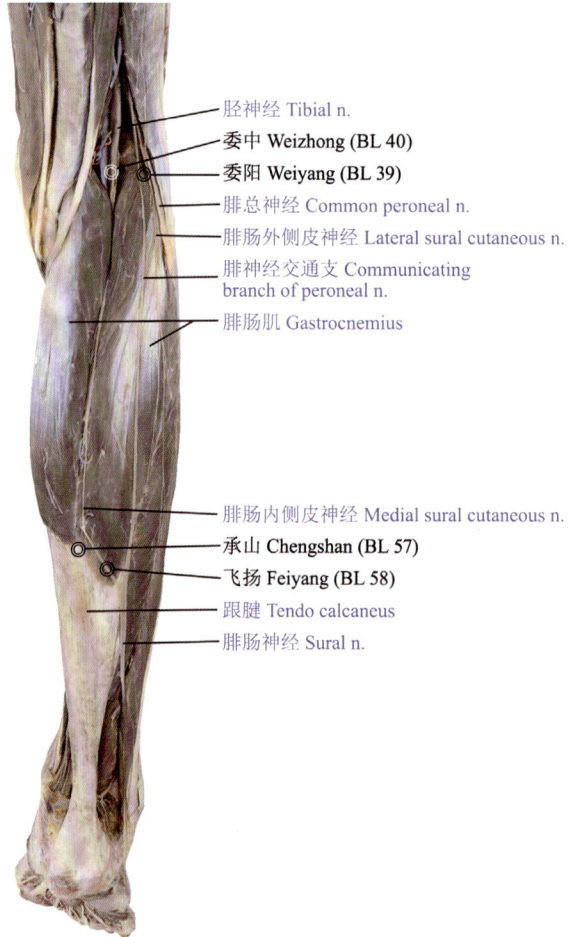

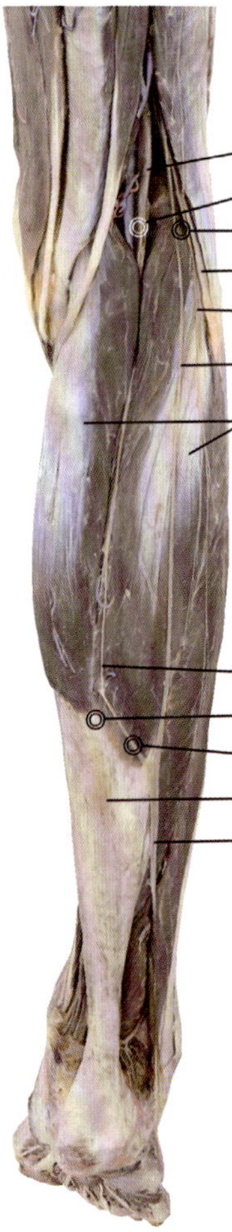
胫神经 Tibial n.
委中 Weizhong (BL 40)
委阳 Weiyang (BL 39)
腓总神经 Common peroneal n.
腓肠外侧皮神经 Lateral sural cutaneous n.
腓神经交通支 Communicating branch of peroneal n.
腓肠肌 Gastrocnemius
腓肠内侧皮神经 Medial sural cutaneous n.
承山 Chengshan (BL 57)
飞扬 Feiyang (BL 58)
跟腱 Tendo calcaneus
腓肠神经 Sural n.

图 6–32　小腿后面腧穴层次解剖（4）

Fig.6-32　Layered anatomy of acupoints on the posterior aspect of the lower leg (4)

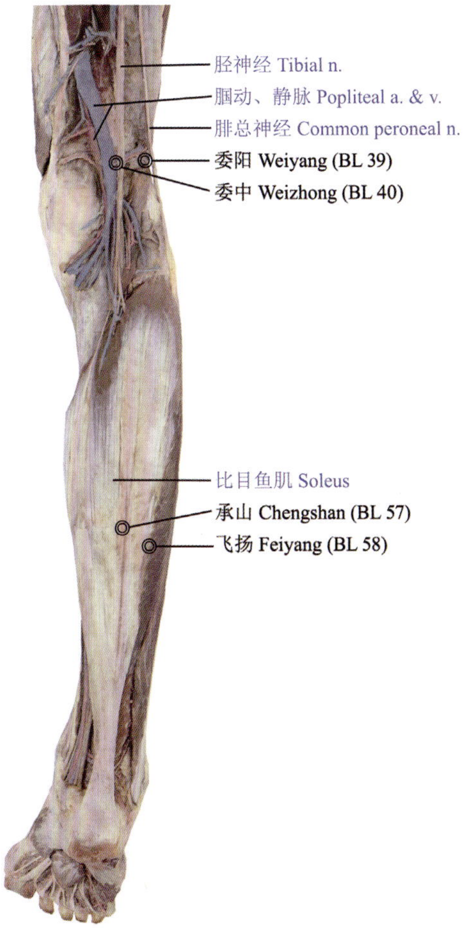
胫神经 Tibial n.
腘动、静脉 Popliteal a. & v.
腓总神经 Common peroneal n.
委阳 Weiyang (BL 39)
委中 Weizhong (BL 40)
比目鱼肌 Soleus
承山 Chengshan (BL 57)
飞扬 Feiyang (BL 58)

图 6–33 小腿后面腧穴层次解剖（5）

Fig.6-33 Layered anatomy of acupoints on the posterior aspect of the lower leg (5)

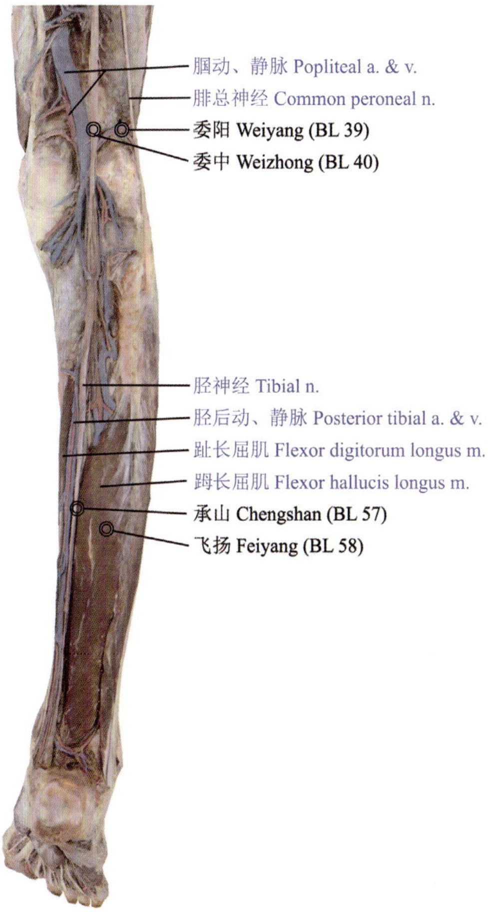
腘动、静脉 Popliteal a. & v.
腓总神经 Common peroneal n.
委阳 Weiyang (BL 39)
委中 Weizhong (BL 40)
胫神经 Tibial n.
胫后动、静脉 Posterior tibial a. & v.
趾长屈肌 Flexor digitorum longus m.
踇长屈肌 Flexor hallucis longus m.
承山 Chengshan (BL 57)
飞扬 Feiyang (BL 58)

图 6–34 小腿后面腧穴层次解剖（6）

Fig.6-34 Layered anatomy of acupoints on the posterior aspect of the lower leg (6)

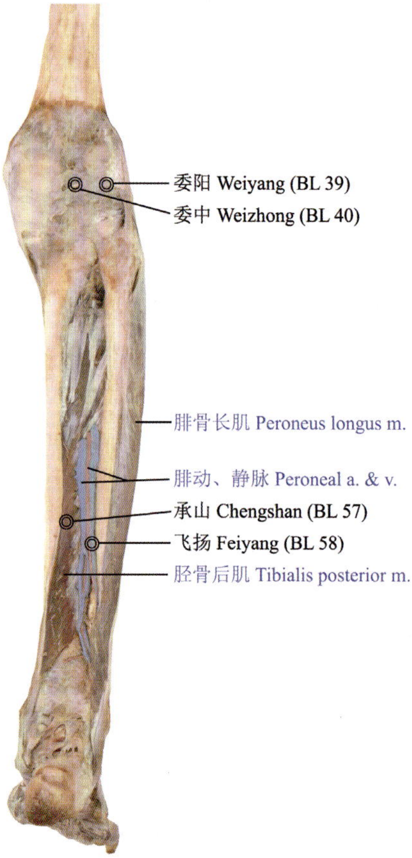
委阳 Weiyang (BL 39)
委中 Weizhong (BL 40)
腓骨长肌 Peroneus longus m.
腓动、静脉 Peroneal a. & v.
承山 Chengshan (BL 57)
飞扬 Feiyang (BL 58)
胫骨后肌 Tibialis posterior m.

图 6–35　小腿后面腧穴层次解剖（7）
Fig.6-35　Layered anatomy of acupoints on the posterior aspect of the lower leg (7)

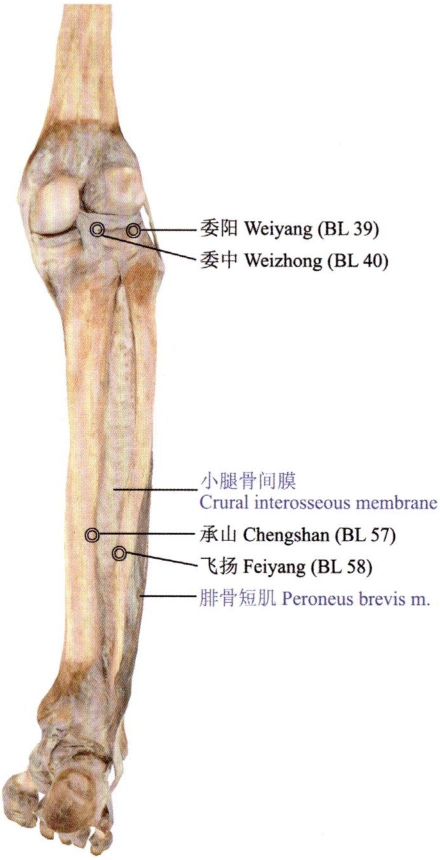
委阳 Weiyang (BL 39)
委中 Weizhong (BL 40)
小腿骨间膜
Crural interosseous membrane
承山 Chengshan (BL 57)
飞扬 Feiyang (BL 58)
腓骨短肌 Peroneus brevis m.

图 6–36　小腿后面腧穴层次解剖（8）
Fig.6-36　Layered anatomy of acupoints on the posterior aspect of the lower leg (8)

第六节　小腿外侧面腧穴

Section 6　Acupoints on the lateral aspect of the lower leg

一、阳陵泉

【定位】腓骨头前下方凹陷中。

【操作】直刺 1 ～ 1.5 寸。

【主治】黄疸，胁痛，口苦，吞酸，下肢麻木、拘急，膝痛，小儿惊风。

【进针层次】①皮肤；②皮下组织（内有腓肠外侧皮神经）；③腓骨长肌；④腓总神经；⑤趾长伸肌（图 6–37 ～图 6–44）。

1. Yanglingquan (GB 34)

【Location】In the depression anteroinferior to the head of the fibula.

【Method】Puncture perpendicularly 1-1.5 cun.

【Indications】Jaundice, pain in the hypochondrium, bitter taste in the mouth, acid regurgitation, numbness and spasm of lower limb, pain in the knee, and infantile convulsions.

【Stratified anatomy】①Skin; ②Subcutaneous tissue (There are lateral sural cutaneous n..); ③Peroneus longus m.; ④Common peroneal n.; ⑤Extensor digitorum longus m. (Fig.6-37 ~ Fig.6-44).

二、光明

【定位】外踝尖上 5 寸，腓骨前缘。

【操作】直刺 1 ～ 1.5 寸。

【主治】目痛，近视，乳房胀痛，乳少，下肢痿痹。

【进针层次】①皮肤；②皮下组织（内有腓肠外侧皮神经的分支和腓浅神经）；③腓骨短肌；④小腿前肌间隔；⑤趾长伸肌；⑥踇长伸肌；⑦腓深神经及胫前动、静脉；⑧小腿骨间膜；⑨胫骨后肌（图 6–37 ～图 6–44）。

2. Guangming (GB 37)

【Location】5 cun above the tip of the external malleolus, and anterior to the fibula.

【Method】Puncture perpendicularly 1-1.5 cun.

【Indications】Eye pain, myopia, breast swelling and pain, hypogalactia, and flaccidity and impediment of lower limb.

【Stratified anatomy】①Skin; ②Subcutaneous tissue (There are branches of the lateral sural cutaneous n., and superficial peroneal n..); ③Peroneus brevis m.; ④Anterior crural intermuscular septum; ⑤Extensor digitorum longus m.; ⑥Extensor hallucis longus m. ⑦Deep peroneal n. and anterior tibial a. and v.; ⑧Crural interosseous membrane; ⑨Posterior tibial m. (Fig.6-37 ~ Fig.6-44).

三、悬钟

【定位】外踝尖上 3 寸，腓骨前缘。

【操作】直刺 1 ～ 1.5 寸。

【主治】痴呆，中风，颈项强痛，胸胁胀满，下肢痿痹。

【进针层次】①皮肤；②皮下组织（内有腓肠外侧皮神经的分支）；③趾长伸肌；④小腿骨间膜（图 6–37 ～图 6–44）。

3. Xuanzhong (GB 39)

【Location】3 cun above the tip of the external malleolus, and anterior to the fibula.

【Method】Puncture perpendicularly 1-1.5 cun.

【Indications】Dementia, wind stroke, stiffness and pain in the neck, distension and pain in the chest and hypochondrium, and flaccidity and impediment of lower limb.

【Stratified anatomy】①Skin; ②Subcutaneous tissue (There are branches of the lateral sural cutaneous n..); ③Extensor digitorum longus m.; ④Crural interosseous membrane (Fig.6-37 ~ Fig.6-44).

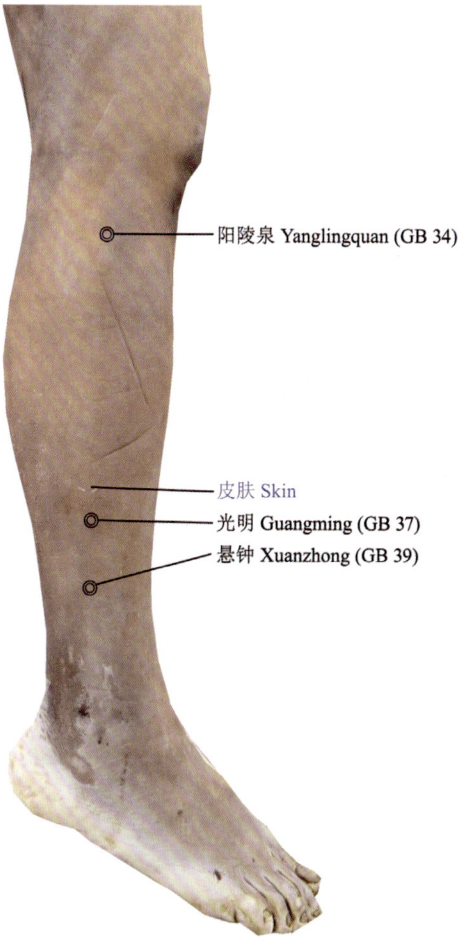

图 6–37 小腿外侧面腧穴层次解剖（1）
Fig.6-37 Layered anatomy of acupoints on the lateral aspect of the lower leg (1)

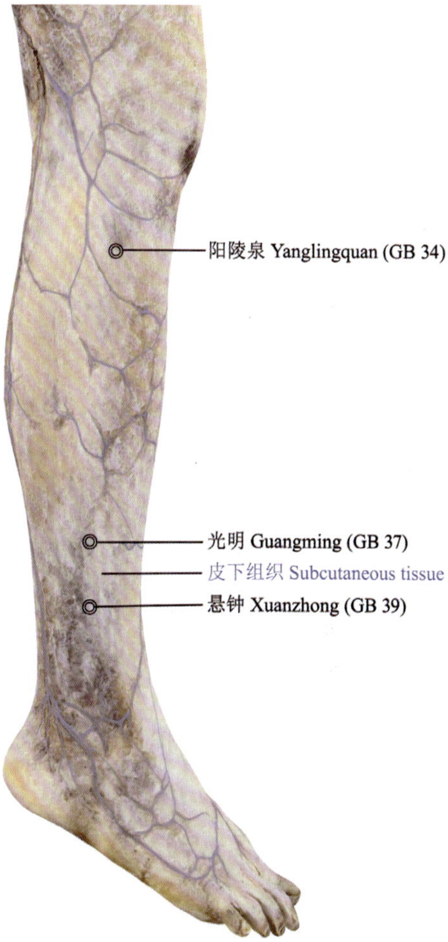

图 6–38 小腿外侧面腧穴层次解剖（2）
Fig.6-38 Layered anatomy of acupoints on the lateral aspect of the lower leg (2)

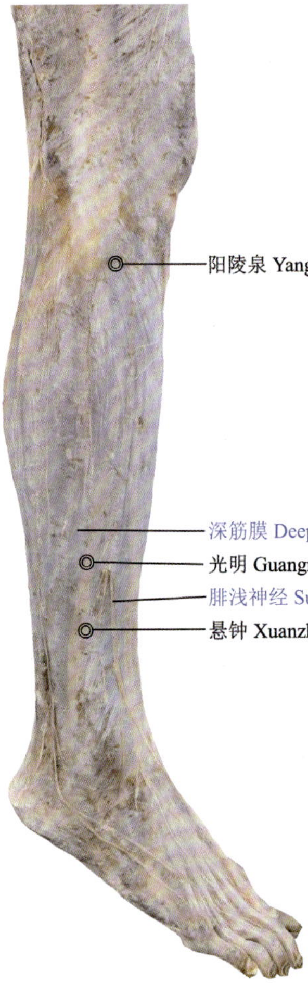
阳陵泉 Yanglingquan (GB 34)
深筋膜 Deep fascia
光明 Guangming (GB 37)
腓浅神经 Superficial peroneal n.
悬钟 Xuanzhong (GB 39)

图 6–39　小腿外侧面腧穴层次解剖（3）

Fig.6-39　Layered anatomy of acupoints on the lateral aspect of the lower leg (3)

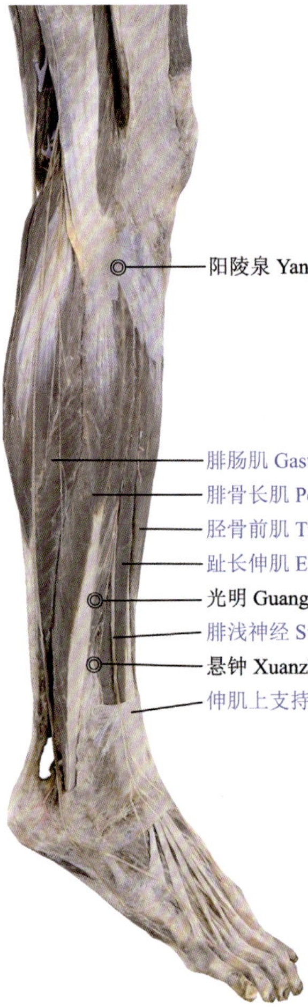
阳陵泉 Yanglingquan (GB 34)
腓肠肌 Gastrocnemius
腓骨长肌 Peroneus longus m.
胫骨前肌 Tibialis anterior m.
趾长伸肌 Extensor digitorum longus m.
光明 Guangming (GB 37)
腓浅神经 Superficial peroneal n.
悬钟 Xuanzhong (GB 39)
伸肌上支持带 Superior extensor retinaculum

图 6–40　小腿外侧面腧穴层次解剖（4）

Fig.6-40　Layered anatomy of acupoints on the lateral aspect of the lower leg (4)

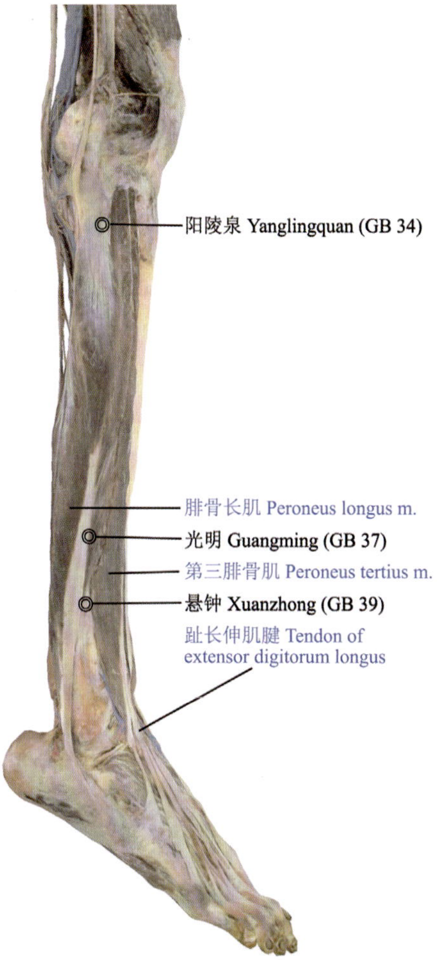
阳陵泉 Yanglingquan (GB 34)
腓骨长肌 Peroneus longus m.
光明 Guangming (GB 37)
第三腓骨肌 Peroneus tertius m.
悬钟 Xuanzhong (GB 39)
趾长伸肌腱 Tendon of extensor digitorum longus

图 6–41　小腿外侧面腧穴层次解剖（5）
Fig.6-41　Layered anatomy of acupoints on the lateral aspect of the lower leg (5)

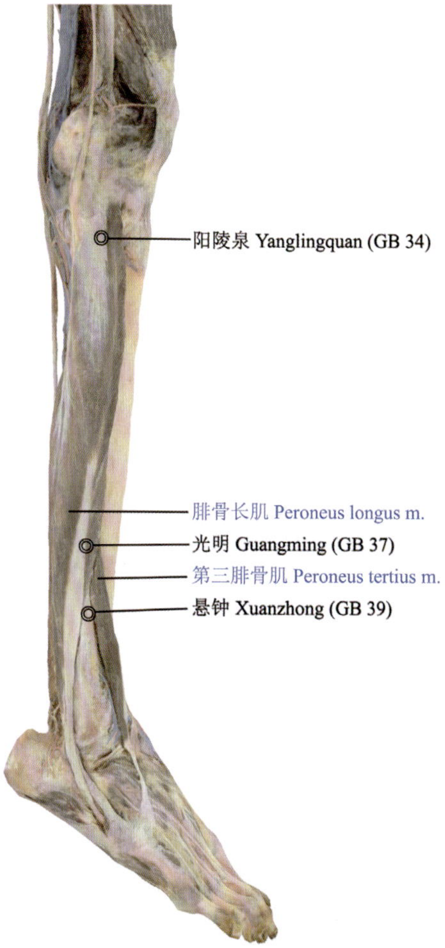
阳陵泉 Yanglingquan (GB 34)
腓骨长肌 Peroneus longus m.
光明 Guangming (GB 37)
第三腓骨肌 Peroneus tertius m.
悬钟 Xuanzhong (GB 39)

图 6–42　小腿外侧面腧穴层次解剖（6）
Fig.6-42　Layered anatomy of acupoints on the lateral aspect of the lower leg (6)

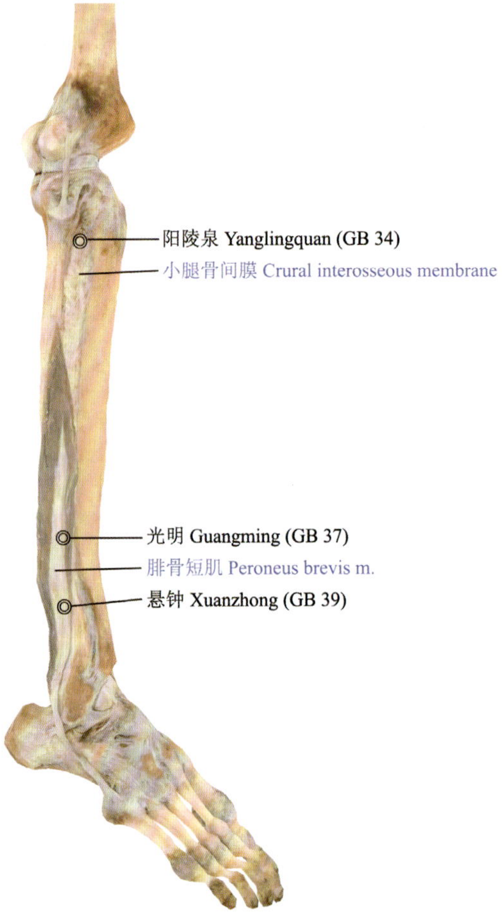
阳陵泉 Yanglingquan (GB 34)
小腿骨间膜 Crural interosseous membrane
光明 Guangming (GB 37)
腓骨短肌 Peroneus brevis m.
悬钟 Xuanzhong (GB 39)

图 6–43　小腿外侧面腧穴层次解剖（7）
Fig.6-43　Layered anatomy of acupoints on the lateral aspect of the lower leg (7)

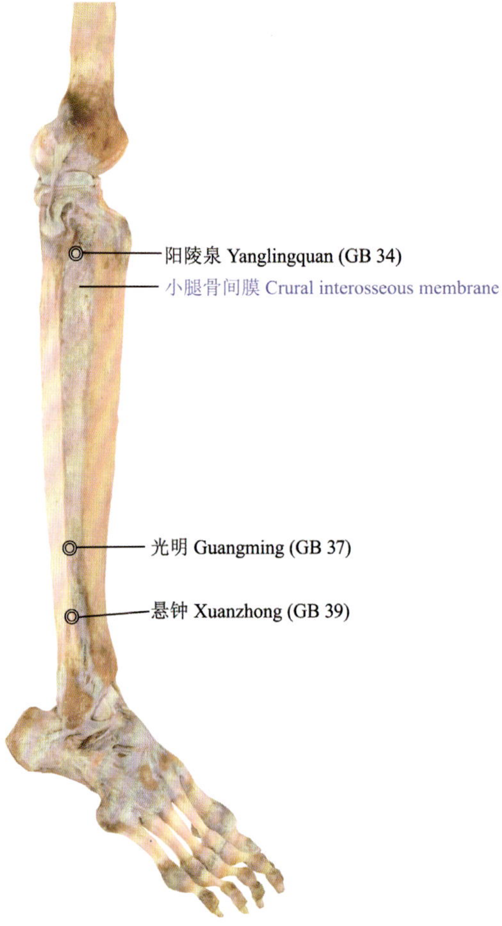
阳陵泉 Yanglingquan (GB 34)
小腿骨间膜 Crural interosseous membrane
光明 Guangming (GB 37)
悬钟 Xuanzhong (GB 39)

图 6–44　小腿外侧面腧穴层次解剖（8）
Fig.6-44　Layered anatomy of acupoints on the lateral aspect of the lower leg (8)

第七节 小腿内侧面腧穴

Section 7 Acupoints on the medial aspect of the lower leg

一、曲泉

【定位】当膝关节内侧端，股骨内侧髁的后缘，半腱肌、半膜肌止端的前缘凹陷处。

【操作】屈膝，直刺 1 ～ 1.5 寸。

【主治】月经不调，痛经，带下，阴挺，阴痒，产后腹痛，遗精，阳痿，疝气，小便不利，膝痛，下肢痿痹，癫痫，头痛，目眩，目赤。

【进针层次】①皮肤；②皮下组织（内有隐神经髌下支和隐神经的分支和大隐静脉）；③缝匠肌和股薄肌腱；④半膜肌腱；⑤腓肠肌内侧头（图 6–45 ～图 6–52）。

1. Ququan (LR 8)

【Location】At the medial end of the knee joint, and the posterior edge of the condylus medialis femoris, and in the depression of the anterior edge of the terminus of the semitendinosus m. and semimembranosus m..

【Method】Puncture perpendicularly 1-1.5 cun with the knee flexed.

【Indications】Irregular menstruation, dysmenorrhea, leukorrhea, prolapse of uterus, pruritus vulvae, postpartum abdominal pain, nocturnal emission, impotence, hernia, dysuria, pain in the knee, flaccidity and impediment of lower limb, epilepsy, headache, blurred vision, and redness in the eye.

【Stratified anatomy】①Skin; ②Subcutaneous tissue (There are subpatellar branch and branches of the saphenous n. and great saphenous v..); ③Sartorius and gracilis tendon; ④Semimembranosus tendon; ⑤Medial head of gastrocnemius (Fig.6-45 ~ Fig.6-52).

二、阴陵泉

【定位】胫骨内侧髁后下缘与胫骨内侧缘之间的凹陷中。

【操作】直刺 1 ～ 2 寸。

【主治】腹胀，水肿，黄疸，泄泻，小便不利，阴茎痛，遗精，妇人阴痛，带下，膝痛，半身不遂，下肢痿痹，虚劳。

【进针层次】①皮肤；②皮下组织（内有隐神经和大隐静脉）；③半腱肌腱；④腓肠肌内侧头和半膜肌腱（图 6–45 ～图 6–52）。

2. Yinlingquan (SP 9)

【Location】In the depression between the postero-inferior edge of the condylus medialis tibiae and the medial edge of the tibia.

【Method】Puncture perpendicularly 1-2 cun.

【Indications】Abdominal distension, edema, jaundice, diarrhea, dysuria, pain in the penis, nocturnal emission, pain in the female external genitalia, leukorrhea, pain in the knee, hemiplegia, flaccidity and impediment of lower limb, and deficiency-consumption.

【Stratified anatomy】①Skin; ②Subcutaneous tissue (There are saphenous n. and great saphenous v..); ③Semitendinosus Tendon; ④Medial head of gastrocnemius and semimembranosus tendon (Fig.6-45 ~ Fig.6-52).

三、地机

【定位】阴陵泉下 3 寸，胫骨内侧缘后际。

【操作】直刺 1 ～ 1.5 寸。

【主治】食欲不振，腹胀，腹痛，泄泻，水肿，小便不利，月经不调，痛经，遗精，腰痛，下肢痿痹。

【进针层次】①皮肤；②皮下组织（内有隐神经的分支和大隐静脉）；③腓肠肌；④比目鱼肌（图 6–45 ～图 6–52）。

3. Diji (SP 8)

【Location】3 cun below Yinlingquan (SP 9) acupoint, and at the posterior edge of the medial tibia

【Method】Puncture perpendicularly 1-1.5 cun.

【Indications】anorexia, abdominal distension, abdominal pain, diarrhea, edema, dysuria, irregular menstruation, dysmenorrhea, nocturnal emission, lumbago, and flaccidity and impediment of lower limb.

【Stratified anatomy】①Skin; ②Subcutaneous tissue (There are branches of the saphenous n. and great saphenous v..); ③Gastrocnemius; ④Soleus (Fig.6-45 ~ Fig.6-52).

四、蠡沟

【定位】内踝上 5 寸，胫骨内侧面的中央。

【操作】平刺 0.5 ～ 0.8 寸。

【主治】月经不调，带下，阴挺，阴痒，疝气，睾丸肿痛，阳强，小便不利，腰痛。

【进针层次】①皮肤；②皮下组织（内有隐神经的分支和大隐静脉的属支）（图 6–45 ～图 6–52）。

4. Ligou (LR 5)

【Location】5 cun above the medial malleolus, and in the centre of the medial tibia.

【Method】Puncture subcutaneously 0.5-0.8 cun.

【Indications】Irregular menstruation, leukorrhea, prolapse of uterus, pudendal pruritus, hernia, testicular swelling and pain, priapism, dysuria, and lumbago.

【Stratified anatomy】①Skin; ②Subcutaneous tissue (There are branches of the saphenous n., and tributaries of the great saphenous v..) (Fig.6-45 ~ Fig.6-52).

五、三阴交

【定位】内踝尖上 3 寸，胫骨内侧缘后际。

【操作】直刺 1 ～ 1.5 寸。

【主治】月经不调，崩漏，带下，阴挺，经闭，不孕，难产，恶露不尽，遗精，阳痿，疝气，小便不利，遗尿，水肿，腹痛，肠鸣，泄泻，便秘，失眠，下肢痿痹，湿疹。

【进针层次】①皮肤；②皮下组织（内有隐神经和大隐静脉）；③趾长屈肌；④胫骨后肌；⑤踇长屈肌（图 6–45 ～图 6–52）。

5. Sanyinjiao (SP 6)

【Location】3 cun above the tip of the medial malleolus, and posterior to the medial tibia.

【Method】Puncture perpendicularly 1-1.5 cun.

【Indications】Irregular menstruation, metrorrhagia and metrostaxis, leukorrhea, prolapse of uterus, amenorrhea, sterility, difficult labor, lochiorrhea, nocturnal emission, impotence, hernia, dysuria, enuresis, edema, abdominal pain, borborygmus, diarrhea, constipation, insomnia, flaccidity and impediment of lower limb, and eczema.

【Stratified anatomy】①Skin; ②Subcutaneous tissue (There are saphenous n. and great saphenous v..); ③Flexor digitorum longus m.; ④Tibialis posterior m.; ⑤Flexor hallucis longus m. (Fig.6-45 ~ Fig.6-52).

六、复溜

【定位】内踝尖上 2 寸，跟腱前缘。

【操作】直刺 0.5 ～ 1 寸。

【主治】水肿，腹胀，泄泻，盗汗，热病无汗，下肢痿痹。

【进针层次】①皮肤；②皮下组织（内有隐神经的分支）；③胫神经及胫后动、静脉与跟腱、跖肌腱之间；④踇长屈肌（图 6–45 ～图 6–52）。

6. Fuliu (KI 7)

【Location】2 cun above the tip of the medial malleolus, and anterior to the Achilles tendon.

【Method】Puncture perpendicularly 0.5-1 cun.

【Indications】Edema, abdominal distension, diarrhea, night sweating, febrile disease with anhidrosis, and flaccidity and impediment of lower limb.

【Stratified anatomy】①Skin; ②Subcutaneous tissue (There are branches of the saphenous n..); ③Between tibial n., posterior tibial a. & v. and the Achilles tendon and plantar tendon; ④Flexor hallucis longus (Fig.6-45 ~ Fig.6-52).

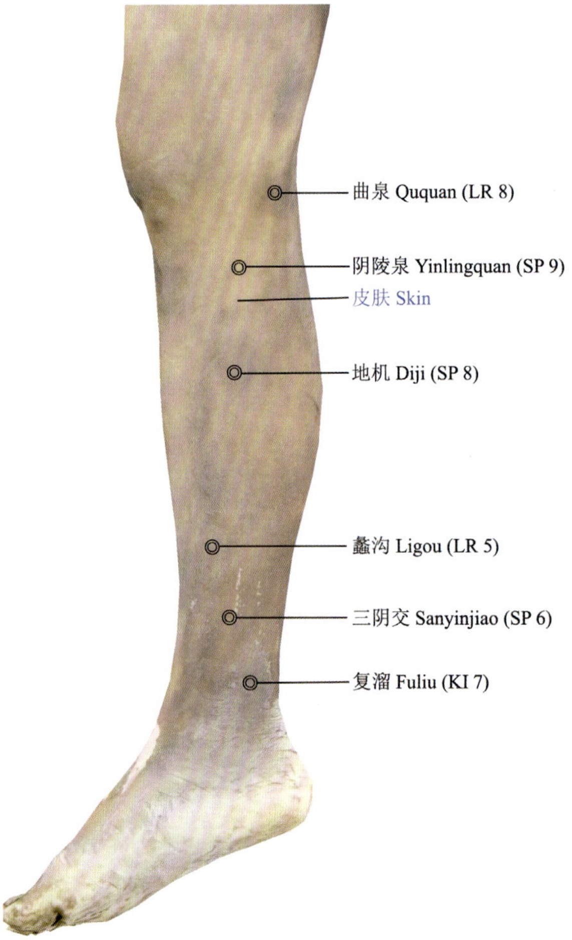

图 6–45　小腿内侧面腧穴层次解剖（1）

Fig.6-45　Layered anatomy of acupoints on the medial aspect of the lower leg (1)

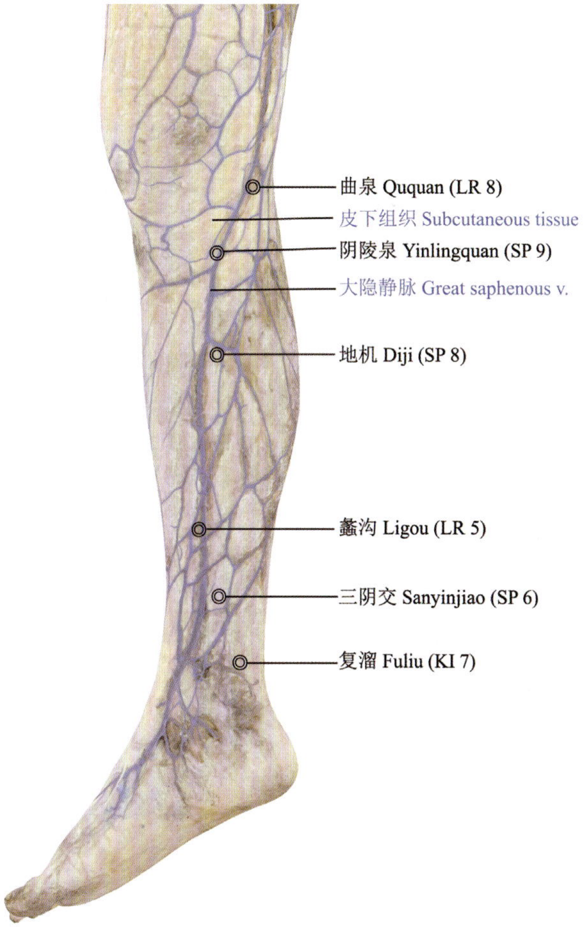
曲泉 Ququan (LR 8)
皮下组织 Subcutaneous tissue
阴陵泉 Yinlingquan (SP 9)
大隐静脉 Great saphenous v.
地机 Diji (SP 8)
蠡沟 Ligou (LR 5)
三阴交 Sanyinjiao (SP 6)
复溜 Fuliu (KI 7)

图 6-46　小腿内侧面腧穴层次解剖（2）
Fig.6-46　Layered anatomy of acupoints on the medial aspect of the lower leg (2)

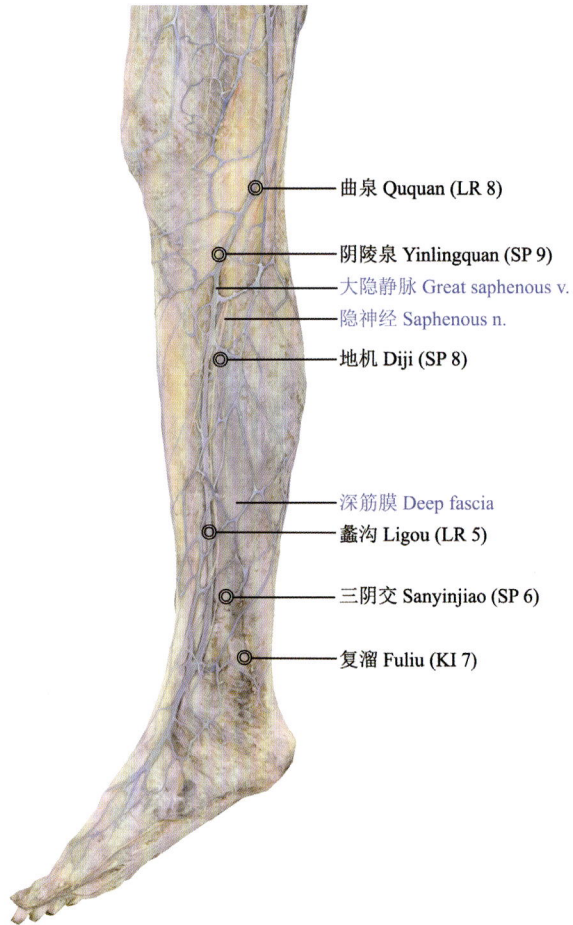

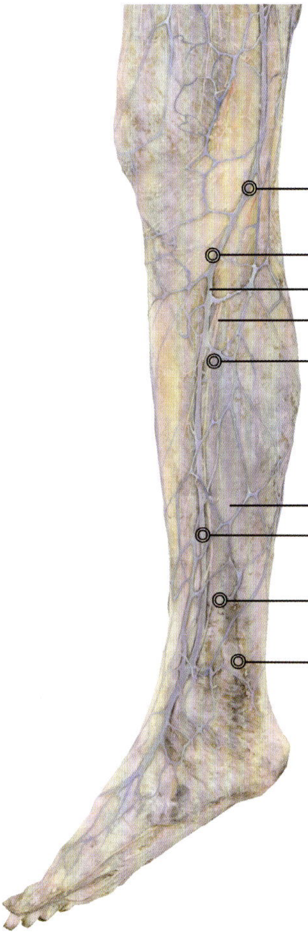
曲泉 Ququan (LR 8)
阴陵泉 Yinlingquan (SP 9)
大隐静脉 Great saphenous v.
隐神经 Saphenous n.
地机 Diji (SP 8)
深筋膜 Deep fascia
蠡沟 Ligou (LR 5)
三阴交 Sanyinjiao (SP 6)
复溜 Fuliu (KI 7)

图 6–47　小腿内侧面腧穴层次解剖（3）
Fig.6-47　Layered anatomy of acupoints on the medial aspect of the lower leg (3)

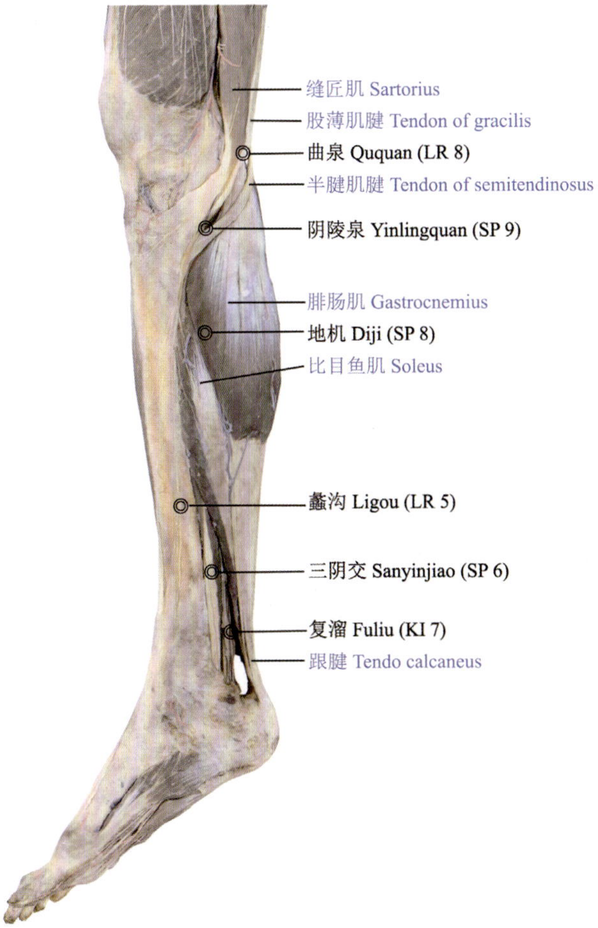
缝匠肌 Sartorius
股薄肌腱 Tendon of gracilis
曲泉 Ququan (LR 8)
半腱肌腱 Tendon of semitendinosus
阴陵泉 Yinlingquan (SP 9)
腓肠肌 Gastrocnemius
地机 Diji (SP 8)
比目鱼肌 Soleus
蠡沟 Ligou (LR 5)
三阴交 Sanyinjiao (SP 6)
复溜 Fuliu (KI 7)
跟腱 Tendo calcaneus

图 6–48　小腿内侧面腧穴层次解剖（4）
Fig.6-48　Layered anatomy of acupoints on the medial aspect of the lower leg (4)

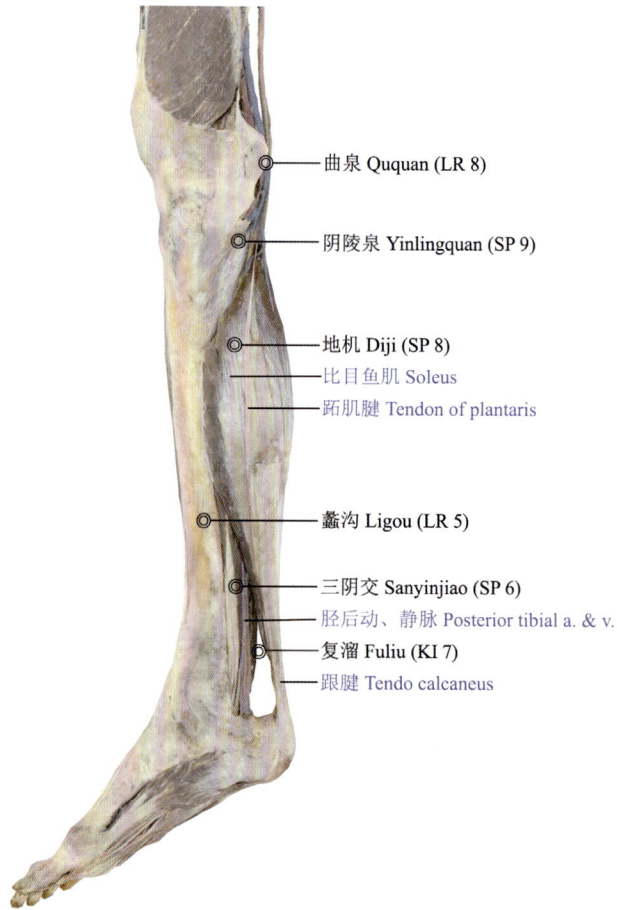

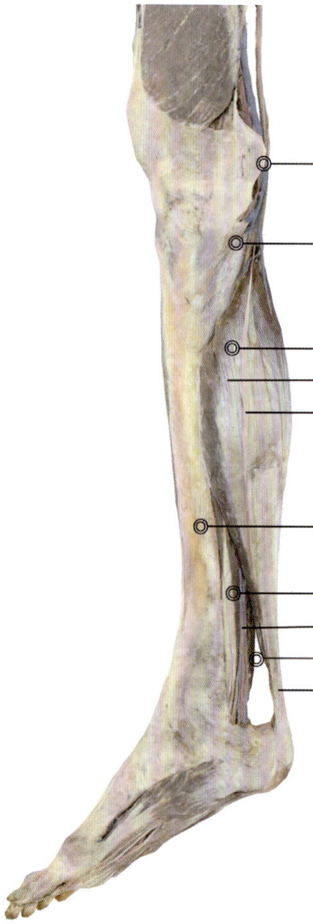
曲泉 Ququan (LR 8)
阴陵泉 Yinlingquan (SP 9)
地机 Diji (SP 8)
比目鱼肌 Soleus
跖肌腱 Tendon of plantaris
蠡沟 Ligou (LR 5)
三阴交 Sanyinjiao (SP 6)
胫后动、静脉 Posterior tibial a. & v.
复溜 Fuliu (KI 7)
跟腱 Tendo calcaneus

图 6–49　小腿内侧面腧穴层次解剖（5）

Fig.6-49　Layered anatomy of acupoints on the medial aspect of the lower leg (5)

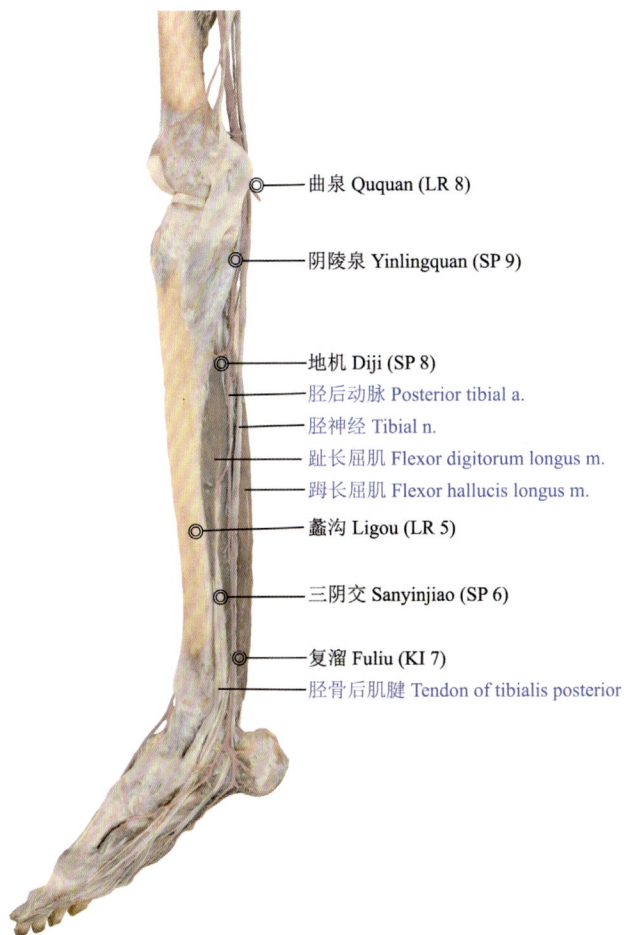

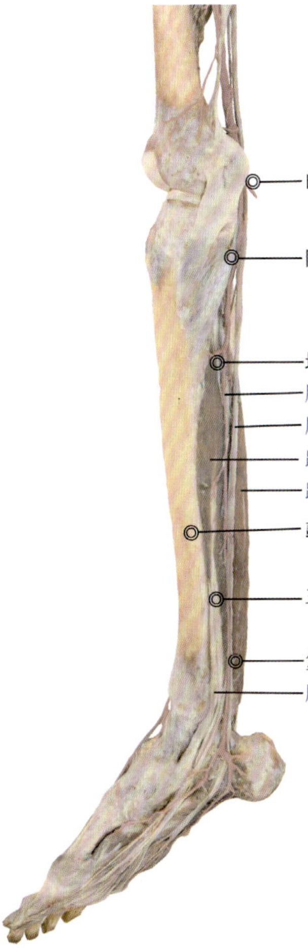
曲泉 Ququan (LR 8)
阴陵泉 Yinlingquan (SP 9)
地机 Diji (SP 8)
胫后动脉 Posterior tibial a.
胫神经 Tibial n.
趾长屈肌 Flexor digitorum longus m.
踇长屈肌 Flexor hallucis longus m.
蠡沟 Ligou (LR 5)
三阴交 Sanyinjiao (SP 6)
复溜 Fuliu (KI 7)
胫骨后肌腱 Tendon of tibialis posterior

图 6–50　小腿内侧面腧穴层次解剖（6）
Fig.6-50　Layered anatomy of acupoints on the medial aspect of the lower leg (6)

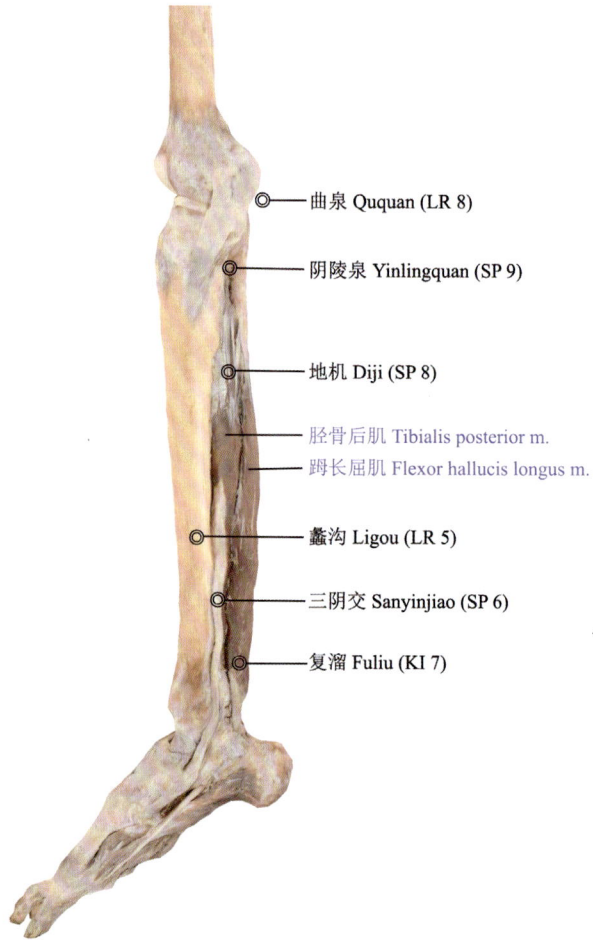

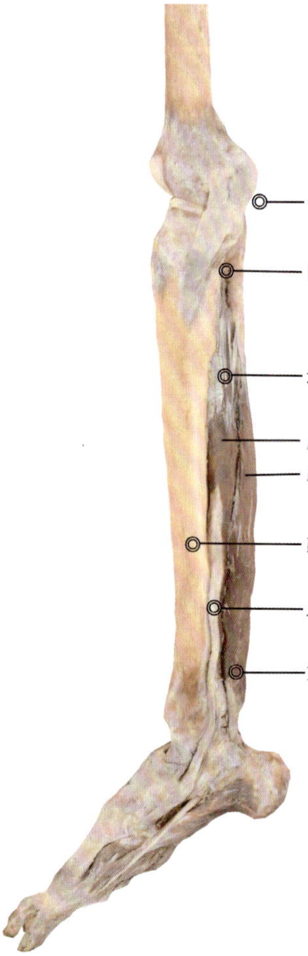

图 6–51　小腿内侧面腧穴层次解剖（7）

Fig.6-51　Layered anatomy of acupoints on the medial aspect of the lower leg (7)

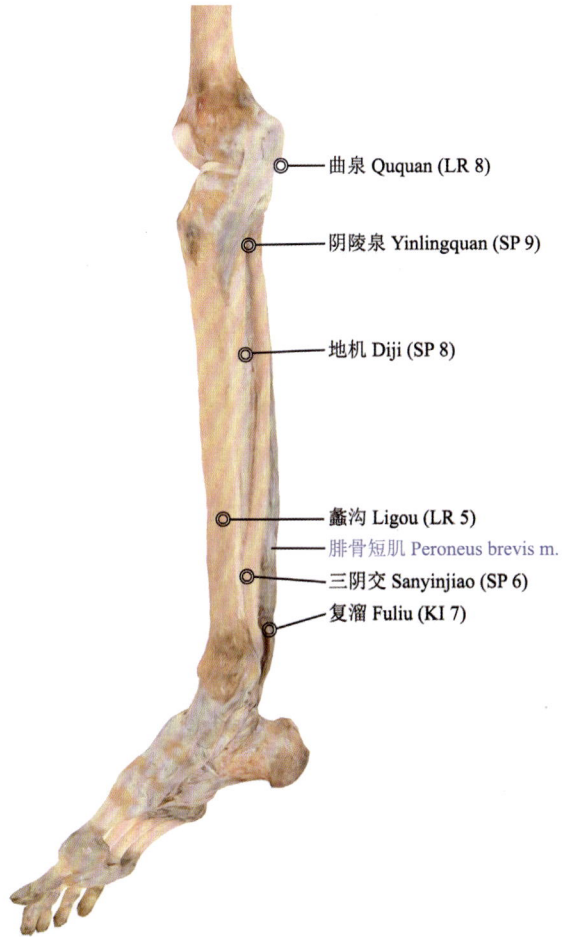

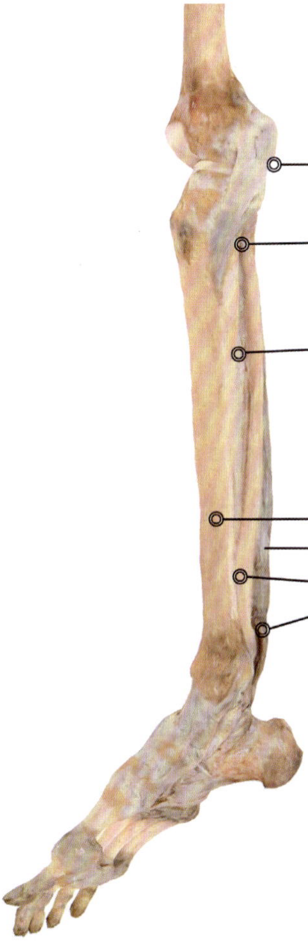
曲泉 Ququan (LR 8)
阴陵泉 Yinlingquan (SP 9)
地机 Diji (SP 8)
蠡沟 Ligou (LR 5)
腓骨短肌 Peroneus brevis m.
三阴交 Sanyinjiao (SP 6)
复溜 Fuliu (KI 7)

图 6–52　小腿内侧面腧穴层次解剖（8）

Fig.6-52　Layered anatomy of acupoints on the medial aspect of the lower leg (8)

第八节　足背腧穴

Section 8　Acupoints on the dorsum of the foot

一、解溪

【定位】踝关节前面中央凹陷中，蹞长伸肌腱与趾长伸肌腱之间。

【操作】直刺 0.5 ～ 1 寸。

【主治】头痛，眩晕，癫狂，腹胀，便秘，下肢痿痹，足踝肿痛。

【进针层次】①皮肤；②皮下组织（内有足背内侧皮神经的分支和足背浅静脉）；③蹞长伸肌与趾长伸肌腱之间；④腓深神经及胫前动、静脉（图 6–53 ～图 6–59）。

1. Jiexi (ST 41)

【Location】In the anterior central depression of the ankle joint, and between the tendon of extensor hallucis longus and tendons of extensor digitorum longus.

【Method】Puncture perpendicularly 0.5-1 cun.

【Indications】Headache, vertigo, insanity and mania, abdominal distension, constipation, flaccidity and impediment of lower limb, and swelling and pain in the ankle.

【Stratified anatomy】①Skin; ②Subcutaneous tissue (There are branches of the medial dorsal cutaneous n., and superficial dorsal v..); ③Between the tendon of extensor hallucis longus and tendons of extensor digitorum longus; ④Deep peroneal n., anterior tibial a. & v. (Fig.6-53 ~ Fig.6-59).

二、太冲

【定位】第 1、第 2 跖骨结合部的前方凹陷中。

【操作】直刺 0.5 ～ 0.8 寸。

【主治】头痛，眩晕，耳聋，耳鸣，口㖞，目赤肿痛，咽干咽痛，胁痛，黄疸，呕吐，月经不调，痛经，经闭，崩漏，带下，遗精，阳痿，早泄，阳强，中风，癫狂痫，小儿惊风，脏躁，郁证，健忘，失眠，癃闭，遗尿，下肢痿痹，足跗肿痛。

【进针层次】①皮肤；②皮下组织（内有足背内侧皮神经和足背静脉弓）；③蹞长、短伸肌腱与趾长伸肌腱之间；④第 1 趾背动、静脉和腓深神经；⑤第 1 骨间背侧肌（图 6–53 ～图 6–59）。

2. Taichong (LR 3)

【Location】In the anterior depression of the junction between the 1st and 2nd metatarsus.

【Method】Puncture perpendicularly 0.5-0.8 cun.

【Indications】Headache, vertigo, deafness, tinnitus, deviated mouth, pain and swelling in the eyes, sore and dry throat, pain in the hypochondrium, jaundice, vomiting, irregular menstruation, dysmenorrhea, amenorrhea, metrorrhagia and metrostaxis, leukorrhea, nocturnal emission, impotence, premature ejaculation, priapism, wind stroke, insanity, mania, epilepsy, infantile convulsions, hysteria, depression, forgetfulness, insomnia, retention of urine, enuresis, flaccidity and impediment of lower limb, and swelling and pain in the dorsum of foot.

【Stratified anatomy】①Skin; ②Subcutaneous tissue (There are medial dorsal cutaneous n. and dorsal venous arch of foot.); ③Between the tendons of extensor hallucis longus & brevis and tendons of extensor digitorum longus; ④The 1st dorsal digital a. & v. and deep peroneal n.; ⑤The 1st dorsal interossei m. (Fig.6-53 ~ Fig.6-59).

三、内庭

【定位】第 2、第 3 趾之间，趾蹼缘后方赤白肉际处。

【操作】直刺或向上斜刺 0.5 ～ 1 寸。

【主治】齿痛，咽喉肿痛，口㖞，鼻衄，热病，腹痛，腹胀，便秘，痢疾，足背肿痛。

【进针层次】①皮肤；②皮下组织（内有足背内侧皮神经的趾背神经和足背浅静脉）；③第 2 趾长、短伸肌腱与第 3 趾长、短伸肌腱之间；④第 2 趾背动、静脉（图 6–53 ～图 6–59）。

3. Neiting (ST 44)

【Location】Between the 2nd and 3rd toes, and at the junction of the red and white skin behind the toe web margin.

【Method】Puncture perpendicularly or obliquely upward 0.5-1 cun.

【Indications】Toothache, sore throat, deviated mouth, epistaxis, febrile disease, abdominal pain, abdominal distension, constipation, dysentery, and swelling and pain on the dorsum of the foot.

【Stratified anatomy】①Skin; ②Subcutaneous tissue (There are dorsal digital n. of the medial dorsal cutaneous n., and dorsal venous rete of foot.); ③Between the 2nd and the 3rd tendons of extensor digitorum longus & brevis; ④The 2nd dorsal digital a. & v. (Fig.6-53 ~ Fig.6-59).

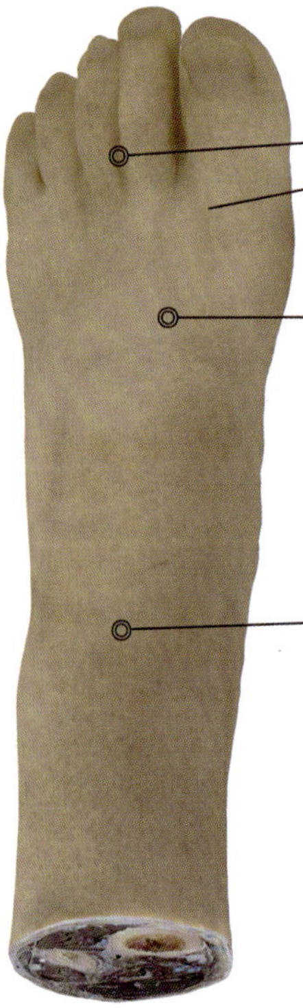
内庭 Neiting (ST 44)
皮肤 Skin
太冲 Taichong (LR 3)
解溪 Jiexi (ST 41)

图 6–53　足背腧穴层次解剖（1）

Fig.6-53　Layered anatomy of acupoints on the dorsum of the foot (1)

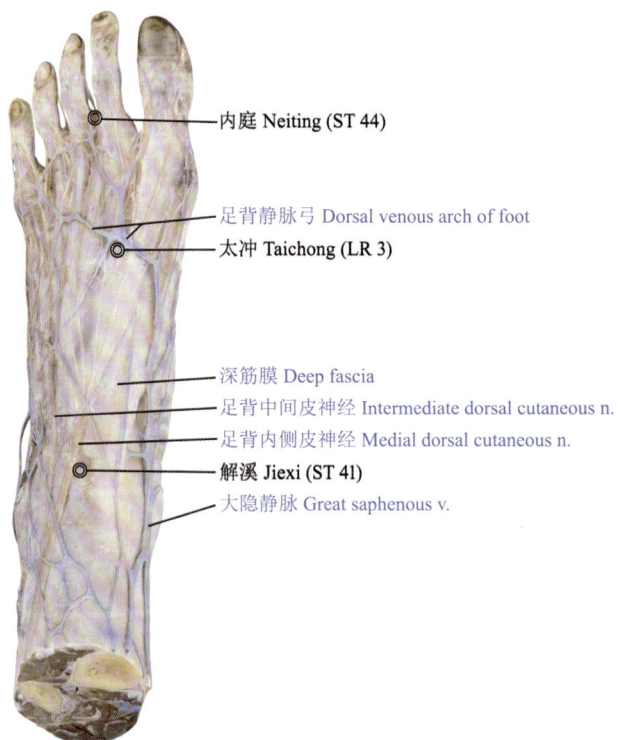

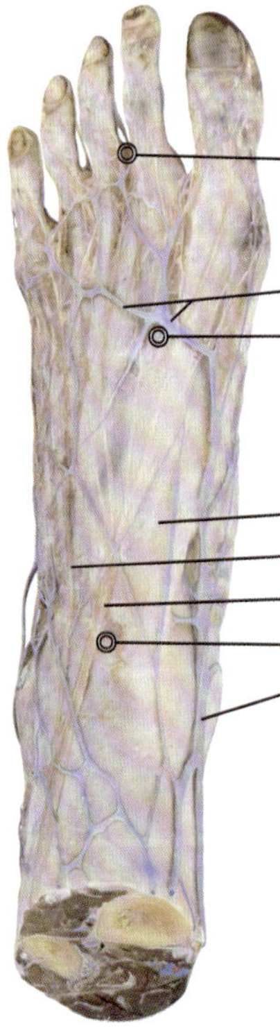
内庭 Neiting (ST 44)
足背静脉弓 Dorsal venous arch of foot
太冲 Taichong (LR 3)
深筋膜 Deep fascia
足背中间皮神经 Intermediate dorsal cutaneous n.
足背内侧皮神经 Medial dorsal cutaneous n.
解溪 Jiexi (ST 41)
大隐静脉 Great saphenous v.

图 6–54　足背腧穴层次解剖（2）

Fig.6-54　Layered anatomy of acupoints on the dorsum of the foot (2)

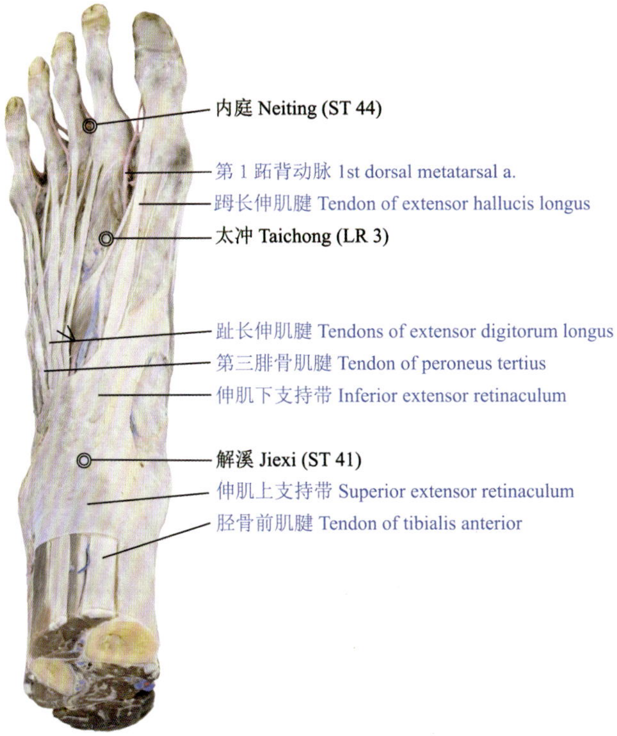
内庭 Neiting (ST 44)
第 1 跖背动脉 1st dorsal metatarsal a.
踇长伸肌腱 Tendon of extensor hallucis longus
太冲 Taichong (LR 3)
趾长伸肌腱 Tendons of extensor digitorum longus
第三腓骨肌腱 Tendon of peroneus tertius
伸肌下支持带 Inferior extensor retinaculum
解溪 Jiexi (ST 41)
伸肌上支持带 Superior extensor retinaculum
胫骨前肌腱 Tendon of tibialis anterior

图 6–55　足背腧穴层次解剖（3）

Fig.6-55　Layered anatomy of acupoints on the dorsum of the foot (3)

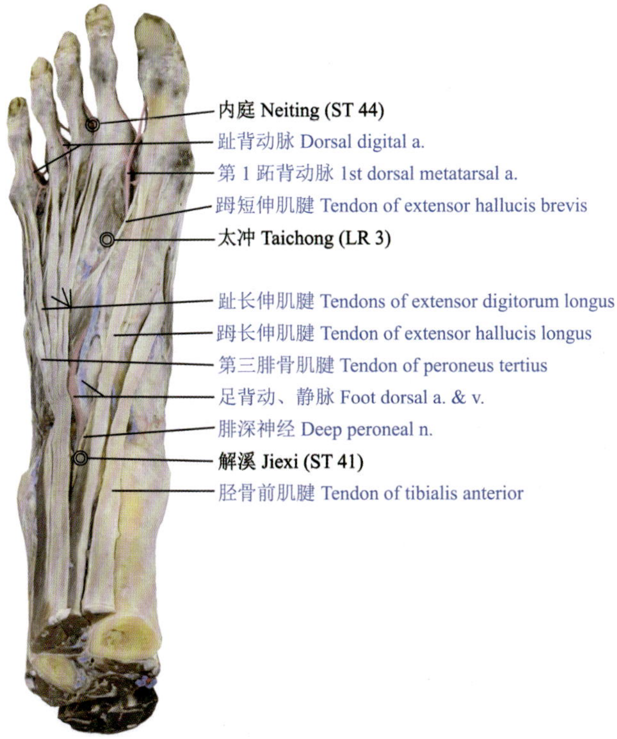
内庭 Neiting (ST 44)
趾背动脉 Dorsal digital a.
第 1 跖背动脉 1st dorsal metatarsal a.
踇短伸肌腱 Tendon of extensor hallucis brevis
太冲 Taichong (LR 3)
趾长伸肌腱 Tendons of extensor digitorum longus
踇长伸肌腱 Tendon of extensor hallucis longus
第三腓骨肌腱 Tendon of peroneus tertius
足背动、静脉 Foot dorsal a. & v.
腓深神经 Deep peroneal n.
解溪 Jiexi (ST 41)
胫骨前肌腱 Tendon of tibialis anterior

图 6–56　足背腧穴层次解剖（4）

Fig.6-56　Layered anatomy of acupoints on the dorsum of the foot (4)

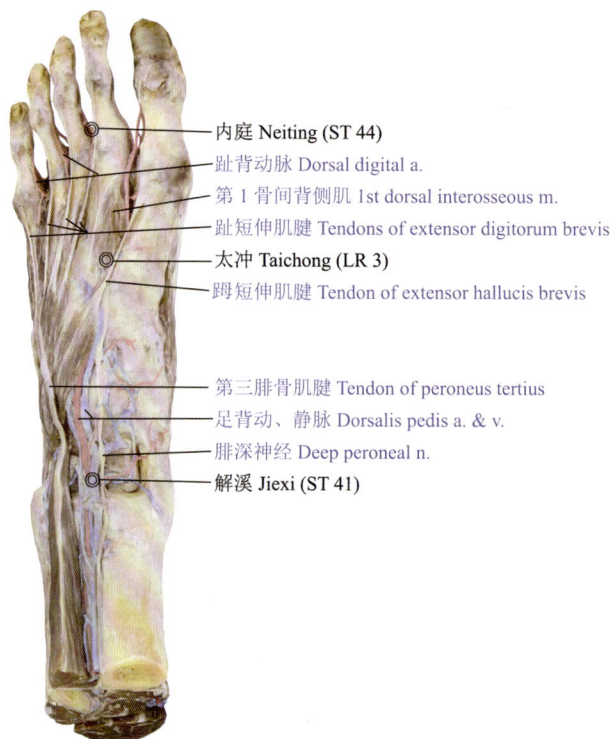

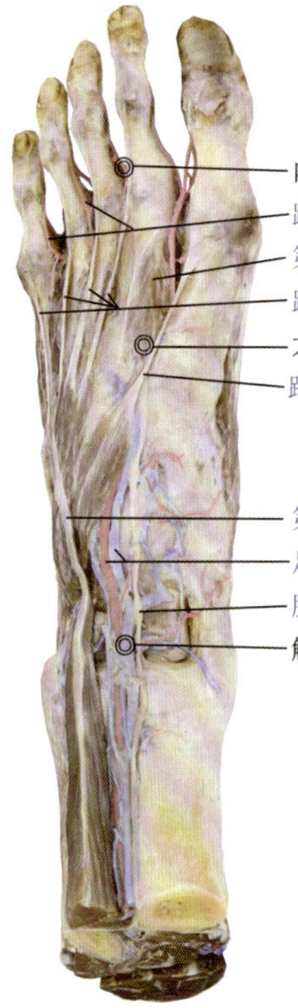
内庭 Neiting (ST 44)
趾背动脉 Dorsal digital a.
第 1 骨间背侧肌 1st dorsal interosseous m.
趾短伸肌腱 Tendons of extensor digitorum brevis
太冲 Taichong (LR 3)
跗短伸肌腱 Tendon of extensor hallucis brevis
第三腓骨肌腱 Tendon of peroneus tertius
足背动、静脉 Dorsalis pedis a. & v.
腓深神经 Deep peroneal n.
解溪 Jiexi (ST 41)

图 6–57　足背腧穴层次解剖（5）

Fig.6-57　Layered anatomy of acupoints on the dorsum of the foot (5)

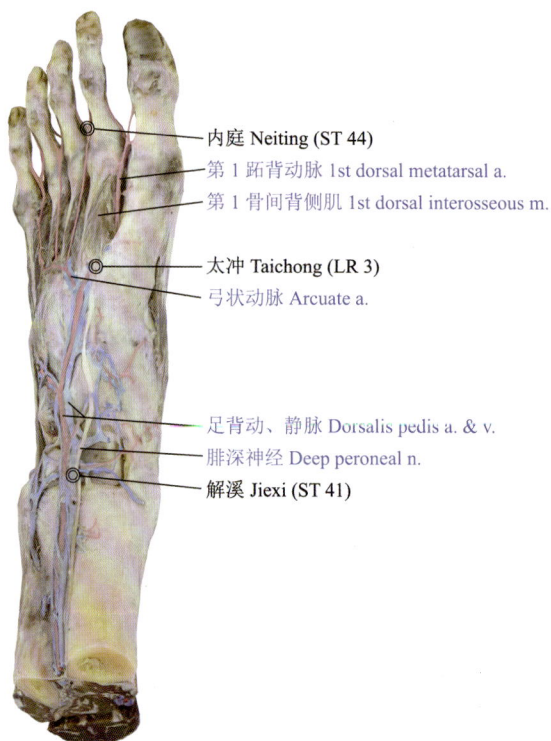

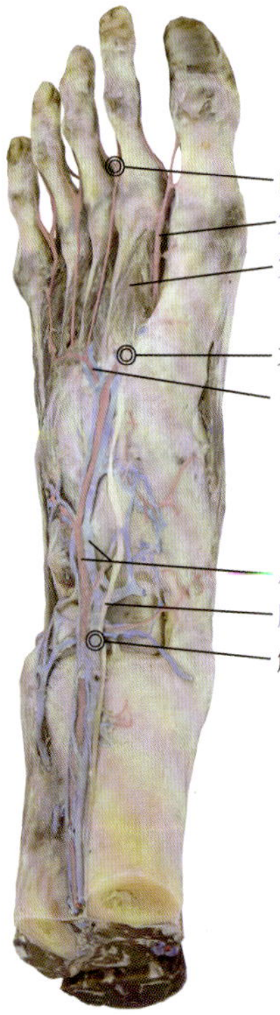
内庭 Neiting (ST 44)
第 1 跖背动脉 1st dorsal metatarsal a.
第 1 骨间背侧肌 1st dorsal interosseous m.
太冲 Taichong (LR 3)
弓状动脉 Arcuate a.
足背动、静脉 Dorsalis pedis a. & v.
腓深神经 Deep peroneal n.
解溪 Jiexi (ST 41)

图 6–58　足背腧穴层次解剖（6）

Fig.6-58　Layered anatomy of acupoints on the dorsum of the foot (6)

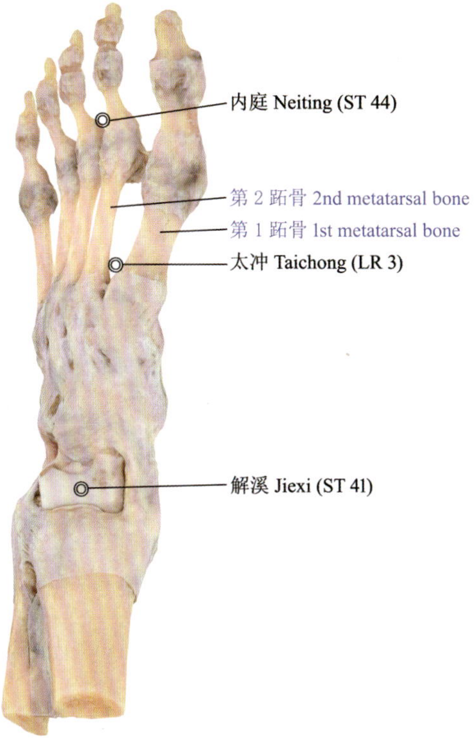
内庭 Neiting (ST 44)
第 2 跖骨 2nd metatarsal bone
第 1 跖骨 1st metatarsal bone
太冲 Taichong (LR 3)
解溪 Jiexi (ST 41)

图 6–59　足背腧穴层次解剖（7）

Fig.6-59　Layered anatomy of acupoints on the dorsum of the foot (7)

第九节　足外侧面腧穴

Section 9　Acupoints on the lateral aspect of the foot

一、昆仑

【定位】外踝尖与跟腱之间的凹陷中。

【操作】直刺 0.5 ～ 1 寸。

【主治】头痛，项强，目眩，鼻衄，腰骶痛，足跟痛，肩背拘急，难产，癫痫。

【进针层次】①皮肤；②皮下组织（内有腓肠神经和小隐静脉）；③疏松结缔组织（图 6–60 ～图 6–67）。

1. Kunlun (BL 60)

【Location】In the depression between the tip of the lateral malleolus and the Achilles tendon.

【Method】Puncture perpendicularly 0.5-1 cun.

【Indications】Headache, stiffness in the neck, dizziness, epistaxis, lumbosacral pain, pain in the heel, spasm in the back and shoulder, difficult labor, and epilepsy.

【Stratified anatomy】①Skin; ②Subcutaneous tissue (There are sural n. and small saphenous v..); ③Loose connective tissue (Fig.6-60 ~ Fig.6-67).

二、申脉

【定位】外踝尖直下，外踝下缘与跟骨之间凹陷中。

【操作】直刺 0.2 ～ 0.3 寸。

【主治】头痛，眩晕，失眠，嗜睡，癫狂痫，腰腿痛，项强，足外翻。

【进针层次】①皮肤；②皮下组织（内有腓肠神经和小隐静脉）；③腓骨长肌腱；④腓骨短肌腱；⑤距跟外侧韧带（图 6–60 ～图 6–67）。

2. Shenmai (BL 62)

【Location】Under the tip of the lateral malleolus directly, and in the depression between the inferior edge of the lateral malleolus and the calcaneus.

【Method】Puncture perpendicularly 0.2-0.3 cun.

【Indications】Headache, vertigo, insomnia, somnolence, insanity, mania, epilepsy, pain in the lower back and leg, stiffness in the neck, and eversion of foot.

【Stratified anatomy】①Skin; ②Subcutaneous tissue (There are sural n. and small saphenous v..); ③Tendon of peroneus longus; ④Tendon of peroneus brevis; ⑤Lateral talocalcaneal lig. (Fig.6-60 ~ Fig.6-67).

三、丘墟

【定位】外踝前下方，趾长伸肌腱外侧凹陷中。

【操作】直刺 0.5 ～ 0.8 寸。

【主治】目赤肿痛，胸胁胀痛，下肢痿痹，中风瘫痪，疝气。

【进针层次】①皮肤；②皮下组织（内有足背外侧皮神经的分支）；③趾短伸肌；④距跟外侧韧带；⑤跗骨窦（图 6–60 ～图 6–67）。

3. Qiuxu (GB 40)

【Location】Anterior and inferior to the lateral malleolus, and in the depression lateral to the tendons of the extensor digitorum longus.

【Method】Puncture perpendicularly 0.5-0.8 cun.

【Indications】Swelling and pain in the eyes, distension and pain in the chest and hypochondrium, flaccidity and impediment of lower limb, paralysis due to apoplexy, and hernia.

【Stratified anatomy】①Skin; ②Subcutaneous tissue (There are branches of the nervus cutaneus dorsalis lateralis pedis.); ③Extensor digitorum brevis m.; ④Lateral talocalcaneal lig.; ⑤Tarsal sinus (Fig.6-60 ~ Fig.6-67).

四、足临泣

【定位】第 4、第 5 跖骨底结合部的前方，第 5 趾长伸肌腱外侧凹陷中。

【操作】直刺 0.3 ～ 0.5 寸。

【主治】偏头痛，目赤肿痛，胁肋疼痛，足跗肿痛，月经不调，乳痈，乳胀。

【进针层次】①皮肤；②皮下组织（内有足背中间皮神经的分支和足背浅静脉）；③第 4 骨间背侧肌和第 3 骨间足底肌（图 6–60 ～图 6–65）。

4. Zulinqi (GB 41)

【Location】Anterior to the junction of the 4th and 5th metatarsals, and in the lateral depression of the 5th extensor digitorum longus tendon.

【Method】Puncture perpendicularly 0.3-0.5 cun.

【Indications】Migraine, swelling and pain in the eyes, pain in the hypochondrium, swelling and pain in the dorsum of foot, irregular menstruation, acute mastitis, and breast distending.

【Stratified anatomy】①Skin; ②Subcutaneous tissue (There are branches of the nervi cutaneus dorsalis intermedius pedis, and superficial dorsalis pedis v..); ③The 4th dorsal interossei m. and the 3rd interosseous plantar m. (Fig.6-60 ~ Fig.6-65).

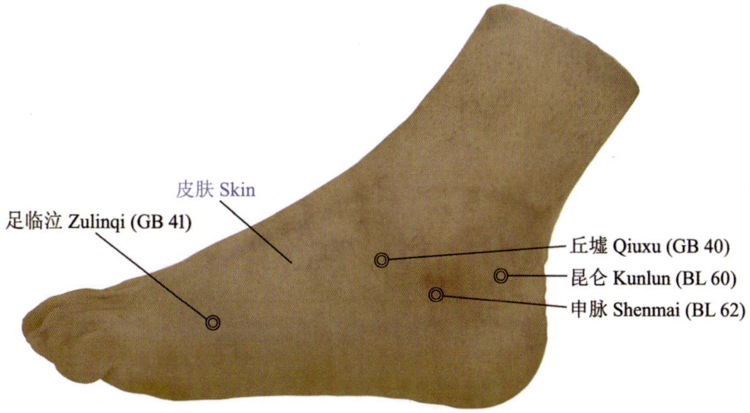

图 6–60　足外侧面腧穴层次解剖（1）

Fig.6-60　Layered anatomy of acupoints on the lateral aspect of the foot (1)

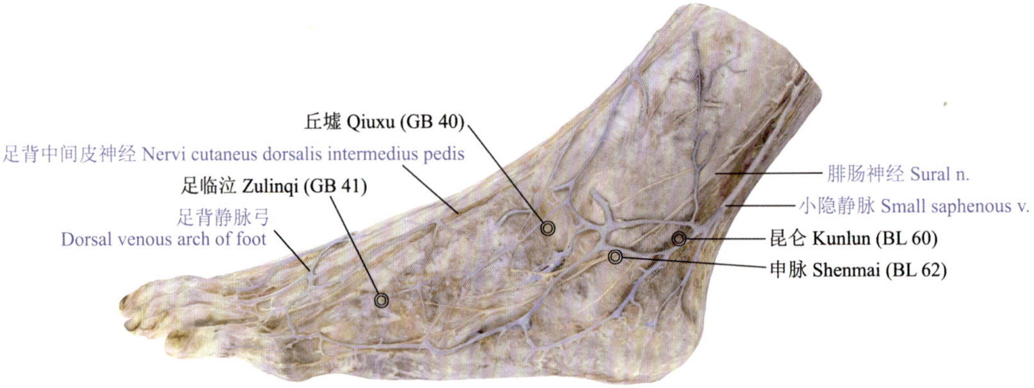
丘墟 Qiuxu (GB 40)
足背中间皮神经 Nervi cutaneus dorsalis intermedius pedis
足临泣 Zulinqi (GB 41)
足背静脉弓
Dorsal venous arch of foot
腓肠神经 Sural n.
小隐静脉 Small saphenous v.
昆仑 Kunlun (BL 60)
申脉 Shenmai (BL 62)

图 6–61　足外侧面腧穴层次解剖（2）

Fig.6-61　Layered anatomy of acupoints on the lateral aspect of the foot (2)

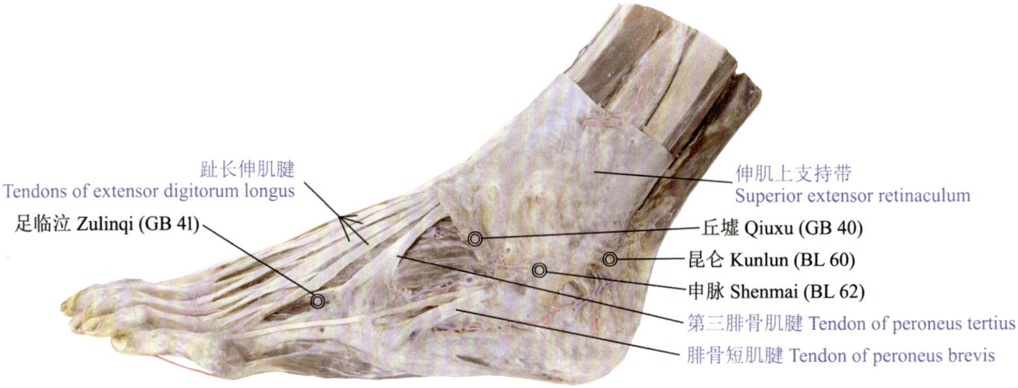
趾长伸肌腱
Tendons of extensor digitorum longus
足临泣 Zulinqi (GB 41)
伸肌上支持带
Superior extensor retinaculum
丘墟 Qiuxu (GB 40)
昆仑 Kunlun (BL 60)
申脉 Shenmai (BL 62)
第三腓骨肌腱 Tendon of peroneus tertius
腓骨短肌腱 Tendon of peroneus brevis

图 6–62　足外侧面腧穴层次解剖（3）

Fig.6-62　Layered anatomy of acupoints on the lateral aspect of the foot (3)

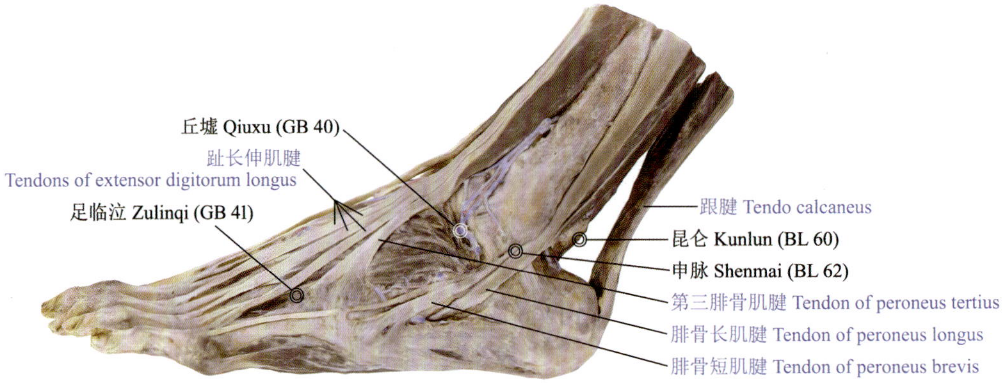
丘墟 Qiuxu (GB 40)
趾长伸肌腱
Tendons of extensor digitorum longus
足临泣 Zulinqi (GB 41)
跟腱 Tendo calcaneus
昆仑 Kunlun (BL 60)
申脉 Shenmai (BL 62)
第三腓骨肌腱 Tendon of peroneus tertius
腓骨长肌腱 Tendon of peroneus longus
腓骨短肌腱 Tendon of peroneus brevis

图 6–63　足外侧面腧穴层次解剖（4）

Fig.6-63　Layered anatomy of acupoints on the lateral aspect of the foot (4)

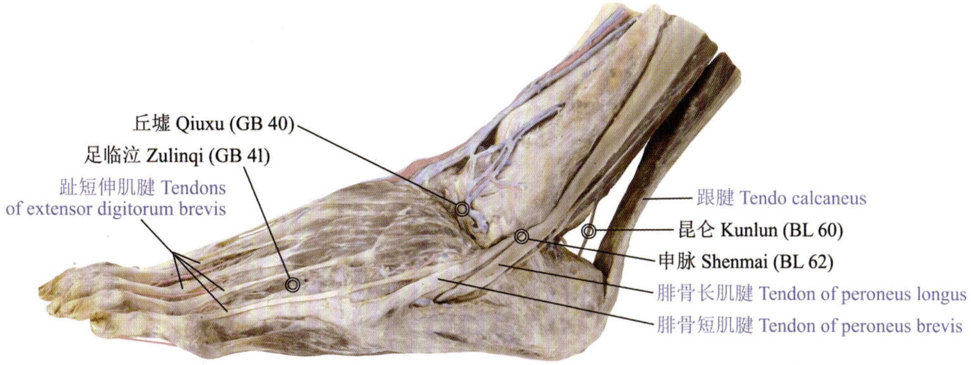
丘墟 Qiuxu (GB 40)
足临泣 Zulinqi (GB 41)
趾短伸肌腱 Tendons of extensor digitorum brevis
跟腱 Tendo calcaneus
昆仑 Kunlun (BL 60)
申脉 Shenmai (BL 62)
腓骨长肌腱 Tendon of peroneus longus
腓骨短肌腱 Tendon of peroneus brevis

图 6–64　足外侧面腧穴层次解剖（5）

Fig.6-64　Layered anatomy of acupoints on the lateral aspect of the foot (5)

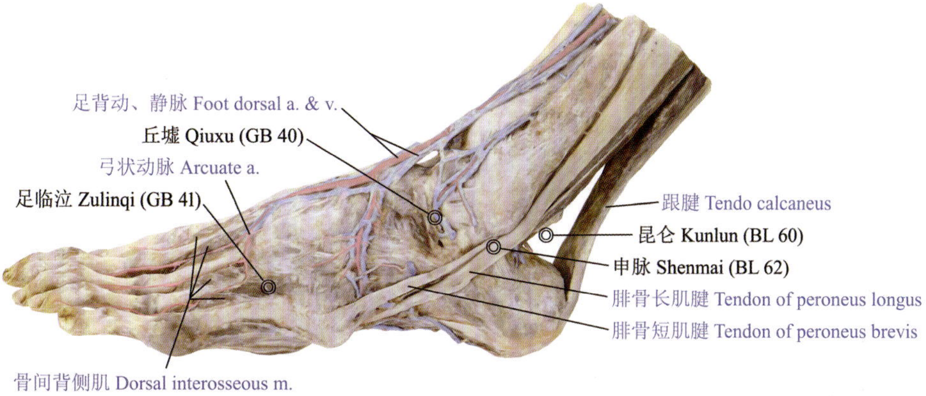
足背动、静脉 Foot dorsal a. & v.
丘墟 Qiuxu (GB 40)
弓状动脉 Arcuate a.
足临泣 Zulinqi (GB 41)
跟腱 Tendo calcaneus
昆仑 Kunlun (BL 60)
申脉 Shenmai (BL 62)
腓骨长肌腱 Tendon of peroneus longus
腓骨短肌腱 Tendon of peroneus brevis
骨间背侧肌 Dorsal interosseous m.

图 6–65　足外侧面腧穴层次解剖（6）

Fig.6-65　Layered anatomy of acupoints on the lateral aspect of the foot (6)

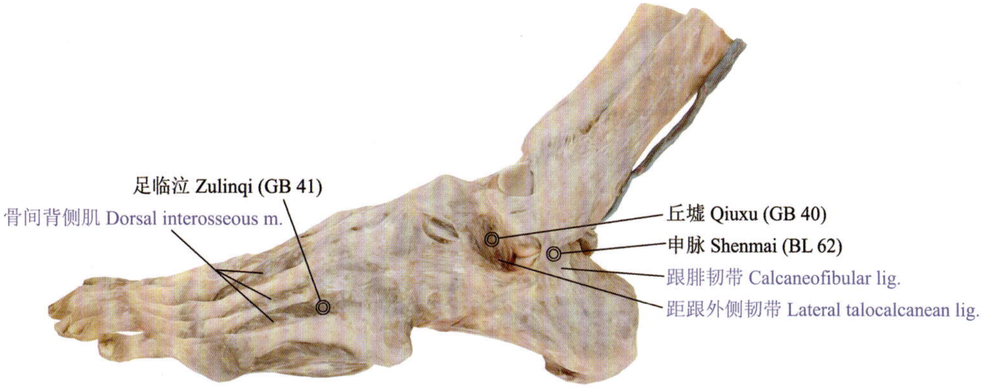
足临泣 Zulinqi (GB 41)
骨间背侧肌 Dorsal interosseous m.
丘墟 Qiuxu (GB 40)
申脉 Shenmai (BL 62)
跟腓韧带 Calcaneofibular lig.
距跟外侧韧带 Lateral talocalcanean lig.

图 6–66　足外侧面腧穴层次解剖（7）

Fig.6-66　Layered anatomy of acupoints on the lateral aspect of the foot (7)

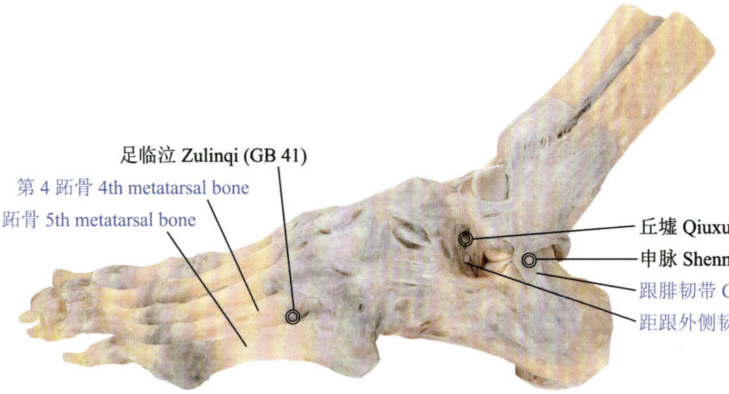

图 6–67　足外侧面腧穴层次解剖（8）
Fig.6-67　Layered anatomy of acupoints on the lateral aspect of the foot (8)

第十节　足内侧面腧穴

Section 10　Acupoints on the medial aspect of the foot

一、太溪

【定位】内踝尖与跟腱之间的凹陷中。

【操作】直刺 0.5 ～ 1 寸。

【主治】月经不调，遗精，阳痿，尿频，消渴，泄泻，腰痛，头晕，目眩，耳聋，耳鸣，咽喉肿痛，齿痛，失眠，咳喘，咳血。

【进针层次】①皮肤；②皮下组织（内有隐神经的分支）；③胫神经及胫后动、静脉与跟腱、跖肌腱之间；④䟆长屈肌（图 6–68 ～图 6–73）。

1. Taixi (KI 3)

【Location】In the depression between the tip of the medial malleolus and the Achilles tendon.

【Method】Puncture perpendicularly 0.5-1 cun.

【Indications】Irregular menstruation, nocturnal emission, impotence, frequent urination, wasting thirst disorder, diarrhea, lumbago, dizziness, blurred vision, deafness, tinnitus, sore throat, toothache, insomnia, asthma, and hemoptysis.

【Stratified anatomy】①Skin; ②Subcutaneous tissue (There are branches of saphenous n..); ③Between tibial n., posterior tibial a. & v. and the Achilles tendon and plantar tendon; ④Flexor hallucis longus m. (Fig.6-68 ~ Fig.6-73).

二、照海

【定位】内踝尖下 1 寸，内踝下缘凹陷中。

【操作】直刺 0.3 ～ 0.5 寸。

【主治】月经不调，痛经，带下，阴挺，阴痒，尿频，癃闭，咽喉干痛，目赤肿痛，失眠，痫证。

【进针层次】①皮肤；②皮下组织（内有隐神经的分支）；③胫骨后肌腱（图 6–68 ～图 6–73）。

2. Zhaohai (KI 6)

【Location】1 cun under the tip of the medial malleolus, and in the depression of the lower edge of the medial malleolus.

【Method】Puncture perpendicularly 0.3-0.5 cun.

【Indications】Irregular menstruation, dysmenorrhea, leukorrhea, prolapse of uterus, pudendal pruritus, frequent urination, retention of urine, sore and dry throat, swelling and pain in the eyes, insomnia, and epilepsy.

【Stratified anatomy】①Skin; ②Subcutaneous tissue (There are branches of the saphenous n..); ③Tibialis posterior tendon (Fig.6-68 ~ Fig.6-73).

三、公孙

【定位】第 1 跖骨底的前下缘赤白肉际处。

【操作】直刺 0.5 ～ 1 寸。

【主治】胃痛，呕吐，完谷不化，腹痛，腹胀，黄疸，肠鸣，泄泻，痢疾，心痛，胸闷，失眠，嗜睡，癫狂，水肿。

【进针层次】①皮肤；②皮下组织（内有隐神经的足内侧缘支和大隐静脉的属支）；③蹞展肌；④蹞短屈肌；⑤蹞长屈肌腱（图 6–68 ～图 6–73）。

3. Gongsun (SP 4)

【Location】At the junction of the red and white skin antero-inferior to the base of the 1st metatarsal bone.

【Method】Puncture perpendicularly 0.5-1 cun.

【Indications】Stomachache, vomiting, diarrhea with undigested food, abdominal pain, abdominal distension, jaundice, borborygmus, diarrhea, dysentery, angina, stuffy chest, insomnia, somnolence, insanity and mania, and edema.

【Stratified anatomy】①Skin; ②Subcutaneous tissue (There are foot medial branch of the saphenous n., and tributaries of the great saphenous v..); ③Abductor hallucis m.; ④Flexor hallucis brevis m.; ⑤Flexor hallucis longus tendon (Fig.6-68 ~ Fig.6-73).

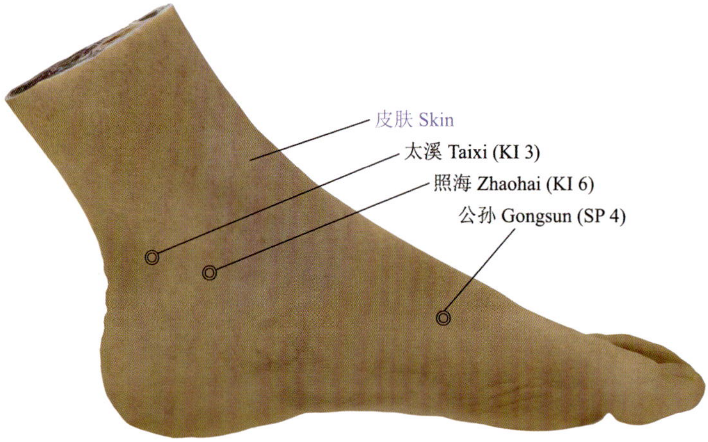
皮肤 Skin
太溪 Taixi (KI 3)
照海 Zhaohai (KI 6)
公孙 Gongsun (SP 4)

图 6-68　足内侧面腧穴层次解剖（1）

Fig.6-68　Layered anatomy of acupoints on the medial aspect of the foot (1)

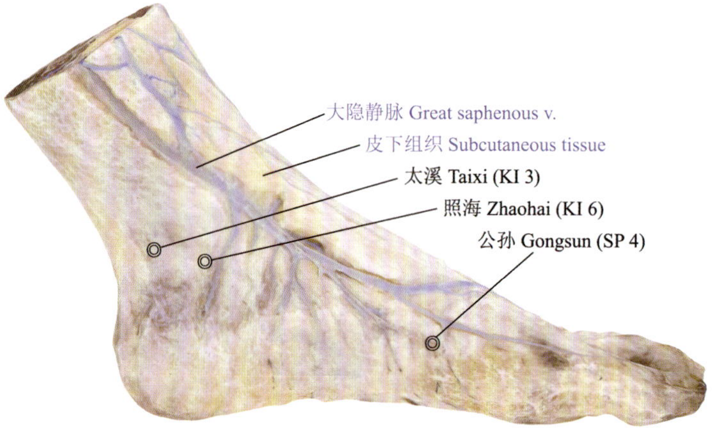
大隐静脉 Great saphenous v.
皮下组织 Subcutaneous tissue
太溪 Taixi (KI 3)
照海 Zhaohai (KI 6)
公孙 Gongsun (SP 4)

图 6-69　足内侧面腧穴层次解剖（2）

Fig.6-69　Layered anatomy of acupoints on the medial aspect of the foot (2)

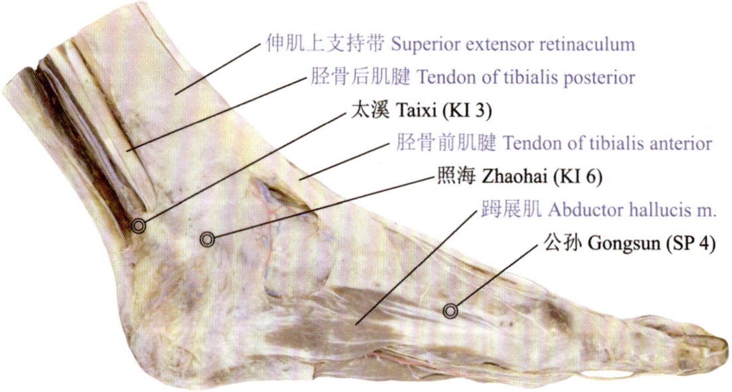
伸肌上支持带 Superior extensor retinaculum
胫骨后肌腱 Tendon of tibialis posterior
太溪 Taixi (KI 3)
胫骨前肌腱 Tendon of tibialis anterior
照海 Zhaohai (KI 6)
踇展肌 Abductor hallucis m.
公孙 Gongsun (SP 4)

图 6-70　足内侧面腧穴层次解剖（3）

Fig.6-70　Layered anatomy of acupoints on the medial aspect of the foot (3)

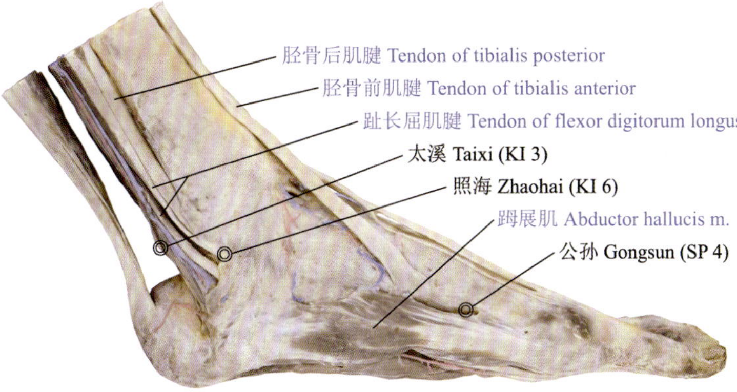
胫骨后肌腱 Tendon of tibialis posterior
胫骨前肌腱 Tendon of tibialis anterior
趾长屈肌腱 Tendon of flexor digitorum longus
太溪 Taixi (KI 3)
照海 Zhaohai (KI 6)
踇展肌 Abductor hallucis m.
公孙 Gongsun (SP 4)

图 6–71　足内侧面腧穴层次解剖（4）

Fig.6-71　Layered anatomy of acupoints on the medial aspect of the foot (4)

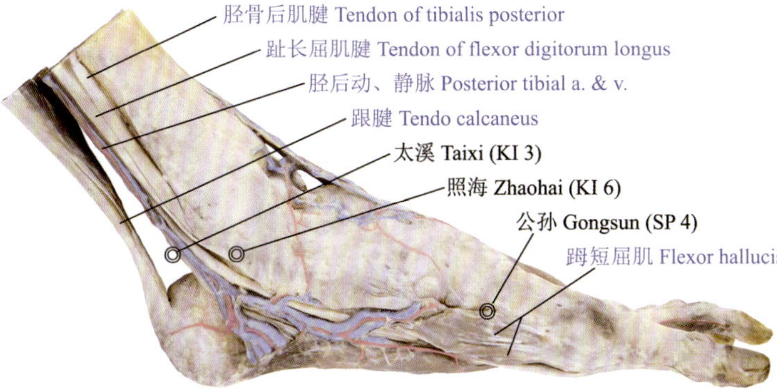
胫骨后肌腱 Tendon of tibialis posterior
趾长屈肌腱 Tendon of flexor digitorum longus
胫后动、静脉 Posterior tibial a. & v.
跟腱 Tendo calcaneus
太溪 Taixi (KI 3)
照海 Zhaohai (KI 6)
公孙 Gongsun (SP 4)
踇短屈肌 Flexor hallucis brevis m.

图 6–72　足内侧面腧穴层次解剖（5）

Fig.6-72　Layered anatomy of acupoints on the medial aspect of the foot (5)

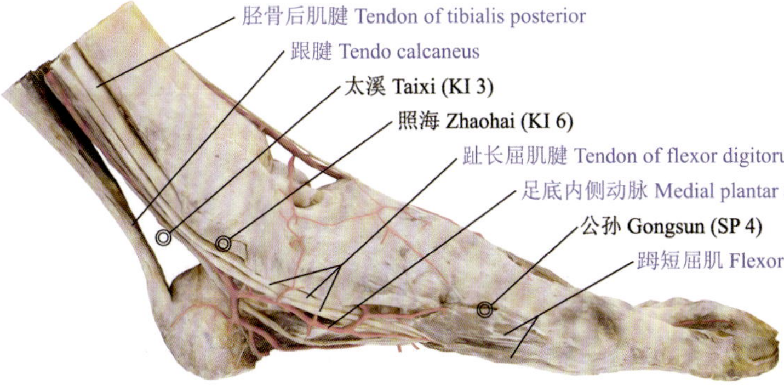
胫骨后肌腱 Tendon of tibialis posterior
跟腱 Tendo calcaneus
太溪 Taixi (KI 3)
照海 Zhaohai (KI 6)
趾长屈肌腱 Tendon of flexor digitorum longus
足底内侧动脉 Medial plantar a.
公孙 Gongsun (SP 4)
踇短屈肌 Flexor hallucis brevis m.

图 6–73　足内侧面腧穴层次解剖（6）

Fig.6-73　Layered anatomy of acupoints on the medial aspect of the foot (6)

第十一节　足底腧穴

Section 11　Acupoints on the sole

涌泉

【定位】蜷足时，足前部凹陷处，约当足底第 2、第 3 趾的趾缝纹头端与足跟连线的前 1/3 与后 2/3 交点处。

【操作】直刺 0.5 ～ 1 寸。

【主治】头顶痛，眩晕，昏厥，癫痫，小儿惊风，失眠，便秘，小便不利，咽喉肿痛，咽干，失音，足心热。

【进针层次】①皮肤；②皮下组织（内有足底内、外侧神经的分支）；③足底腱膜；④第 2 趾足底总神经和第 2 跖足底总动、静脉；⑤第 2 蚓状肌（图 6–74 ～图 6–81）。

Yongquan (KI 1)

【Location】When curling up the foot, the acupoint is located in the depression of the front of the foot, about at the intersection of the anterior 1/3 and the posterior 2/3 of the sole, and on the line connecting the toe webbing end of the 2nd and 3rd toes and the heel.

【Method】Puncture perpendicularly 0.5-1 cun.

【Indications】Pain on the top of the head, vertigo, coma, epilepsy, infantile convulsions, insomnia, constipation, dysuria, sore throat, dry throat, aphonia, and feverish soles.

【Stratified anatomy】①Skin; ②Subcutaneous tissue (There are branches of the lateral and medial plantar n.); ③Plantar aponeurosis; ④Common plantar digital n., a. & v. of the 2nd toe; ⑤The 2nd lumbrical m. (Fig.6-74 ~ Fig.6-81).

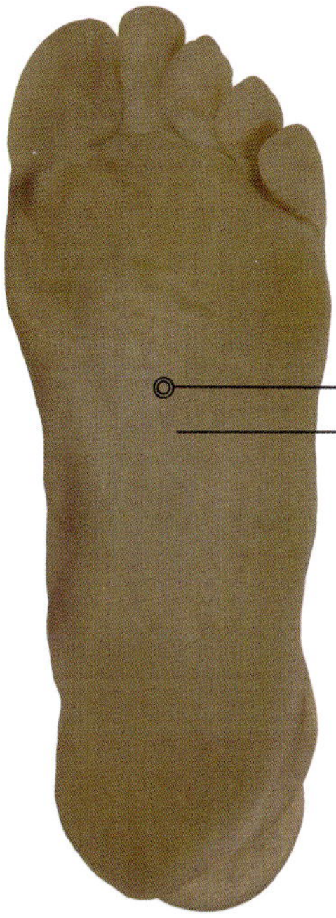

图 6–74　足底腧穴层次解剖（1）
Fig.6-74　Layered anatomy of acupoints on the sole (1)

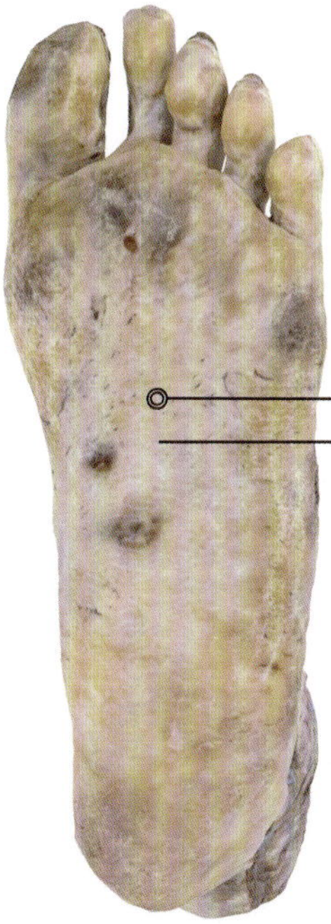

图 6–75　足底腧穴层次解剖（2）
Fig.6-75　Layered anatomy of acupoints on the sole (2)

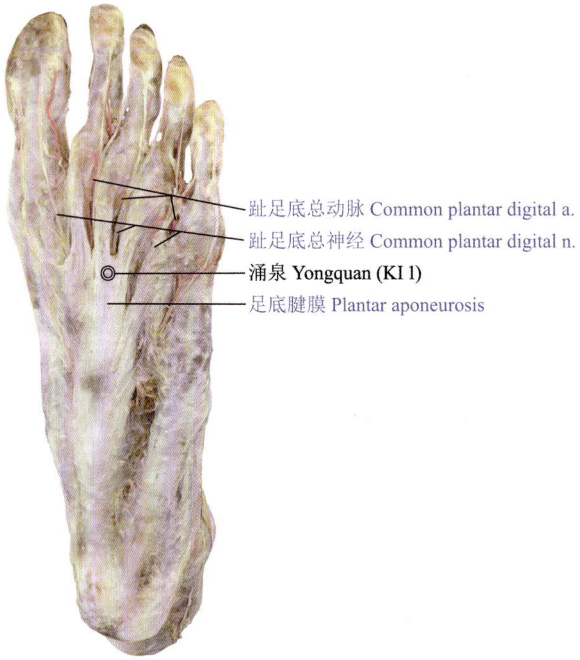
趾足底总动脉 Common plantar digital a.
趾足底总神经 Common plantar digital n.
涌泉 Yongquan (KI 1)
足底腱膜 Plantar aponeurosis

图 6–76　足底腧穴层次解剖（3）

Fig.6-76　Layered anatomy of acupoints on the sole (3)

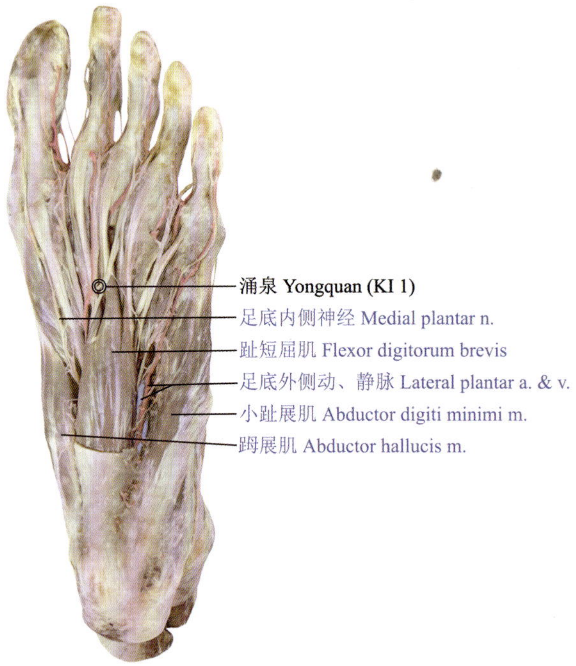
涌泉 Yongquan (KI 1)
足底内侧神经 Medial plantar n.
趾短屈肌 Flexor digitorum brevis
足底外侧动、静脉 Lateral plantar a. & v.
小趾展肌 Abductor digiti minimi m.
踇展肌 Abductor hallucis m.

图 6–77　足底腧穴层次解剖（4）

Fig.6-77　Layered anatomy of acupoints on the sole (4)

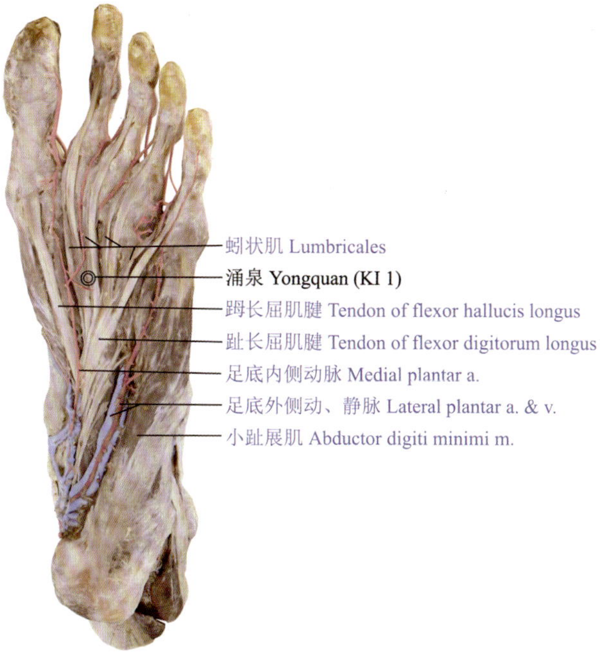
蚓状肌 Lumbricales
涌泉 Yongquan (KI 1)
踇长屈肌腱 Tendon of flexor hallucis longus
趾长屈肌腱 Tendon of flexor digitorum longus
足底内侧动脉 Medial plantar a.
足底外侧动、静脉 Lateral plantar a. & v.
小趾展肌 Abductor digiti minimi m.

图 6-78 足底腧穴层次解剖（5）

Fig.6-78 Layered anatomy of acupoints on the sole (5)

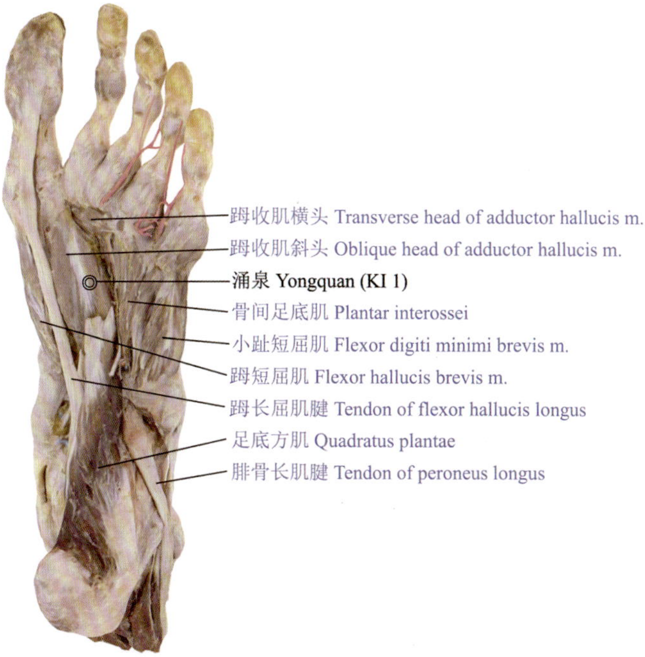
踇收肌横头 Transverse head of adductor hallucis m.
踇收肌斜头 Oblique head of adductor hallucis m.
涌泉 Yongquan (KI 1)
骨间足底肌 Plantar interossei
小趾短屈肌 Flexor digiti minimi brevis m.
踇短屈肌 Flexor hallucis brevis m.
踇长屈肌腱 Tendon of flexor hallucis longus
足底方肌 Quadratus plantae
腓骨长肌腱 Tendon of peroneus longus

图 6-79 足底腧穴层次解剖（6）

Fig.6-79 Layered anatomy of acupoints on the sole (6)

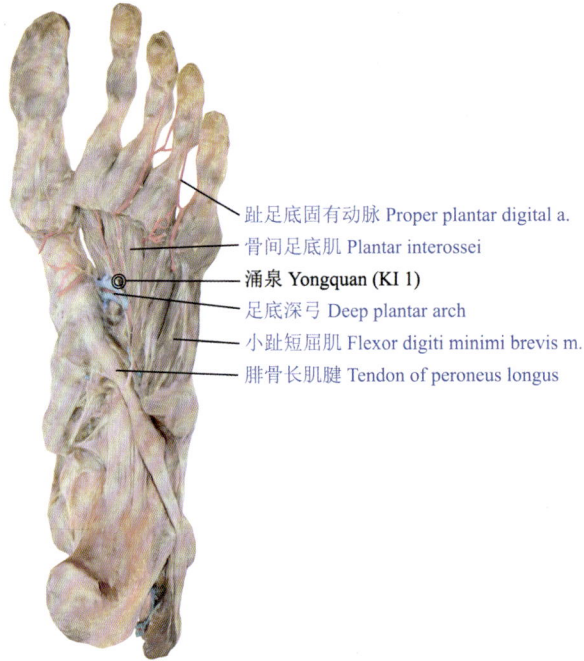

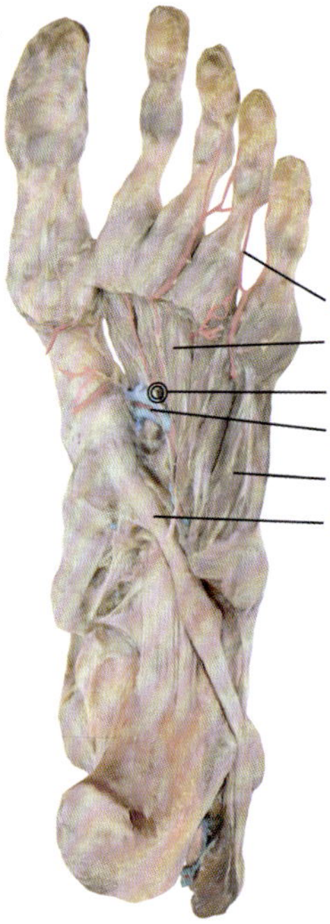
趾足底固有动脉 Proper plantar digital a.
骨间足底肌 Plantar interossei
涌泉 Yongquan (KI 1)
足底深弓 Deep plantar arch
小趾短屈肌 Flexor digiti minimi brevis m.
腓骨长肌腱 Tendon of peroneus longus

图 6–80　足底腧穴层次解剖（7）
Fig.6-80　Layered anatomy of acupoints on the sole (7)

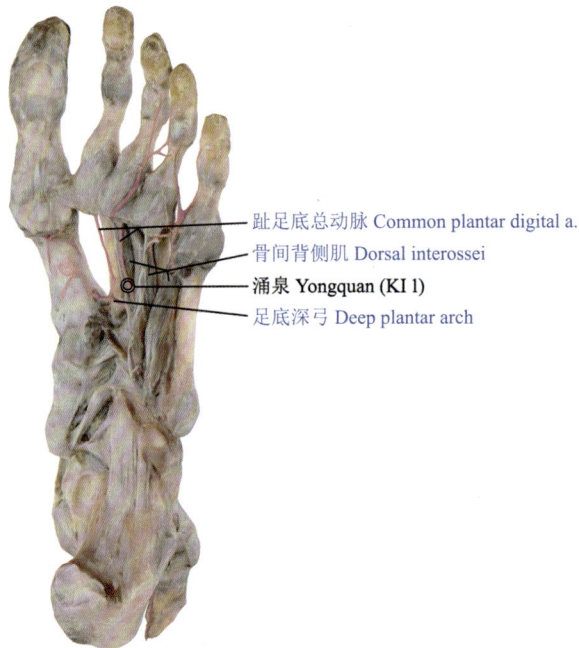

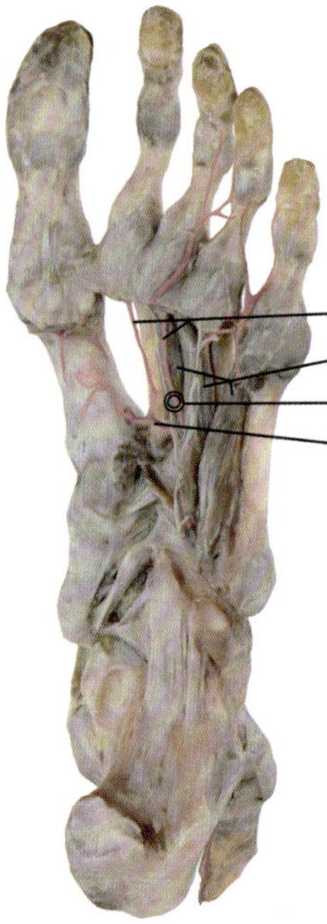
趾足底总动脉 Common plantar digital a.
骨间背侧肌 Dorsal interossei
涌泉 Yongquan (KI 1)
足底深弓 Deep plantar arch

图 6–81　足底腧穴层次解剖（8）
Fig.6-81　Layeredanatomy of acupoints on the sole (8)